Management of Multiple Pregnancies

Management of Multiple Pregnancies

A Practical Guide

Edited by

Leanne Bricker
Corniche Hospital, Abu Dhabi, United Arab Emirates

Julian N. Robinson
Brigham & Women's Hospital, Boston, USA

Basky Thilaganathan
St George's Hospital Medical School, University of London, UK

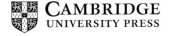

CAMBRIDGE
UNIVERSITY PRESS

CAMBRIDGE
UNIVERSITY PRESS

University Printing House, Cambridge CB2 8BS, United Kingdom

One Liberty Plaza, 20th Floor, New York, NY 10006, USA

477 Williamstown Road, Port Melbourne, VIC 3207, Australia

314–321, 3rd Floor, Plot 3, Splendor Forum, Jasola District Centre,
New Delhi – 110025, India

103 Penang Road, #05–06/07, Visioncrest Commercial, Singapore 238467

Cambridge University Press is part of the University of Cambridge.

It furthers the University's mission by disseminating knowledge in the pursuit of
education, learning, and research at the highest international levels of excellence.

www.cambridge.org
Information on this title: www.cambridge.org/9781108843195
DOI: 10.1017/9781108915038

First published 2023

Printed in the United Kingdom by TJ Books Limited, Padstow Cornwall

A catalogue record for this publication is available from the British Library.

ISBN 978-1-108-84319-5 Hardback

Cambridge University Press has no responsibility for the persistence or accuracy of
URLs for external or third-party internet websites referred to in this publication
and does not guarantee that any content on such websites is, or will remain,
accurate or appropriate.

....

Every effort has been made in preparing this book to provide accurate and up-to-date information
that is in accord with accepted standards and practice at the time of publication. Although case histories
are drawn from actual cases, every effort has been made to disguise the identities of the individuals
involved. Nevertheless, the authors, editors, and publishers can make no warranties that the information
contained herein is totally free from error, not least because clinical standards are constantly
changing through research and regulation. The authors, editors, and publishers therefore disclaim
all liability for direct or consequential damages resulting from the use of material contained
in this book. Readers are strongly advised to pay careful attention to information provided by the
manufacturer of any drugs or equipment that they plan to use.

Contents

The colour plate section can be found between pages 180 and 181

Video content can be found in the resources at www.cambridge.org/multiplepregnancies

Editors

Leanne Bricker undertook undergraduate training in South Africa and then in the UK specialised in OBGYN and subspecialised in Fetomaternal Medicine. She was Director of Fetal Medicine at Liverpool Women's Hospital in the UK (2003–2014) and served on the British Maternal and Fetal Medicine Society executive committee (2009–2014). Since 2014 she has been Chair of Fetal Medicine at Corniche Hospital, Abu Dhabi, UAE. She has published over sixty papers, abstracts and book chapters. She is an expert in the management of multiple pregnancy and was involved in the development of the UK NICE guidelines for the management of multiple pregnancy and the RCOG green top guideline for the management of monochorionic twin pregnancy. She is a Fellow of the Royal College of Obstetrics and Gynaecology

Julian N. Robinson trained at Guy's Hospital, London and the Nuffield Department of Obstetrics and Gynaecology in Oxford. He completed a fellowship in Maternal Fetal Medicine (MFM) at the Brigham and Women's Hospital, Harvard Medical School. Faculty appointments include MFM attending posts at the New York Presbyterian Hospital, New York and the Brigham and Women's Hospital, Boston. Julian was an Associate Professor of Obstetrics and Gynecology at Columbia Medical School, New York, and is currently an Associate Professor of Obstetrics, Gynecology, and Reproductive Biology at Harvard Medical School. His clinical interests include obstetrics, prenatal diagnosis and the management of multiple pregnancy. He has approximately 150 peer-reviewed academic publications.

Basky Thilaganathan was appointed Director of Fetal Medicine at St George's Hospital in 1999. He has authored over 300 peer-reviewed publications in indexed journals. His major research interest is placental dysfunction leading to pre-eclampsia, fetal growth restriction and stillbirth (TED talk: http://bit.ly/2i1SqDk). He has led on the implementation of algorithm-based screening at St George's which has led to an 80% reduction in preterm pre-eclampsia – the severest form of the disease (https://vimeo.com/rcog/authorinsights16361). He is the Clinical Director of the Tommy's National Centre for Maternity Improvement (https://vimeo.com/638468663/23d205d029) located at the RCOG and is Editor Emeritus of Ultrasound in Obstetrics and Gynaecology, the medical journal affiliated to ISUOG. He is a Council Member on the Royal College of Obstetrics and Gynaecology (RCOG) and represents the RCOG on the UK National Screening Committee and the DH Saving Babies Lives Care Bundle oversight committee. He is also the Clinical Lead for the first dedicated high-throughput cfDNA screening NHS lab to undertake cfDNA aneuploidy screening (NIPT) in pregnancy (www.theSAFEtest.co.uk).

Contributors

Abdallah Adra
Division of Maternal Fetal Medicine
Department of Obstetrics and
Gynecology
American University of Beirut
Beirut, Lebanon

Ranjit Akolekar
Clinical Lead for Fetal Medicine
Clinical Lead for Research and Innovation
Fetal and Obstetric Medicine Centre
Medway NHS Foundation Trust
Kent, UK

Tarek Ansari
Consultant Anaesthetist
Corniche Hospital
Abu Dhabi, UAE

Nikolaos Antonakopoulos
Fetal Medicine Unit
St George's Hospital
St George's University of London
London, UK

Amir Aviram
Associate Professor
Sunnybrook Health Sciences Centre
Department of Obstetrics and Gynecology
Division of Maternal-Fetal Medicine,
affiliated to the University of Toronto
Toronto, Ontario, Canada

Adam Balen
Professor of Reproductive Medicine and
Surgery and Clinical Lead
Leeds Fertility, Leeds Teaching Hospitals
NHS Trust, Leeds, UK

Christian Bamberg
Consultant in Fetal and Maternal Medicine
University Medical Center Hamburg
Hamburg, Germany

Caitlin D. Baptiste
Gynecology, Maternal Fetal Medicine
Columbia University Irving Medical Center
New York, New York, USA

Alejandra Barrero-Castillero
Attending Neonatologist
Beth Israel Deaconess Medical Center
Instructor in Pediatrics
Harvard Medical School
Boston, Massachusetts, USA

Jon F. R. Barret
Sunnybrook Health Sciences Centre
Department of Obstetrics and
Gynecology, Division of Maternal–Fetal
Medicine, affiliated to the University of
Toronto
Toronto, Ontario, Canada

Michael A. Belfort
Departments of Obstetrics and
Gynecology, Surgery, Anesthesia and
Neurosurgery
Baylor College of Medicine
Obstetrician and Gynecologist-in-Chief,
Texas Children's Hospital
Medical Director, Texas Children's Fetal
Center, Houston, Texas, USA

Beryl Benacerraf
Department of Radiology and Obstetrics
and Gynecology
Brigham and Women's Hospital
Boston, Massachusetts, USA

Vincenzo Berghella
Maternal Fetal Medicine Division

Obstetrics and Gynecology Department
Sidney Kimmel Medical College at Thomas
Jefferson University
Philadelphia, Pennsylvania, USA

Carolina Bibbo
Department of Obstetrics and Gynecology
Division of Maternal Fetal Medicine
Brigham and Women's Hospital
Boston, Massachusetts, USA

Werner Diehl
Chief of Fetal Medicine
Corniche Hospital
Abu Dhabi, UAE

Sarah Rae Easter
Division of Maternal–Fetal Medicine
Division of Critical Care Medicine
Brigham and Women's Hospital
Boston, Massachusetts, USA

Natasha Fenwick
Twins Trust Research Officer

Mike Foley
Department of Obstetrics and Gynecology
Banner University Medical Center
University of Arizona College of Medicine
Phoenix, Arizona, USA

Nathan S. Fox
Associate Clinical Professor
Maternal Fetal Medicine Associates, PLLC
Icahn School of Medicine at Mount Sinai
New York, New York, USA

Janice L. Gibson
Ian Donald Fetal Medicine Centre
Queen Elizabeth University Hospital
Glasgow, UK

Maria del Mar Gil
Obstetrics and Gynecology Department
Hospital Universitario de Torrejón,
Torrejón de Ardoz, Madrid, Spain

School of Medicine
Universidad Francisco de Vitoria (UFV)
Pozuelo de Alarcón, Madrid, Spain
Fetal Medicine Research Institute
King's College Hospital, London, UK

Jane Gorringe
Twins Trust Maternity Engagement Project
Manager

Leo Gurney
West Midlands Fetal Medicine Centre
Birmingham Women's and Children's
NHS Foundation Trust, Edgbaston, UK

Guillermo Gurza
Maternal Fetal Medicine Division
Obstetrics and Gynecology Department
Sidney Kimmel Medical College at Thomas
Jefferson University
Philadelphia, Pennsylvania, USA

Kurt Hecher
Professor of Obstetrics and Fetal Medicine
Department of Obstetrics and Fetal Medicine
University Medical Center Hamburg-
Eppendorf, Hamburg, Germany

Jon Hyett
Clinical Professor
Discipline of Obstetrics, Gynaecology and
Neonatology
Faculty of Medicine
University of Sydney
Sydney, Australia

Johannes Keunen
Ontario Fetal Centre
Toronto, Ontario, Canada

Asma Khalil
Fetal Medicine Unit
St George's Hospital
St George's University of London
London, UK
Vascular Biology Research Centre

Molecular and Clinical Sciences Research
Institute, St George's University of London
London, UK

Mark D. Kilby
Institute of Metabolism and Systems
Research, College of Medical and
Dental Sciences
University of Birmingham
Birmingham, UK
The Fetal Medicine Centre
Birmingham Women's and Children's
Foundation Trust, Birmingham, UK

Alice King
Assistant Professor
Department of Surgery
Baylor College of Medicine
Texas Children's Fetal Center
Houston, Texas, USA

Christop C. Lees
Queen Charlotte's and Chelsea
Hospital, Imperial Healthcare NHS Trust
Institute of Reproductive and
Developmental Biology
Imperial College, London, UK
Department of Development and
Regeneration
KU Leuven, Leuven, Belgium

Liesbeth Lewi
Department of Obstetrics and Gynaecology
University Hospitals Leuven
Department of Development and
Regeneration Biomedical Sciences
KU Leuven, Leuven, Belgium

Enrico Lopriore
Department of Neonatology
Leiden University Medical Center
Leiden, The Netherlands

Pierre Macé
Service de Gynécologie-Obstétrique
Hôpital Necker-Enfants Malades

Assistance Publique
Hôpitaux de Paris (AP-HP)
Université Paris Descartes
Paris, France

Houman Mahallati
Department of Radiology
University of Calgary
Calgary, Alberta, Canada

Fergal Malone
Master/CEO
Rotunda Hospital Dublin
Professor of Obstetrics and Gynaecology
Royal College of Surgeons in Ireland
Dublin, Ireland

Mariano Mascarenhas
Postdoctoral Fellowship in Reproductive
Medicine
Clinical Fellow
Leeds Fertility, Leeds Teaching Hospitals
NHS Trust
Leeds, UK

Ann McHugh
Royal College of Surgeons in Ireland,
Rotunda Hospital,
Dublin, Ireland

Elad Mei-Dan
North York General Hospital
Department of Obstetrics and Gynecology,
affiliated to the University of Toronto
Toronto, Ontario, Canada

Nir Melamed
Sunnybrook Health Sciences Centre
Department of Obstetrics and Gynecology
Division of Maternal–Fetal Medicine,
affiliated to the University of Toronto
Toronto, Ontario, Canada

Tim van Mieghem
Fetal Medicine Unit
Department of Obstetrics and
Gynaecology

Mount Sinai Hospital and University of
Toronto, Toronto, Ontario, Canada

R. Katie Morris
West Midlands Fetal Medicine Centre
Birmingham Women's and Children's
NHS Foundation Trust
Edgbaston, UK
Institute of Applied Health Research
College of Medical and Dental Sciences
University of Birmingham
Birmingham, UK

Rajit Narayan
Staff Specialist
Maternal Fetal Medicine
RPA Women and Babies
Royal Prince Alfred Hospital
Sydney, Australia

Kypros Nicolaides
Fetal Medicine Research Institute
King's College Hospital
London, UK

Laure Noël
Fetal Medicine Unit
St George's University Hospitals
NHS Foundation Trust
London, UK

Errol R. Norwitz
Department of Obstetrics and Gynecology
Tufts University School of Medicine
Mother Infant Research Institute
Tufts Medical Center
Boston, Massachusetts, USA

Vagisha Pruthi
Ontario Fetal Centre
Toronto, Ontario, Canada

DeWayne M. Pursley
Neonatologist-in-Chief
Beth Israel Deaconess Medical Center
Associate Professor of Pediatrics
Harvard Medical School
Boston, Massachusetts, USA

Alexandra Ramirez
Maternal Fetal Medicine Division
Obstetrics and Gynecology Department
Sidney Kimmel Medical College at Thomas
Jefferson University
Philadelphia, Pennsylvania, USA

Andrei Rebarber
President, Maternal Fetal Medicine
Associates, PLLC
President, Carnegie Imaging for
Women, PLLC
Codirector and Clinical Professor
Ichan School of Medicine at Mount Sinai
Division of Maternal Fetal Medicine
Englewood Hospital, Englewood, New
Jersey, USA

Amanda Roman
Department of Obstetrics and Gynecology
Division of Maternal-Fetal Medicine
Thomas Jefferson University
Philadelphia, Pennsylvania, USA

Greg Ryan
Ontario Fetal Centre
Toronto, Ontario, Canada

Laurent J. Salomon
Service de Gynécologie-Obstétrique
Hôpital Necker-Enfants Malades
Assistance Publique - Hôpitaux de Paris
EA 7328 FETUS and LUMIERE
Platform, Université Paris Descartes
Paris, France

Waldo Sepulveda
Director
FETALMED–Maternal-Fetal Diagnostic
Center, Santiago, Chile

Caroline J. Shaw
Queen Charlotte's and Chelsea
Hospital
Imperial Healthcare NHS Trust
Institute of Reproductive and
Developmental Biology

Imperial College London
London, UK

Shiri Shinar
Ontario Fetal Centre
Toronto, Ontario, Canada

Lynn Simpson
Hillary Rodham Clinton Professor of
Women's Health, Department of Obstetrics
and Gynecology
Division Director, Maternal Fetal Medicine
Columbia University Irving Medical Center
New York, New York, USA

Simi Gupta Talati
Assistant Clinical Professor
Maternal Fetal Medicine Associates/
Carnegie Imaging for Women
Icahn School of Medicine at Mount Sinai

New York, New York,
USA

Hong-Thao Thieu
Department of Obstetrics and Gynecology
Tufts University School of Medicine
Boston, Massachusetts, USA

Lala Langtry White
Perinatal Parent Support Specialist
Doula
Childbirth Educator Mother of Twins
Founding Partner, Love Through Loss,
Small and Mighty Babies,
TwinsPlus Arabia, UAE

Amy E. Wong
Department of Maternal–Fetal Medicine
Palo Alto Medical Foundation
Mountain View, California, USA

Chapter 1

Epidemiology of Multiple Pregnancy

Hong-Thao Thieu and Errol R. Norwitz

The Facts

Overall Incidence of Multifetal Pregnancies

From the introduction of modern record-keeping in the early 1900s until the 1970s, the combined incidence of multiple births in the United States was stable at around 2%. Of these, twins occurred in 18.9 per 1,000 live births and higher-order multiples (triplets and above) in 32.3 per 100,000 births.[1] In the 1980s, the widespread introduction of assisted reproductive technologies (ART) and shifting maternal demographics led to a steady increase in multiple pregnancies. From 1980 to 2009, twin births in the United States rose 76% to 33.2 per 1,000 births among women of all ages. Higher-order multiples increased 400%, peaking at 193.5 per 100,000 births in 1998.[2] In the late 1990s, concerns over the rising rates of multiple pregnancies led to the introduction of professional societal guidelines to reduce the number of multifetal gestations attributable to ART. Higher-order multiple pregnancy rates began to fall shortly thereafter and, in 2018, higher-order multiples occurred in only 93.0 per 100,000 births, a 52% decrease from 1998, but still nearly threefold higher than during the pre-ART era.[3] The twin birth rate was slower to stabilise, settling at around 33 per 1,000 births between 2007 and 2014. In 2014, for the first time in three decades, the twin birth rate began to decline and, in 2018, represented 32.6 out of 1,000 live births (Figure 1.1).[3-6]

Incidence of Twin Pregnancies

Twin pregnancies are classified according to their zygosity (genetic make-up) and chorionicity (anatomic arrangement of the placentas and fetal membranes).

- **Dizygous (non-identical) twins** arise from the fertilisation of two separate oocytes ovulated during the same menstrual cycle and comprise ~70% of spontaneous twin pregnancies. The dizygous (DZ) twin rate is impacted by numerous risk factors (discussed later in this chapter). While data regarding pregnancies conceived by in vitro fertilisation (IVF) are collected nationally, pregnancies arising from clomiphene citrate treatment or ovulation induction/intrauterine insemination (OI/IUI) are not. As such, the true rate of spontaneous DZ twins is difficult to determine. All DZ twins have dichorionic-diamniotic placentation (Figure 1.2).[6]
- **Monozygous (identical) twins** arise from the fertilisation of a single oocyte followed by a fission event shortly thereafter. Monozygous (MZ) twins represent the remaining 30% of twin pregnancies or around 0.45% of all gestations. Monozygotic twinning is a random event that occurs once every 250 to 300 conceptions. Such pregnancies are

1

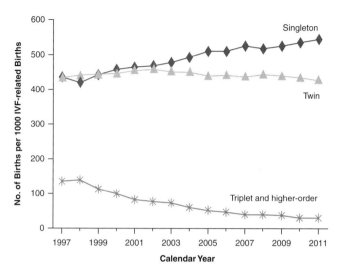

Figure 1.1 Changing incidence of multiple pregnancies
(Kulkarni AD, Jamieson DJ, Jones HW Jr, Kissin DM, Gallo MF, Macaluso M, Adashi EY. Fertility treatments and multiple births in the United States. *N Engl J Med* 2013; 369(23):2218–25. doi: 10.1056/NEJMoa1301467). (A black and white version of this figure will appear in some formats. For the colour version, please refer to the plate section.)

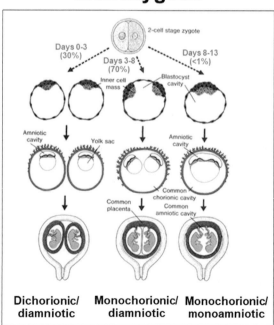

Figure 1.2 Zygosity and chorionicity of twin pregnancies. (A black and white version of this figure will appear in some formats. For the colour version, please refer to the plate section.)

classified according to their chorionicity, which is the single most important determinant of pregnancy outcome in MZ twins and dictates management.[7] If the zygote divides before day 3 post conception, which occurs in 30% of MZ twins, the placentation is dichorionic-diamniotic, identical to that in DZ twins. If the zygote divides between days 3 and 8 post conception, which is the most common timing, occurring in ±70% of MZ twins, the placentation is monochorionic-diamniotic. This means that the twins share a single blood supply. Division between days 8 and 13 post conception results in monochorionic-monoamniotic placentation, which occurs in only <1% of MZ twins (Figure 1.2).[6] Division after day 13 results in incomplete separation and conjoined twins. This is a rare condition complicating only 1 out of 60,000 pregnancies.

- **'Vanishing twin'** refers to a singleton pregnancy that began as twins with a subsequent spontaneous reduction so early in pregnancy that no evidence of the twin remains. Close monitoring during IVF has shown that this phenomenon is far more common than previously recognised, occurring in 10.4–18.8% of twin pregnancies. Because 80% of these losses occur prior to 9 weeks' gestation and thus prior to ultrasound examination, the rate of vanishing twins is likely under-reported in spontaneous pregnancies. Interestingly, male fetuses are at higher risk of spontaneous reduction than female fetuses. This may explain the difference in male-to-female gender ratios between singleton (1.05), twin (0.98) and triplet pregnancies (0.82).[8]

Incidence of Higher-Order Multiples

Triplets constitute more than 90% of higher-order multiples and occur spontaneously in approximately 1 in 8,000 pregnancies. Pregnancies with four or more fetuses occur spontaneously in only 1 out of 70,000 pregnancies. The vast majority of higher-order multiple pregnancies arise from ART.

Types and Incidence of Atypical Twinning

Several atypical forms of twins have been reported.[9] **Heterotopic pregnancies** occur when twins implant in different locations, most commonly one intrauterine and one ectopic. With ART, approximately 1 in 3,900 pregnancies are heterotopic. **Superfetation** refers to the fertilisation and implantation of a second conceptus during an existing pregnancy. Although well documented in other animal species, superfetation has not been definitively demonstrated in humans. **Complete moles** with a coexisting twin occur in 1 out of 22,000–100,000 pregnancies. **Fetus in fetu** is extremely rare (1 in 500,000 births) and results when a partially formed fetus is enveloped within the body of its surviving twin. It can be distinguished from a teratoma by the presence of vertebrae and limb alignment.

Risk Factors for Monozygotic Twinning

Monozygotic twinning is a random event that occurs once every 250 to 300 conceptions for an overall incidence of 0.45% of spontaneous conceptions. There are no historic or demographic risk factors, and the incidence of MZ twins is the same throughout the world. The only known risk factor for MZ twinning is ART, which increases the rate threefold (range 2–12 fold) to around 1.2%.[10] The precise mechanism by which ART leads to MZ twinning is not clear. One theory is that embryos cultured in vitro in artificial media have a hardened zona pellucida and that when the embryo hatches from the zona between days 4 and 5 post conception, it is more likely to get caught on the zona and divide. This is most obvious clinically following a single embryo transfer during IVF, but accounts for only 0.5% of IVF twins. Monozygotic twinning is likely a significant contributor to IVF higher-order multiples, with up to 28.8% of triplets and 64.7% of quadruplets following the transfer of fewer than three and four embryos, respectively.[10] This risk appears to be elevated even further with blastocyst transfer and remains a significant area of ongoing research.

Risk Factors for Dizygotic Twinning

- **Race/ethnicity.** Spontaneous multiple pregnancy rates vary greatly worldwide, ranging from a low of 1.3 per 1,000 births in Japan to a high of approximately 50 per 1,000 births in Nigeria. Pre-ART era data indicate that the spontaneous DZ twinning rate in African-American women is 1 in 80 pregnancies as compared with 1 in 100 pregnancies in Caucasian women and 1 in 155 pregnancies in Asian women.

- **Maternal age.** Even after controlling for ART, increasing maternal age is a major risk factor for DZ twinning. Women aged 35 are twofold to threefold more likely to conceive DZ twins than their 15-year-old counterparts. This is thought to be due to increasing circulating levels of follicle-stimulating hormone (FSH) and diminishing ovarian reserve with increasing maternal age, leading to the recruitment of more follicles each month and the potential for multiple ovulation events. As the maternal population in the United States ages, maternal age is becoming an increasingly important contributor to the total number of multiple gestations. Between 1980 and 2009, the percentage of total births to women older than age 30 rose from 20% to 35%. In 2016, it was estimated that delayed childbearing accounted for 24% and 38% of the national plural birth excess for non-Hispanic white and black women, respectively. Approximately one-third of the total increase in twin pregnancy rates from 1980 to 2009 is attributed to delayed childbearing independent of ART.[11,12]

- **Endogenous levels of gonadotropins.** Circulating levels of FSH and luteinising hormone (LH) are elevated in women who delivered DZ twins as compared to those who delivered singletons. The underlying cause of elevated gonadotropins is not well understood and is a focus of ongoing research.

- **Parity**. Increasing parity is associated with an increased likelihood of DZ twinning independent of maternal age.

- **Family and personal history.** Dizygotic twinning is known to run in families. Although the precise mode of inheritance remains unknown, the risk appears to be conferred through both the maternal and paternal lineages. Women with sisters who have DZ twins have a risk of 1.7 compared to the general population, and the offspring of female DZ twins have a risk of 2.5.[13] A family history of DZ twins in the male partner or sperm donor is also a risk factor for DZ twins, but the effect appears to be much weaker.

- **Genetic factors.** Taken together, the risk of recurrent DZ twins, the association with a positive family history and the racial/ethnic disparity suggest that genetic factors are involved. However, the identification of the 'twin gene(s)' remains elusive. The *FSH* and *FSH receptor* genes have been energetically investigated given the known contribution of gonadotropins to follicular development, but studies thus far have failed to show such an association. A number of other genes have been identified through familial genome mapping and genome-wide association studies. These include the *growth differentiation factor 9 (GDF9)* gene variant that appears to double the risk of DZ twinning. However, this variant is found in less than 4% of the population and as such is not believed to be a significant driver of twinning.[13] The *fragile X mental retardation 1 (FMR1)* gene has also been implicated in DZ twinning, though this association is confounded by the premature ovarian failure phenotype and elevated FSH levels in *FMR1 gene* carriers. In sum, no clinically significant or actionable genes for twinning have thus far been identified, although this is a focus of intense study with particular interest in genes encoding components of the hypothalamic-pituitary-ovarian axis.

- **Maternal body composition.** Both increased maternal height and body mass index (BMI) have been found to independently increase the risk of DZ twinning.[14] Much of these data were gleaned from pre-ART-era databases and prior to the obesity epidemic in the United States, which suggests that such factors may be increasingly important in years to come.

- **Seasonal variation.** Rates of DZ twinning appear to vary in a predictable fashion through the year with more twins conceived in summer/autumn and more twins born in winter, although not all studies have confirmed this association. Interestingly, of the studies that demonstrated seasonal variation, the impact appears to have been stronger in the 19th century as compared with the 20th.

- **Diet.** A number of nutritional factors have been associated with higher rates of multiple pregnancies, such as folic acid supplementation and β-carotene. However, these associations are relatively weak and not consistent in the literature.

- **Assisted reproductive technology.** By far the most important driver of DZ twinning is ART. In the United States, infertility affects 15.5% of reproductive-aged couples and approximately 1.7% of births result from ART. Currently, 36% of twin and 77% of triplet pregnancies occur in the setting of infertility treatment, and two-thirds of the plural birth excess in the United States is attributable to ART. Initially, the high incidence of multiple pregnancies was due to the transfer of two or more embryos in a given IVF cycle. As IVF technology developed, the risk of multiple pregnancies increased dramatically, particularly in association with gamete intrafallopian transfer (GIFT) and zygote intrafallopian transfer (ZIFT), procedures now abandoned. After the release of the first set of practice guidelines aimed at reducing ART-related multiple gestations in 1998, the rate of higher-order multiple pregnancies decreased, although the absolute numbers continued to climb due to increased use of ART.[15] More recently, use of pre-implantation genetic screening (PGS) has been shown to reduce the risk of multiple gestation, primarily by promoting the use of single embryo transfer in older patients. Ovulation induction using clomiphene citrate, letrozole (a non-steroidal aromatase inhibitor) or exogenous gonadotropins also increases the risk of multifetal gestation. This is due to ovarian hyper-stimulation leading to multiple ovulation. The risk of DZ twinning with OI/IUI is higher than that with traditional IVF, although pregnancy outcomes with OI/IUI are not tracked as closely as IVF and, as a result, multiple rates may be underreported.

- **Other risk factors.** Factors such as smoking, lower socio-economic status, oral contraceptives and coital frequency have been associated with a higher rate of DZ twinning. However, the evidence in support of these associations is inconsistent and frequently confounded.

Risk Factors for Higher-Order Multiple Pregnancies

Similarly to DZ twinning, triplet and higher-order multiple rates are affected by race/ethnicity, family history, maternal age and parity. However, the vast majority of such pregnancies are attributable to ART. Despite a significant decline in the rate of higher-order multiples since the implementation of practice guidelines a decade ago, the rate of higher-order multiple pregnancies is still threefold higher than that before the ART era.

The Issues

Most of the risk factors for twin and higher-order multiple pregnancies are not modifiable and as such cannot be actively managed. The one exception is ART, which has been the major driver of the increase in multiple pregnancies over the past 30 years (Figure 1.1). In the United States, the American Society for Reproductive Medicine (ASRM) and the Society for Reproductive Technology (SART) first reported ART practice data in 1988. Until 1992, submission of ART outcome data to the SART registry was voluntary. In 1992, Congress passed the Fertility Clinic Success Rate and Certification Act, which mandated creation of a federal data registry of pregnancy success rates from all ART centres as well as the certification status of embryo laboratories. In collaboration with the ASRM/SART, the US Centers for Disease Control and Prevention (CDC) is responsible for implementing the Fertility Clinic Success Rate and Certification Act. To be a member of the ASRM/SART, an ART programme must agree to submit their IVF procedure activity data to the registry and make them publicly available. This is not necessarily true of other infertility procedures, such as OI/IUI. In the United Kingdom, the Human Fertilisation and Embryo Authority (HFEA) collects the data and statistics of all the IVF treatment cycles on a yearly basis and publishes them for the use of patients, researchers and clinicians. The last year for which data were published was 2018 (published in June 2020). Data are currently available from all years, from the first year of collection of 1991 to 2018.

The major rate-limiting factor for ART is implantation. Although critical to survival of the species, implantation in humans is relatively inefficient. Maximal fecundity (the likelihood of getting pregnant each cycle) peaks at 30%. Only 50% of conceptions advance beyond 20 weeks' gestation, and of all unsuccessful pregnancies, 75% represent a failure of implantation. Despite exhaustive research, the factors responsible for optimal implantation are not well understood. Interestingly, humans are one of only a few mammalian viviparous species in which endometrial decidualisation (priming) occurs spontaneously during each menstrual cycle and is therefore independent of the conceptus. This suggests that the health of a pregnancy is determined even before the blastocyst arrives, which offers physicians a unique opportunity for intervention. Research in this area is ongoing at the population and cellular levels. A better understanding of these factors may help to further reduce multiple gestations arising from ART.

Management Options

As discussed, most risk factors for multiple pregnancies are not modifiable with the exception of ART. The goal of ART is a single, healthy, take-home baby. The ASRM recognises that multifetal gestations, particularly higher-order multiples, should not be regarded as a success but as a failure of ART. The Committee on Ethics of the American

College of Obstetricians and Gynecologists (ACOG) states that 'the first approach to the problem of multifetal pregnancies should be prevention'.[16,17]

Assisted Reproductive Technology Methodology

A number of precautions can be taken to reduce the risk of multifetal gestation with ART. The use of low-dose ovarian stimulation protocols whenever possible will reduce the risk of superovulation. Regardless of the stimulation protocol used, the patient should be followed with serial serum estradiol-17β levels and follicle number by transvaginal ultrasound and the cycle cancelled if too many follicles develop to minimise the risk of ovarian hyper-stimulation syndrome (OHSS). The ASRM consensus guidelines also offer recommendations for embryo transfer number based on predicted IVF success rates with the stated goal of reducing rates of higher-order multiple pregnancy.[15,17] These recommendations are based on characteristics associated with a more favourable prognosis, including embryo number and quality, first IVF cycle, prior IVF success and donor oocytes from women younger than 35 years of age. Women younger than 35 with favourable prognostic indicators should be offered single embryo transfer and should not have more than two embryos transferred. A third embryo may be transferred in women older than age 35, especially if they have poor-quality embryos or have suffered multiple failed IVF cycles, but this should be the exception, not the rule.[15] In the United Kingdom, the HFEA, working with other British obstetrics and scientific governing bodies, updated its advice in 2019 for IVF to ideally limit embryo transfer to one per treatment cycle to minimise the risk of multiple pregnancy. In older women or in those with poor-quality embryos, two may be transferred with a maximum of three in those older than 40 years. Care should be taken to avoid financial influences when making decisions around embryo transfer.[16] In the United States, in states with no mandate for health insurance coverage of infertility treatments, patients must pay out of pocket. They are therefore often incentivised to maximise the success rate of each cycle, leading them to advocate for the transfer of more embryos and driving up the multiples rate. Strategies to reduce these barriers include petitioning state governments to change their insurance mandates and/or offering alternative payment plans through the clinics.

Multifetal Pregnancy Reduction

The ASRM and the ACOG recognise the increase in morbidity and mortality associated with multifetal gestation for both the pregnant patient and the fetuses (Table 1.1).[1,7,12,13,15,16] Moreover, medical costs for twins quadruple that of their singleton counterparts, while triplet costs are tenfold higher.[18] Higher rates of maternal depression and child abuse have also been reported with multiples. Given the potential adverse consequences of multiples, multifetal pregnancy reduction (MFPR) is sometimes recommended. This refers to the termination of one or more fetuses in the setting of a multifetal gestation with a view to optimising the outcome for the surviving fetuses. It is most typically performed in higher-order multiple pregnancies and involves the intra-cardiac injection of potassium chloride. Multifetal pregnancy reduction has been shown to significantly reduce spontaneous pregnancy loss, preterm birth and neonatal death for the surviving fetus(es) as well as maternal medical complications associated with higher-order pregnancy. Multifetal pregnancy reduction is in contrast to selective fetal reduction, in which one or more fetuses are selectively terminated due to an underlying structural, genetic or metabolic disorder.

Table 1.1 Maternal and perinatal complications associated with multiple pregnancies

Characteristic	Single	Twins	Triplets	Quads
Preterm birth	10–12%	40–50%	85–95%	100%
Gestational age (week)	39.5	35.3	32.2	29.9
Birth weight (gram)	3,500	2,347	1,687	1,309
Fetal growth restriction	10%	15–25%	50–60%	50–60%
NICU admission	5–10%	25%	75%	100%
NICU length of stay	1–3 days	18 days	38 days	58 days
Congenital anomalies	3–4%	6–15%	20%	-
Major handicap	< 1%	7%	20%	40–50%
Risk of cerebral palsy	reference	4 × singles	17 × singles	-
Risk of neonatal death	reference	7 × singles	20 × singles	-

Data from references 1, 7, 12, 13, 15, and 16

Multifetal pregnancy reduction raises a host of complex and deeply personal social, economic, ethical and medical issues. Appropriate counselling is critical. The ACOG recommends that 'nondirective patient counselling should be offered to all women with higher-order multifetal pregnancies and should include discussion of the risks unique to multifetal pregnancy as well as the option to continue or reduce the pregnancy'.[1,16] Consultation with experts in maternal fetal medicine, neonatology, support groups and family planning or other providers with expertise in the procedure is advised. The ACOG further recommends that if MFPR is not in alignment with a provider's personal beliefs, a timely referral should be offered.

Key Points

- Widespread introduction of ART and shifting maternal demographics led to a steady increase in multiple pregnancies, which plateaued after the 2010s with the implementation of societal guidelines aimed at reducing multifetal gestations.
- Dizygotic (non-identical) twins comprise approximately 70% of spontaneous twin pregnancies; the remaining 30% are MZ (identical).
- Monozygotic twinning is a random event occurring in 1 out of 250 to 300 pregnancies.
- Dizygotic twinning is influenced by many factors, including maternal age, race/ethnicity, parity, family history and use of ART. The only risk factor for MZ twinning is IVF.
- Both IVF and OI/IUI increase the risk of multifetal gestation, with OI/IUI carrying a slightly higher risk.
- Multifetal pregnancy, particularly higher-order multiple pregnancy, is recognised as an undesirable outcome by both the ASRM and the ACOG due to increased maternal and fetal morbidity and mortality.
- Providers should seek to prevent multifetal gestation by using low-dose ovarian stimulation protocols and carefully monitoring ovulation induction cycles.

- When performing IVF, single embryo transfer should be considered whenever possible.
- When a higher-order multifetal gestation is encountered, the patient should be offered non-directive and multidisciplinary counselling regarding MFPR.

References

1. American College of Obstetricians and Gynecologists. Multifetal pregnancy reduction. ACOG Committee Opinion No. 719. Obstet Gynecol 2017;**130**(3):670–1. https://doi.org/10.1097/aog .0000000000002302

2. Martin JA, Hamilton BE, Osterman MJK. Three decades of twin births in the United States, 1980–2009. NCHS Data Brief. 2012;**80**:1–8.

3. Martin JA, Hamilton BE, Osterman MJK, Driscoll AK. Births: final data for 2018. Natl Vital Stat Rep 2019;**68**(13):1–55.

4. Martin JA, Osterman MJK. Is twin childbearing on the decline? Twin births in the United States, 2014–2018. NCHS Data Brief 2019;**351**:1–8.

5. Martin JA, Osterman MJK, Thoma ME. Declines in triple and higher-order multiple births in the United States, 1998–2014. NCHS Data Brief 2016;**243**:108.

6. Norwitz ER. Multiple pregnancies: trends past, present and future. In The Infertility and Reproductive Medicine Clinics of North America, Diamond M, DeCherney A (eds.). Philadelphia: W. B. Saunders, 1998;chapter 9, pp. 351–69.

7. Lee YM, Wylie BJ, Simpson LL, D'Alton ME. Twin chorionicity and the risk of stillbirth. Obstet Gynecol 2008;**111** (1):301–8. https://doi.org/10.1097/AOG .0b013e318160d65d

8. Ein-Mor E, Mankuta D, Hochner-Celnikier D, Hurwitz A, Haimov-Kochman R. Sex ratio is remarkably constant. Fertil Steril 2010;**93**(6):1961–5. https://doi.org/10.1016/j .fertnstert.2008.12.036

9. Mcnamara HC, Kane SC, Craig JM, Short RV, Umstad MP. A review of the mechanisms and evidence for typical and atypical twinning. Am J Obstet Gynecol 2016;**214**(2):172–91. https://doi.org/10.1016/ j.ajog.2015.10.930

10. Gee RE, Dickey RP, Xiong X, Clark LS, Pridjian G. Impact of monozygotic twinning on multiple births resulting from in vitro fertilization in the United States, 2006–2010. Am J Obstet Gynecol 2014;**210** (5):468.e1–6. https://doi.org/10.1016/j .ajog.2013.12.034

11. Adashi EY, Gutman R. Delayed childbearing as a growing, previously unrecognized contributor to the national plural birth excess. Obstet Gynecol 2018;**132**(4):999–1006. https://doi.org/10 .1097/aog.0000000000002853

12. American College of Obstetricians and Gynecologists. Multifetal gestations: twin, triplet and higher-order multifetal pregnancies. ACOG Practice Bulletin No. 169. Obstet Gynecol 2016;**128**(4): 926–8. https://doi.org/10.1097/aog .0000000000001709

13. Hoekstra C, Zhao ZZ, Lambalk CB, Willemsen G, Martin NG, Boomsma DI, Montgomery GW. Dizygotic twinning. Hum Reprod Update 2008;**14**(1):37–47. https://doi.org/10.1093/humupd/dmm036

14. Reddy U, Branum A, Klebanoff M. Relationship of maternal body mass index and height to twinning. Obstet Gynecol 2005;**105**(3):593–7. https://doi.org/10.1097/ 01.aog.0000169607.78155.7f

15. American Society for Reproductive Medicine. Multiple gestation associated with infertility therapy: an American Society of Reproductive Medicine Practice Committee Opinion. Fertil Steril 2012;**97** (4):825–34. https://doi.org/10.1016/j .fertnstert.2011.11.048

16. American College of Obstetricians and Gynecologists. Perinatal risks associated with assisted reproductive technology. ACOG Committee Opinion No 671. Obstet Gynecol 2016;**128**(3).e61–8. https://doi.org/10.1097/aog .0000000000001643

17. American Society for Reproductive Medicine and Society for Assisted Reproductive Technology. Criteria for number of embryos to transfer: a committee opinion. Practice Committees of ASRM and SART. Fertil Steril 2013; **99**(1):44–6. https://doi.org/10.1016/j.fertnstert.2012.09.038

18. Callahan TL, Hall JE, Ettner SL, Christiansen CL, Greene MF, Crowley WF Jr. The economic impact of multiple-gestation pregnancies and the contribution of assisted-reproduction techniques to their incidence. N Engl J Med 1994;**331**(4):244–9. https://doi.org/10.1056/NEJM199407283310407

Assisted Conception and Multiple Pregnancy
Strategies to Reduce Rates

Mariano Mascarenhas and Adam Balen

The Facts

Multiple pregnancy rates are higher following assisted conception than after natural conceptions, thus forming, along with ovarian hyper-stimulation syndrome (OHSS), one of the two main iatrogenic risks of treatment for infertility. The reproductive medicine specialist has to often run a tightrope between the risks of multiple pregnancy (which have been well illustrated in other chapters in this book) and improving the efficacy of fertility treatment – and meeting patient expectations.

A study from our group which attempted to assess the mode of conceptions of all births (n = 7,015) within a span of a week in 2003 in the United Kingdom noted that the multiple birth rate was significantly greater in assisted (13.5%) than in natural conception (1.2%). Of the multiple births following fertility treatment, 17% resulted from clomiphene citrate therapy, 72% from in vitro fertilisation (IVF) or frozen embryo replacements (FET) and 6% from superovulation with intrauterine insemination (IUI).[1] As we describe in this chapter, multiple pregnancy rates following IVF have fallen significantly since that study was performed. The maternal risks due to multiple pregnancy have been covered in Chapter 18 and neonatal risks in Chapter 26 of this volume.

Assisted conception appears to amplify the adverse maternal and fetal outcomes of twin pregnancies. Dichorionic twin pregnancies conceived following IVF have a higher risk of placenta praevia, preterm birth, very preterm birth, low birthweight and congenital malformations.[2] A retrospective study noted that IVF increases the risk of preterm birth in twin pregnancies complicated with pre-eclampsia and that this increased risk persists after adjusting for confounders, including maternal age.[3]

For the purposes of discussing strategies to reduce multiple pregnancy rates, infertility treatments have been classified into ovulation induction (OI) (with/without IUI) and IVF as the prevalence, aetiology and risk-reduction strategies for multiple pregnancy differ according to the infertility treatment strategy employed.

Ovulation Induction for Anovulatory Infertility with/without Intrauterine Insemination

Ovulation induction is the primary infertility treatment for women with World Health Organization (WHO) type 1 (hypogonadotrophic hypogonadism) and type 2 (which includes polycystic ovary syndrome (PCOS)) anovulatory infertility. Women with hypogonadotrophic hypogonadism are ideally treated with pulsatile gonadotrophin-releasing hormone (GnRH) provided through a mini-infusion pump, which provides a physiological restoration of the cycle with a low risk of multiple pregnancy.[4] Unfortunately, this method has fallen out of use due to the lack of availability of the medication in recent years. Instead, gonadotrophin preparations with both follicle-stimulating hormone (FSH) and luteinising hormone (LH) bioactivity are used. Ovulation induction for PCOS can be achieved via a spectrum of medications, but the primary drugs in use include clomiphene citrate (CC) (a selective anti-oestrogen), letrozole (an aromatase inhibitor) and gonadotrophins (from either urinary or recombinant sources).[5]

The primary aetiology behind multiple pregnancies in OI (irrespective of whether it is combined with IUI) is the ovulation of multiple follicles, thereby leading to multiple fertilisation events leading to multiple embryos. The multiple pregnancies ensuing from OI are primarily of the multi-zygotic type. There is no clear evidence that OI increases the risk of monozygotic twinning.

The incidence of multiple pregnancies was reported as high as 15% following OI with CC and 30% following OI with gonadotrophins in the 1970s.[6] The advent of first real-time and then transvaginal ultrasound monitoring techniques and accumulating clinical expertise has led to a steady decline in the incidence of multiple pregnancies with OI with data from the turn of the century indicating a multiple pregnancy rate of 8% with CC and 11% with gonadotrophins.[7] This is further illustrated by data from the latest Cochrane reviews on the topic. Despite data from the initial randomised controlled trials (RCTs) indicating a lower risk of multiple pregnancies with letrozole than with CC, recent data appear to indicate that both methodologies have a similar low risk for multiple pregnancy rates. At this time, it is unclear whether this can be taken as a 'real-world picture' or whether it is a phenomenon unique to the 'RCT environment' with its stringent requirements for safety and therefore strict cancellation criteria in cases of multi-follicular recruitment.

The incidence of multiple pregnancy as outlined in the latest Cochrane literature appears to be not significantly different between CC and letrozole (1.7% with CC versus 1.3% with letrozole; OR 0.69, 95% CI 0.41 to 1.16; 17 RCTs; n = 3,579; I^2 = 0%; high-quality evidence).[8] There was also no significant difference noted in multiple pregnancy rates between recombinant and urinary gonadotrophins (RR 0.86, 95% CI 0.46 to 1.61; eight RCTs; n = 1,368; I^2 = 0%; low-quality evidence). Surprisingly, the Cochrane review also did not note a significant difference between gonadotrophins and CC in multiple pregnancy rates, but the data were more limited (RR 0.89, 95% CI 0.33 to 2.44; one RCT; n = 661; I^2 = 0%; moderate-quality evidence).[9]

The principle of minimising multiple pregnancy rates with OI for women with PCOS is relatively straightforward, and the criteria for cancellation can be strict as OI is, in principle, to be used for women with anovulation and therefore uni-follicular ovulation should be all that is required to restore fertility. Current guidelines suggest that ultrasound monitoring is provided for OI with CC and letrozole for at least the first one or two cycles at each dose used or until it can be established that there is an appropriate ovarian response.[5] Ultrasound monitoring is mandatory for every cycle of gonadotrophin OI, and we propose strict criteria before the administration of the pre-ovulatory trigger of human chorionic gonadotrophin (hCG), which initiates the release of the eggs, namely no more than a total of two follicles greater than 14 mm in diameter, with the largest follicle usually at least 17 mm.[5] Furthermore, it is necessary to provide at least six-day if not seven-day service for ultrasound monitoring, as follicle growth can be unpredictable and scans may be required alternate days or even daily once the follicles reach a mature size.

Laparoscopic ovarian diathermy ('drilling') is a second-line OI method for women with PCOS which commonly involves multiple needle diathermies (usually four per ovary) targeted at the ovarian stroma. The aim of laparoscopic ovarian drilling is to induce spontaneous ovulation without the need for exogenous medications or the attendant monitoring. Randomised controlled trials have suggested that the incidence of multiple pregnancy is lower with laparoscopic ovarian drilling than with gonadotrophins (OR 0.13; 95% CI 0.03 to 0.52; five RCTs; n = 166; I^2 = 0%).[10]

Ovulation Induction with Intrauterine Insemination for Unexplained Infertility

Ovulation induction agents such as clomiphene, letrozole and gonadotrophins have also been employed as ovarian stimulation agents for women with natural ovulation. Ovarian stimulation with IUI is employed as a strategy in unexplained infertility and mild male factor infertility as an alternative to IVF where there are good patient prognostic factors (young age, a moderate duration of infertility) or where resources for IVF are limited and expectant management is not an acceptable option.

There does not appear to be a clear risk of increased multiple pregnancies with ovarian stimulation with IUI as compared with expectant management for unexplained infertility (OR 2.00, 95% CI 0.18 to 22.34; two RCTs; n = 304; moderate-quality evidence), but neither was there a difference in live birth rates (OR 0.82, 95% CI 0.45 to 1.49; one RCT; n = 253; moderate-quality evidence).[11] There was insufficient evidence whether ovarian stimulation with IUI made a significance difference to live birth rates or multiple pregnancy rates as compared with expectant management of mild male factor infertility.[12]

A recent three-armed RCT comparing ovarian stimulation with IUI with conventional IVF with single embryo transfer and modified natural cycle IVF noted no significant difference in multiple pregnancy rates. It is pertinent to note that strict cancellation criteria were utilised with IUI cancelled if there were more than three follicles with a diameter of at least 16 mm, or more than five follicles with a diameter of 12 mm.[13]

When it comes to women with unexplained infertility who are already having natural uni-follicular recruitment, the goal of ovarian stimulation is multi-follicular recruitment.[14] A balance therefore has to be found between minimising multiple pregnancy rates and maintaining an acceptable success rate for superovulation. Suggested recommendations have included cycle cancellation when more than two follicles greater than 16 mm are visualised on ultrasound or when the serum estradiol levels are higher than 1,000 pg/ml.[15] However, the published literature indicates that none of these criteria can be effective in eliminating higher-order multiple pregnancy[16] and that intermediate follicles of size 12 mm or greater could contribute to multiple pregnancy.[17]

Superovulation for In Vitro Fertilisation

In vitro fertilisation rather than OI (or superovulation) contributes to the majority of multiple births following assisted conception. It is therefore important for multiple birth reduction strategies to maximise focus on this aspect. Multiple births after IVF place an inordinate burden on public health care systems. A 2006 modelling study noted that the cost to the health service was £3,313 for a singleton birth following IVF, but rose to £9,122 for a twin birth. The costs due to a triplet birth following IVF were far higher at £32,354.[18] The authors suggested that redirecting the cost incurred in managing multiple gestations to instead broaden public health funding for IVF to be linked to limiting the number of embryos transferred would be a cost-effective approach. Public funding, including partial reimbursement where single embryo transfer is performed, has been shown to be cost-effective with the savings in birth-admission costs alone recuperating more than half the cost spent on IVF cycles in Australia.[19] Furthermore, the publication of IVF outcomes in the UK by the Human Fertilisation and Embryology Authority (HFEA) presents data per number of embryos transferred, which consequently favours those clinics with a strict elective single embryo transfer policy.

The incidence of multiple pregnancies following IVF is primarily due to the transfer of more than one embryo. Among couples having IVF, there appears to be a preference to have a double embryo transfer as demonstrated in a trial comparing elective single embryo transfer with double embryo transfer where 40% of women in the elective single embryo transfer arm chose to have double embryo transfer instead.[20] More than half of infertile couples (58%) surveyed in a 2014 Spanish study stated that they would prefer to have twin pregnancies with the most common reason being 'to avoid a new IVF attempt'.[21] However, acceptance of single embryo transfer is improved when patients are educated regarding the risks of multiple pregnancy with oral, written and/or electronic information.[22]

Strict regulations by organisations such as the British Fertility Society, the National Institute for Health and Care Excellence (NICE) and the HFEA have resulted in a drop in multiple live birth rates from 24% in 2008 to 10% in 2017.[23] This drop in multiple live birth rates has been primarily due to elective single embryo transfer, the acceptability of which has increased due to two laboratory factors:

1. Better embryo selection through
   a. Blastocyst culture
   b. Improvement in embryo selection techniques

2. Improvements in embryo cryopreservation techniques so that surplus good-quality embryos can be frozen, thereby enabling further attempts at embryo transfer without the need to go through a full cycle with ovarian stimulation.

Data from RCTs indicate that the cumulative live birth rates are not significantly different between double embryo transfer and transfer of a single embryo with elective cryopreservation followed by frozen embryo transfer of the second embryo at a later date (OR 1.22, 95% CI 0.92 to 1.62, three RCTs; n = 811, I^2 = 0%, low-quality evidence). However, the multiple pregnancy rate is significantly higher with the former approach (OR 30.54, 95% CI 7.46 to 124.95, three RCTs, n = 811, I^2 = 23%, low-quality evidence).[24]

Based on such evidence, NICE recommends elective single embryo transfer where a top-quality blastocyst is available for transfer.[25] In other cases, the recommendation is to consider a single embryo transfer (dependent of embryo quality) for women younger than the age of 40 years having their first or second full cycle of IVF (a full cycle includes all fresh and frozen embryo transfers from a single oocyte retrieval attempt).

Monozygotic Twins

Some of the latest laboratory techniques such as pre-implantation genetic testing[26] and extended culture to blastocyst stage[27] appear to increase the risk of monozygotic twinning. Monozygotic twins have a poorer prognosis than dizygotic twins. Furthermore, the limited literature on monozygotic twins following IVF appears to indicate that their prognosis may be poorer than the naturally conceived monozygotic twins.[28,29]

Twin Pregnancies after Egg Donation

Pregnancies after egg donation (provided to women with premature ovarian insufficiency) have a higher risk of preterm birth and low birthweight as compared with IVF pregnancies using a woman's own eggs.[30] A pilot RCT comparing a single double embryo transfer with two sequential elective single embryo transfer in egg donation cycles noted no significant difference in cumulative live birth rate, but a significant increase in the risk of twin pregnancies.[31] Therefore single embryo transfer needs to be considered for egg donation cycles, especially for women aged 45 years or older, who have a 65% risk of preterm birth, a 15% risk of early preterm birth (<32 weeks) and an 18% risk of life-threatening complications such as requirement for blood product transfusion or admission to intensive care if they have twin pregnancies.[32]

Key Points

- Reducing multiple pregnancy rates can be achieved clinically by:
  - Strict cycle cancellation criteria for OI and ovarian stimulation for intrauterine insemination and careful monitoring with serial ultrasounds (ideally with a seven-day service).
  - Single embryo transfer in IVF.
- For acceptance of these techniques, it is essential to have:
  - Appropriate education of reproductive medicine specialists.
  - Proper counselling of patients.
  - Public funding/reimbursement of IVF linked to single embryo transfer.
- Public health commissioning bodies need to be aware that:
  - Multiple pregnancies pose a significant strain on public health care services.
  - These costs could be reduced by a blanket public funding of IVF linked to single embryo transfer.

References

1. Bardis N, Maruthini D, Balen AH. Modes of conception and multiple pregnancy: a national survey of babies born during one week in 2003 in the United Kingdom. Fertil Steril 2005 Dec;**84**(6):1727–32.

2. Qin JB, Wang H, Sheng X, Xie Q, Gao S. Assisted reproductive technology and risk of adverse obstetric outcomes in dichorionic twin pregnancies: a systematic review and meta-analysis. Fertil Steril 2016 May;**105** (5):1180–92.

3. Okby R, Harlev A, Sacks KN, Sergienko R, Sheiner E. Preeclampsia acts differently in in vitro fertilization versus spontaneous twins. Arch Gynecol Obstet 2018;**297** (3):653–8.

4. Yasmin E, Davies M, Conway G, Balen AH. British Fertility Society null. British Fertility Society. 'Ovulation induction in WHO Type 1 anovulation: guidelines for practice'. Produced on behalf of the BFS Policy and Practice Committee. Hum Fertil Camb Engl 2013 Dec;**16**(4):228–34.

5. Balen AH, Morley LC, Misso M, Franks S, Legro RS, Wijeyaratne CN et al. The management of anovulatory infertility in women with polycystic ovary syndrome: an analysis of the evidence to support the development of global WHO guidance. Hum Reprod Update 2016;**22**(6):687–708.

6. Schenker JG, Yarkoni S, Granat M. Multiple pregnancies following induction of

ovulation. Fertil Steril 1981 Feb;**35**(2):105–23.

7. Mitwally MF, Biljan MM, Casper RF. Pregnancy outcome after the use of an aromatase inhibitor for ovarian stimulation. Am J Obstet Gynecol 2005 Feb;**192**(2):381–6.

8. Franik S, Eltrop SM, Kremer JA, Kiesel L, Farquhar C. Aromatase inhibitors (letrozole) for subfertile women with polycystic ovary syndrome. Cochrane Database Syst Rev 2018 24;5:CD010287.

9. Weiss NS, Kostova E, Nahuis M, Mol BWJ, Van der Veen F, Van Wely M. Gonadotrophins for ovulation induction in women with polycystic ovary syndrome. Cochrane Database Syst Rev [Internet]. 2019 [cited 2019 Aug 23];(**1**). Available from www.cochranelibrary.com/cdsr/doi/10.1002/14651858.CD010290.pub3/full

10. Farquhar C, Brown J, Marjoribanks J. Laparoscopic drilling by diathermy or laser for ovulation induction in anovulatory polycystic ovary syndrome. Cochrane Database Syst Rev [Internet]. 2012 [cited 2019 Aug 23];(**6**). Available from www.cochranelibrary.com/cdsr/doi/10.1002/14651858.CD001122.pub4/full

11. Veltman-Verhulst SM, Hughes E, Ayeleke RO, Cohlen BJ. Intra-uterine insemination for unexplained subfertility. Cochrane Database Syst Rev 2016;**2**(100909747):CD001838.

12. Cissen M, Bensdorp A, Cohlen BJ, Repping S, De Bruin JP, Van Wely M. Assisted reproductive technologies for male subfertility. Cochrane Database Syst Rev 2016 Feb **26**;2:CD000360.

13. Tjon-Kon-Fat RI, Bensdorp AJ, Bossuyt PMM, Koks C, Oosterhuis GJE, Hoek A et al. Is IVF – served two different ways – more cost-effective than IUI with controlled ovarian hyperstimulation? Hum Reprod. 2015 Oct 1;**30**(10):2331–9.

14. Van Rumste MME, Custers IM, Van der Veen F, Van Wely M, Evers JLH, Mol BWJ. The influence of the number of follicles on pregnancy rates in intrauterine insemination with ovarian stimulation: a meta-analysis. Hum Reprod Update 2008 Nov 1;**14**(6):563–70.

15. Practice Committee of American Society for Reproductive Medicine. Use of exogenous gonadotropins in anovulatory women: a technical bulletin. Fertil Steril 2008 Nov;90(5Suppl):S7–12.

16. Fong SA, Palta V, Oh C, Cho MM, Loughlin JS, McGovern PG. Multiple pregnancy after gonadotropin-intrauterine insemination: an Unavoidable event? ISRN Obstet Gynecol [Internet]. 2011 [cited 2019 Dec 29]. Available from www.ncbi.nlm.nih.gov/pmc/articles/PMC3255317

17. Giles J, Cruz M, González-Ravina C, Caligara C, Prados N, Martínez JC et al. Small-sized follicles could contribute to high-order multiple pregnancies: outcomes of 6552 intrauterine insemination cycles. Reprod Biomed Online 2018 Nov;**37**(5):549–54.

18. Ledger WL, Anumba D, Marlow N, Thomas CM, Wilson ECF. Cost of Multiple Births Study Group (COMBS Group): the costs to the NHS of multiple births after IVF treatment in the UK.BJOG Int J Obstet Gynaecol 2006 Jan;**113**(1):21–5.

19. Chambers GM, Illingworth PJ, Sullivan EA. Assisted reproductive technology: public funding and the voluntary shift to single embryo transfer in Australia. Med J Aust 2011;**195**(10):594–8.

20. Prados N, Quiroga R, Caligara C, Ruiz M, Blasco V, Pellicer A et al. Elective single versus double embryo transfer: live birth outcome and patient acceptance in a prospective randomised trial. Reprod Fertil Dev 2015 Jun;**27**(5):794–800.

21. Mendoza R, Jáuregui T, Diaz-Nuñez M, De la Sota M, Hidalgo A, Ferrando M et al. Infertile couples prefer twins: analysis of their reasons and clinical characteristics related to this preference. J Reprod Infertil 2018 Sep;**19**(3):167–73.

22. Sunderam S, Boulet SL, Jamieson DJ, Kissin DM. Effects of patient education on desire for twins and use of elective single embryo transfer procedures during ART

treatment: a systematic review. Reprod Biomed Soc Online 2018 Aug;6:102–19.

23. Human Fertilisation and Embryology Authority. Fertility treatment 2017: trends and figures. 2019. www.hfea.gov.uk/about-us/publications/research-and-data/fertility-treatment-2019-trends-and-figures

24. Pandian Z, Marjoribanks J, Ozturk O, Serour G, Bhattacharya S. Number of embryos for transfer following in vitro fertilisation or intra-cytoplasmic sperm injection. Cochrane Database Syst Rev 2013 Jul 29;(7):CD003416.

25. National Institute for Health and Care Excellence. (2013). Fertility problems: assessment and treatment (NICE Quality Standard No. 156). Retrieved from www.nice.org.uk/guidance/cg156.

26. Kamath MS, Antonisamy B, Sunkara SK. Zygotic splitting following embryo biopsy: a cohort study of 207 697 single embryo transfers following IVF treatment. BJOG Int J Obstet Gynaecol [Internet]. [cited 2019 Dec 29];n/a(n/a). Available from https://obgyn.onlinelibrary.wiley.com/doi/abs/10.1111/1471-0528.16045

27. Knopman JM, Krey LC, Oh C, Lee J, McCaffrey C, Noyes N. What makes them split? Identifying risk factors that lead to monozygotic twins after in vitro fertilization. Fertil Steril 2014 Jul;102(1):82–9.

28. Hack KEA, Vereycken MEMS, Torrance HL, Koopman-Esseboom C, Derks JB. Perinatal outcome of monochorionic and dichorionic twins after spontaneous and assisted conception: a retrospective cohort study. Acta Obstet Gynecol Scand 2018 Jun;97(6):717–26.

29. Mascarenhas M, Kamath MS, Muthukumar K, Mangalaraj AM, Chandy A, Aleyamma T. Obstetric outcomes of monochorionic pregnancies conceived following assisted reproductive technology: a retrospective study. J Hum Reprod Sci 2014;7(2):119–24.

30. Mascarenhas M, Sunkara SK, Antonisamy B, Kamath MS. Higher risk of preterm birth and low birth weight following oocyte donation: a systematic review and meta-analysis. Eur J Obstet Gynecol Reprod Biol 2017 Nov;218:60–7.

31. Clua E, Tur R, Coroleu B, Rodríguez I, Boada M, Gómez MJ et al. Is it justified to transfer two embryos in oocyte donation? A pilot randomized clinical trial. Reprod Biomed Online 2015 Aug;31(2):154–61.

32. Laskov I, Michaan N, Cohen A, Tsafrir Z, Maslovitz S, Kupferminc M et al. Outcome of Twin pregnancy in women ≥45 years old: a retrospective cohort study. J Matern Fetal Neonatal Med 2013 May 1;26(7):669–72.

Zygosity, Chorionicity and Amnionicity

Waldo Sepulveda and Amy E. Wong

There is NO diagnosis of twins. There are only monochorionic twins or dichorionic twins. This diagnosis should be written in capital red letters across the top of the patient's chart.

Kypros H. Nicolaides[1]

Introduction

Spontaneous multiple pregnancy occurs with a frequency of approximately 1 in 90 for twins, 1 in 8,000 for triplets and 1 in 700,000 for quadruplets. With the development of assisted reproductive techniques, however, the incidence of multiple pregnancy has increased dramatically over the past several decades due to the use of ovulatory medications and the transfer of multiple embryos during in vitro fertilisation procedures.[2] The increase in the rate of multiple pregnancies has tremendous clinical and logistic implications because these pregnancies are at risk for multiple perinatal complications, including pregnancy loss and severe prematurity. Indeed, although twin pregnancies account for about 1% of all pregnancies, they contribute disproportionally to more than 10% of all neonatal intensive care admissions, with considerable burden on the family, caregivers and society as a whole.[2]

To optimise perinatal care and outcomes, timely diagnosis of a twin pregnancy and tailoring management according to its chorionicity – that is, the number of implantation sites and therefore the number of placentas – and its amnionicity are essential.[3] An integral part of antenatal management of twins includes the routine determination of chorionicity and amnionicity and knowledge of their clinical implications as one of the critical steps of prenatal care. With the widespread availability and use of prenatal ultrasound, most twin pregnancies are currently diagnosed sonographically early in pregnancy, providing the opportunity to accurately classify multiple pregnancies and to monitor them for specific complications depending on their chorionicity. Because appropriate management depends so crucially on chorionicity, every professional performing obstetric ultrasound should be prepared to diagnose a twin gestation and be familiar with the sonographic signs to classify the pregnancy according to chorionicity.

While chorionicity is sonographically identified based on the appearance of placentation, it does not always define the genetic composition of the pregnancy or zygosity. Twin pregnancies are classified into two groups, as dizygotic or monozygotic, based on the type of conception. Dizygotic twins result from two fertilised eggs, each one fertilised by different sperm, and are therefore associated with two different genotypes and invariably with dichorionic-diamniotic placentation. Monozygotic twins, on the other hand, develop from a single egg that is fertilised by a single sperm. The resulting morula, blastula or gastrula subsequently divides into two separate embryonic structures. Therefore these twins will have the same genotype, although placentation can vary depending on the timing of the division (Figure 3.1). If the splitting

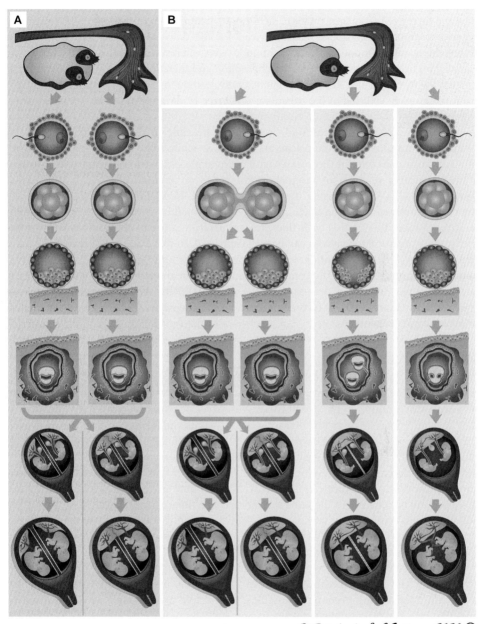

WSepulveda & CGutierrez 2020 ©

Figure 3.1 Classical representation of the three types of placentation in twin pregnancies according to zygosity. **(A)** Dizygotic twins develop from two separate eggs that are fertilised by two sperm; all have dichorionic-diamniotic placentation. **(B)** Monozygotic twins develop from a single zygote that subsequently splits and forms two embryos. Depending on the timing of splitting, they can be dichorionic-diamniotic, monochorionic-diamniotic or monochorionic-monoamniotic. (A black and white version of this figure will appear in some formats. For the colour version, please refer to the plate section.)

process occurs within the first 3 days after conception while the morula is still in the fallopian tube and therefore before implantation, dichorionic-diamniotic twins will result. If the splitting process occurs at the blastocyst stage, between 4 and 8 days after conception and therefore during implantation, monochorionic-diamniotic twins will result. If the division occurs during gastrulation between 9 and 12 days after conception and therefore after the amniotic cavity is formed, the twins will also share the amniotic cavity, leading to monochorionic-monoamniotic twins. Incomplete splitting of the trilaminar disk after 12 days will result in conjoined twins, which are all monochorionic-monoamniotic.[2,4]

Before the advent of ultrasound, it was only possible to determine chorionicity by postpartum examination of the placenta(s). This was achieved by determining the number of placental masses and, in those cases with a single placental mass – which can represent a single placenta of a set of monochorionic twins or anatomically fused placentas of dichorionic twins – by assessing the characteristics of the dividing membrane. Although the pathogenesis of twinning in humans is poorly explained, basic human embryology is well understood. It is on this basis that prenatal determination of chorionicity and amnionicity and its relation to zygosity can be well explained. In this chapter, we review the main embryologic, clinical and sonographic factors to determine zygosity, chorionicity and amnionicity prenatally. Specific complications of twin pregnancies in both monochorionic and dichorionic twins are discussed in the other chapters of this book. We focus on chorionicity and amnionicity in twin pregnancies, as the same principles apply to higher-order multiple pregnancies.

Zygosity

Zygosity refers to the similarity of genetic material in specific loci or alleles (homozygotic or heterozygotic) and is specifically used to describe the genetic similarity or dissimilarity between twins (monozygotic or dizygotic). Monozygotic twins are genetically identical as they develop from a single zygote that subsequently splits and forms two embryos. However, they can have any of the three types of placentation: dichorionic-diamniotic, monochorionic-diamniotic or monochorionic-monoamniotic. Dizygotic twins, on the other hand, are genetically different as they develop from two separate eggs that are fertilised by two sperm; all are dichorionic-diamniotic (Figure 3.2). The genome of these dizygotic conceptuses therefore will be different in the same way siblings are, theoretically sharing only 50% of the parental genes. Monozygotic twins are also known as 'identical' twins and dizygotic twins as 'fraternal' twins. It is generally accepted that approximately two-thirds of spontaneously conceived twins are dizygotic and one-third are monozygotic.

Prenatal determination of zygosity has limited clinical application. Nevertheless, parental curiosity and future medical and social implications make the question of zygosity a relevant issue during prenatal counselling of multiple pregnancies.[2] It is important to note that zygosity can only be determined prenatally by ultrasound under two conditions. Firstly, dizygosity can be established when the fetuses have different sexes (theoretically in 50% of the cases). We should mention, however, the exceptionally rare occurrence of opposite-sex twins in the context of a monochorionic twin pregnancy, known as hetero-karyotypic twins, which are thought to be due to either a discordant chromosomal abnormality or an unequal distribution of mosaic embryonic cells during twinning of the embryos.[2,4] Secondly, when a monochorionic placenta is present, the twins are known to be monozygotic. In contrast, it is not possible to establish zygosity prenatally by ultrasound

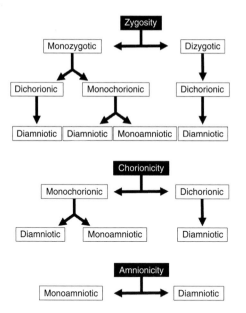

Figure 3.2 Flowchart diagrams illustrating the relationships between zygosity, chorionicity and amnionicity in twin pregnancies

in same-sex twins from dichorionic-diamniotic twin pregnancies; only DNA testing can determine if the twins are identical or fraternal. This can be done by analysing cells directly obtained from both twins, either chorionic villi or amniocytes, and comparing the genetic molecular profiles between them. This has the disadvantage of requiring an invasive procedure to obtain the fetal samples. In recent years, the analysis of cell-free DNA and evaluation of single-nucleotide polymorphisms in maternal circulation has made it possible to examine the zygosity of twin pregnancies prenatally in a non-invasive manner.[5] Nevertheless, the application of cell-free DNA for this sole purpose is not usually necessary because it is chorionicity, not zygosity, that guides proper obstetric management.[3] However, with the increasing use of non-invasive prenatal screening for aneuploidy using molecular biology techniques in maternal plasma, many more twin pregnancies will undergo genetic analysis and antenatal knowledge of zygosity will be more common.

Chorionicity

In multiple pregnancies, the term 'chorionicity' is used to refer to the number of implant-ation sites and therefore the number of chorionic cavities and placentas. This terminology comes from 'chorion' (Greek *khorion*, 'membrane surrounding the fetus'), which is the tissue that is embryologically derived from the trophoblast and that forms the outermost fetal membrane that surrounds the embryo. During initial stages of embryogenesis, the fertilised ovum undergoes rapid cell division, forming the morula. At around four to five days after conception, the morula undergoes cavitation, forming the blastocyst and a fluid-filled cavity or blastocele. Simultaneously, two types of differentiated cells develop. One is an internal accumulation of cells forming a compact structure called the inner cell mass or embryoblast, from which the embryo and fetus originate. The other is the outer layer of cells that surrounds both the blastocele and embryoblast, called the trophoblast, from which the placenta and chorionic membrane originate. The trophoblast together with maternal decidua develops into the chorionic villi. Chorionic villi in contact with the decidua basalis proliferate quickly to form the chorion frondosum that fuses with the decidua basalis and becomes the placental plate and future placenta. In contrast, growth of the chorionic villi in contact with the decidua capsularis arrests, forming the chorion leave, which then fuses with the decidua capsularis and becomes the chorionic membrane or chorion. The chorion forms the outer boundary of the entire conceptus that surrounds the amniotic sac and subsequently fuses with the amnion to form the chorio-amniotic membrane.

Depending on the number of placentas, twin pregnancies are classified as dichorionic, if there are two chorionic cavities and therefore two placentas, or monochorionic, if there is only one chorionic cavity and the twins share a single placenta. Dichorionic twins therefore are independent anatomically as well as functionally in relation to each other, whereas twins with monochorionic placentation are hemodynamically connected through vascular anastomoses within the placenta (chorioangiopagus). Each dichorionic twin has its own placenta, chorionic cavity and amniotic cavity, similar to singleton pregnancies. Monochorionic twins, on the other hand, share a single placenta and may or may not share an amniotic sac.

In clinical practice, determination of chorionicity is relevant to all multiple pregnancies, as this is one of the most important factors that determines the prognosis of the pregnancy. Monochorionic twins are associated with higher rates of pregnancy loss, prematurity, congenital anomalies, intrauterine growth restriction and perinatal death compared to dichorionic twins.[6] In addition, monochorionic placentation is associated with specific conditions including twin–twin transfusion syndrome, twin-reversed arterial perfusion sequence (acardiac twinning), abnormal placental sharing with selective intrauterine growth restriction, single intrauterine demise of one twin with cerebral hypoperfusion of the surviving twin and twin anemia-polycythemia sequence, which are all consequences of the shared circulation.[3,6] In the setting of monoamnionicity, entanglement of the umbilical cords and conjoined twins are also well-recognised, although rare complications. Monochorionic twins also pose specific diagnostic and management challenges in cases of discordant malformation and selective termination of pregnancy or embryo reduction.[2,3,6] Perinatal complications in pregnancies with monochorionic placentation and the corresponding management are discussed in the other chapters of this book.

Prenatal Determination of Chorionicity

In dichorionic pregnancies, chorionicity can be established by prenatal ultrasound as early as the twin pregnancy is identified sonographically by the presence of two or more gestational sacs. Monochorionic pregnancies, on the other hand, can only be diagnosed as such after more than one embryonic structure, such as multiple yolk sacs or embryos, are visualised within a single gestational sac. During each trimester of pregnancy, specific sonographic features are present that can be used to determine chorionicity.[7] The first trimester, especially before the 11th week, is the optimal time to diagnose and classify twin pregnancies based on chorionicity and amnionicity. In a dichorionic pregnancy, two gestational sacs are clearly seen as distinct from each other with a thick interposing chorion and maternal decidua. However, as pregnancy progresses, this separation becomes less evident with the progressive increase in size of the gestational sacs and the corresponding compression of the dividing membrane between the sacs. Therefore, establishing chorionicity using this criterion becomes more difficult with advancing gestational age.

Early determination of chorionicity is especially relevant to pregnancies achieved by assisted reproductive techniques as they are at high risk for not only twin gestation but also for higher-order multiple pregnancies. Fortunately, these pregnancies are typically monitored with close serial sonographic evaluation beginning in the early first trimester by sonologists familiar with these types of pregnancies and accurate determination of chorionicity is successfully performed in most cases.[7,8] In spontaneous pregnancies, on the other hand, the diagnosis of twins is often not made until the 11th to 13th week at the time of routine first-trimester ultrasound screening for chromosomal abnormalities and structural defects. These two periods have distinct ultrasound features based on their chorionicity and are analysed separately.

Early First Trimester

The first sonographic evidence of a gestational sac can be identified with transvaginal ultrasound at around the 4th to 5th week. It appears as a round, anechoic structure surrounded by a relatively thick echoic rim representing the developing chorion and maternal decidual reaction. At the 6th week, the first embryonic structures are visible within the sac, including the amnion and yolk sac. Later this week, the first evidence of an embryo appears as a small echoic pole in close relation to the wall of the yolk sac (the 'engagement ring' sign). Definitive evidence of a viable embryo is the visualisation of cardiac activity within the fetal pole, which is detected using conventional real-time ultrasound with or without Doppler technology between the 6th and 7th week. In the 7th week, a living embryo can be clearly identified separate from the yolk sac and both the amniotic and chorionic cavities are visible.

Dichorionic twins: Dichorionicity can be detected using ultrasound from the moment the implanted gestational sacs are visualised. Using high-resolution transvaginal ultrasound, a dichorionic twin pregnancy is seen as the presence of two gestational sacs within the uterine cavity from the 4th to 5th week onwards. Each sac contains the same structures as the ones present in a developing singleton fetus. Rarely, heterotopic twins develop, the most frequent presentation being one intrauterine pregnancy and another ectopic pregnancy in the fallopian tube.[2] During the 5th to 6th weeks, the yolk sac appears, and in the 6th to 7th weeks, an embryo can be visualised in each sac. Definite proof of chorionicity can be established at the time confident identification of live embryos is observed (Figure 3.3). All dichorionic twin pregnancies have two amniotic sacs and are by definition diamniotic. However, during the classification of twins, both descriptors (dichorionic and diamniotic) and also the number of fetuses should be used to clearly state the presence of two fetuses. As a dichorionic pregnancy can also occur in a triplet pregnancy, its placentation therefore should be classified as a dichorionic-triamniotic or dichorionic-diamniotic triplet pregnancy, indicating that one of the triplets has its own placenta and amniotic sac, whereas the other two are monochorionic and share a single placenta with two or one amniotic sacs, respectively.

Monochorionic twins: Monochorionic twins are frequently overlooked during the early first trimester. However, meticulous examination of the gestational sac can reveal the

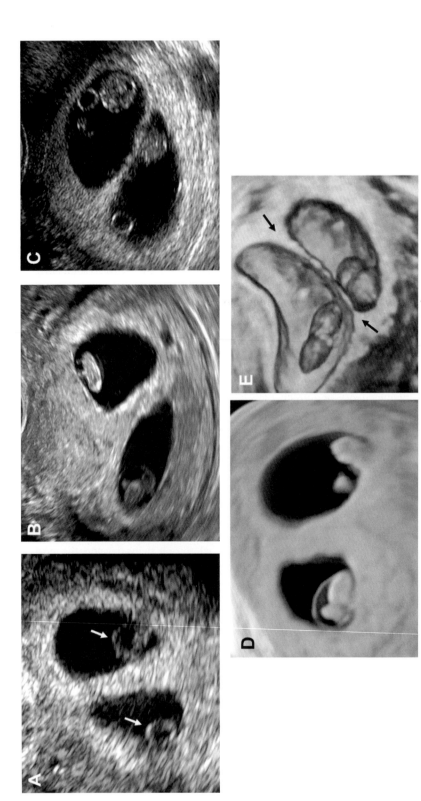

Figure 3.3 Representative early first-trimester ultrasound views of dichorionic-diamniotic twin pregnancies. **(A)** At 6 weeks 5 days, two gestational sacs, each containing a yolk sac and an embryo (arrows), are clearly seen separated by thick echoic tissue representing the chorion and maternal decidual reaction. **(B)** At 7 weeks 4 days, two embryos are seen in their own gestational sac and separated by a thick septum. **(C)** At 8 weeks 6 days, each amniotic sac contains an embryo. The extra-amniotically located yolk sacs are also visualised. Note that the interposing chorion is getting thinner with advancing gestation, with the exception of the base of the membrane where the chorion remains thick, displaying the 'lambda' or 'twin peak' sign. **(D)** Three-dimensional ultrasound in the case shown in B. Two distinct gestational sacs separated by a thick septum are seen. **(E)** Three-dimensional ultrasound in the case shown in C. Note that the 'lambda' sign is clearly seen at the two ends of the dividing membrane (arrows).

presence of a monochorionic twin pregnancy at the 6th to 7th week by detecting two different fetal poles within the same gestational sac. After the 7th week, the identification of two embryos sharing the same chorionic sac and having one or two amniotic cavities and yolk sacs becomes more evident (Figure 3.4). The criteria for the determination of amnionicity in these cases are described in the corresponding section that follows.

Late First Trimester

The period between the 11th and 13th weeks is an important window in which to diagnose twins and determine their chorionicity and amnionicity, especially in undiagnosed spontaneous twin pregnancies. If the diagnosis of twin pregnancy has been already made, this window also provides the opportunity to confirm the chorionicity assigned by previous examiners. The most predictive sonographic feature at this gestational age is the presence or absence of the chorionic tissue projection at the base of the dividing membrane (Figure 3.5). The presence of this projection, which is called the 'lambda' sign due to its close resemblance to the Greek letter λ, is particularly prominent at the site of contact between two fused placentas. Initially described in 1981 by Bessis and Papiernik,[9] who should be credited as the first ones to determine chorionicity prenatally, it was subsequently also named the 'twin peak' sign by Finberg,[10] who confirmed its reliability as pathognomonic of dichorionicity in the second- and third-trimester twin pregnancies. During the scan at the 11th to the 13th week, the lambda sign is easily identified in all dichorionic twin pregnancies regardless of the position of the placentas; at this gestational age, dichorionic placentas will display the lambda sign at the inter-twin membrane–placental junction whether they are fused or separate (Figure 3.6).[11] The absence of the lambda sign, also known as the 'T' sign (Figure 3.7),[7,8] means that there is no interposing chorion and that therefore the dividing membrane is formed only by the two amnions, indicating monochorionicity (Figure 3.8). Several studies have confirmed that the use of the lambda sign alone, classified subjectively as present or absent, is almost 100% accurate at determining chorionicity in twin pregnancies at this gestational age. Placental location is also an important factor that should be considered; if anatomically separate placentas are observed during the scan, dichorionicity can also be established. However, due to the size of the placentas and the relatively small uterine cavity at this gestational age, the vast majority of placentas are positioned close to each other, which can give dichorionic placentas the false appearance of a single placenta rather than fused placentas. Thickness of the dividing membrane is also another ultrasound feature, but this relies on subjective rather than objective assessment because a cut-off in the first trimester has not been established. Finally, although fetal sex can usually be determined in the first trimester, the accuracy of sex assignment is not sufficient to be used as a reliable factor in determining dichorionicity if presumably opposite-sex twins are suspected.

Second and Third Trimesters of Pregnancy

Determination of chorionicity in the second and third trimesters relies on several sonographic features, some of which are similar to the ones already present at the scan performed at the 11th to 13th week. These include determination of fetal sex, examination of the location and number of placentas, assessment of the inter-twin membrane–placental junction for the presence or absence of the lambda versus the T sign and evaluation of the thickness of the dividing membrane (Figure 3.9).[7] As all of these

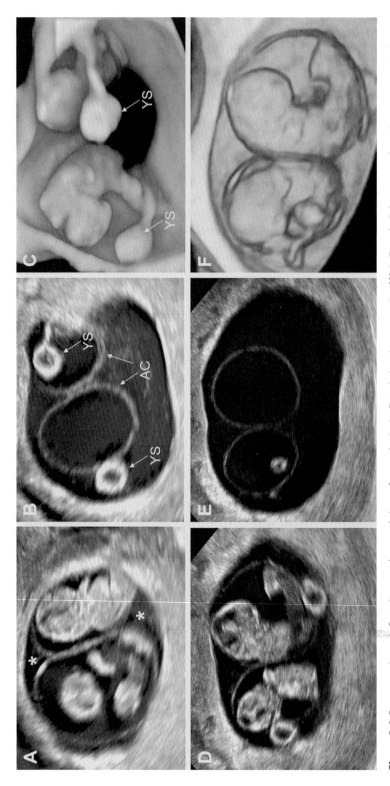

Figure 3.4 Representative early first-trimester ultrasound views of monochorionic-diamniotic twin pregnancies. **(A)** At 7 weeks 5 days, two embryos in separate amniotic cavities are seen sharing a single chorionic sac. The 'black lambda' sign is displayed at the corners of the chorionic sac (asterisks). **(B)** Two amniotic cavities (AC) and two yolk sacs (YS) are clearly seen. Note that there is no interposing chorion between the amnions. **(C)** Three-dimensional ultrasound shows the two embryos in two distinct amniotic sacs. Although the thin dividing membrane is hard to visualise with this technology, the presence of two yolk sacs (YS) is highly suggestive of diamnionicity. **(D, E, and F)** Similar sonographic findings at 9 weeks 3 days in a different monochorionic-diamniotic twin pregnancy. Note the dividing membrane with no interposing chorion.

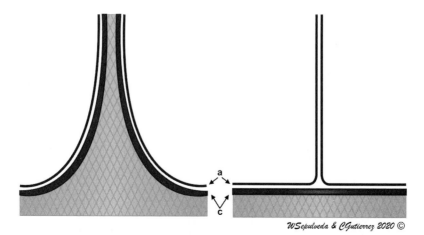

WSepulveda & CGutierrez 2020 ©

Figure 3.5 Schematic representation of the inter-twin membrane–placental junction in dichorionic-diamniotic (left panel) and monochorionic-diamniotic (right panel) twin pregnancies. In dichorionic-diamniotic twin pregnancy, there is a triangular projection of chorionic tissue into the base of the dividing membrane ('lambda' sign). In monochorionic-diamniotic twin pregnancy, the projection is absent as there is no interposing chorion between the amnions ('T' sign). a, amnion; c, chorion.

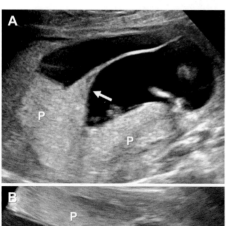

Figure 3.6 Late first-trimester ultrasound views of dichorionic-diamniotic twin pregnancies. At the inter-twin membrane–placental junction, the chorion is thicker than in the rest of the dividing membrane, giving this area the appearance of the Greek letter λ ('lambda' sign, arrows). **(A)** Fused dichorionic placentas giving the appearance of a single placental mass. **(B)** Separate dichorionic placentas. Note the thick dividing membrane between the twins. P, placenta.

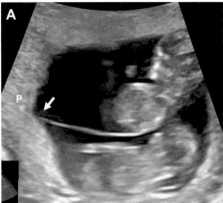

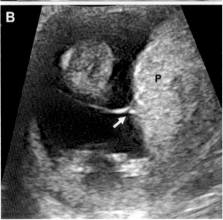

Figure 3.7 Late first-trimester ultrasound views of monochorionic-diamniotic twin pregnancies. At the inter-twin membrane–placental junction, the chorionic projection ('lambda' sign) is absent. The amnions arise perpendicularly from the fetal surface of the placenta, giving this area the appearance of the letter T ('T' sign, arrows). **(A)** Single placenta with the 'T' sign, indicative of monochorionicity. **(B)** 'T' sign at the base of the membrane. Note the thin dividing membrane between the twins P, placenta.

techniques have limitations, it is important to assess as many of these features as possible during the obstetric scan.

- Determination of fetal sex: Sonographic determination of fetal gender is almost 100% accurate after the 13th week. If the fetuses are of different sex, there is compelling evidence of dizygosity and therefore of a dichorionic twin pregnancy. Sex discordance in monochorionic twins is extremely rare, but it is possible in a heterokaryotypic twin pregnancy. Therefore, the detection of opposite-sex twins in the context of a sonographically identified monochorionic placentation should prompt genetic testing of both twins to evaluate for heterokaryotypic twinning. When same-sex twins are detected, additional assessment is required as chorionicity cannot be determined; although 100% of monochorionic twins are of the same sex, so are theoretically 50% of dichorionic twins.
- Determination of the number of placentas: With careful examination of the location of the placenta(s), it is possible to identify those that are separate from those that conform a single placental mass. Separate placentas can be taken as strong evidence of

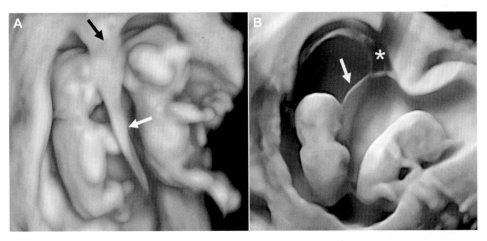

Figure 3.8 Surface-rendering three-dimensional ultrasound views of first-trimester twin pregnancies show the differences between dichorionic-diamniotic and monochorionic-diamniotic twins at the level of the dividing membrane (white arrows). **(A)** In dichorionic twins, the dividing membrane is thicker than in monochorionic-diamniotic twins and the 'lambda' sign is clearly seen at the inter-twin membrane–placental junction (black arrow). **(B)** In monochorionic-diamniotic twins, the dividing membrane is thin and is devoid of interposing chorion, which is also reflected at the level of the chorionic cavity (asterisk). (A black and white version of this figure will appear in some formats. For the colour version, please refer to the plate section.)

a dichorionic twin pregnancy. However, due to the large size of the placentas, many dichorionic placentas that are in close proximity fuse with growth and can be mistaken for a single monochorionic placenta. Dichorionic placentas may be so tightly fused that even the pathologist may be unable to separate them postnatally. Monochorionic placentation therefore cannot be necessarily diagnosed based on the identification of a single placental mass.

- Assessment of the inter-twin membrane–placental junction: Sonographic examination of the area where the dividing membrane arises from the fetal surface of the placenta provides important information about chorionicity, especially during the first and second trimesters of pregnancy.[7,8,10,11] In dichorionic pregnancies, the interposing chorion is significantly thicker at this location immediately adjacent to the placenta compared to the rest of the dividing membrane (Figure 3.10). This prominence at the base of the membrane can be identified in almost all dichorionic twins as a sonographically echoic structure resembling a pyramid, known as the lambda or twin peak sign.[7,8,10,11] However, the prominence of the lambda sign decreases as pregnancy progresses; a longitudinal study reported that after the 20th week, the sign was no longer seen in 26% of pregnancies with separate placentas and in 7% of pregnancies with fused placentas.[12] Therefore, while the lambda sign is easily detected at the scan taken in the 11th to 13th week and can be confidently used to determine chorionicity in the first trimester, its absence should not be used in the second and third trimesters with the same predictive value.[11,12]

Monochorionic placentation, on the other hand, does not have an interposing chorion between the amnions, so the dividing membrane is thin starting from the point at which it arises from the placenta and has the same thickness through its entire length. In these cases, the inter-twin membrane–placental junction appears as a perpendicular angle resembling the shape of the letter T, hence the name of T sign to describe this feature.[7,8]

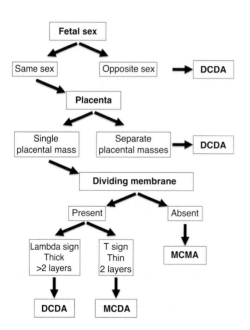

Figure 3.9 Flowchart diagram to determine chorionicity and amnionicity in the second and third trimesters. DCDA, dichorionic-diamniotic; MCDA, monochorionic-diamniotic; MCMA, monochorionic-monoamniotic

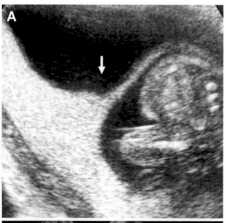

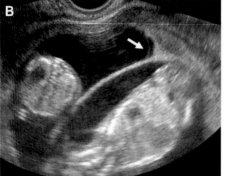

Figure 3.10 The 'lambda' sign in second-trimester dichorionic twin pregnancies (arrows). **(A)** The echoic projection of chorionic tissue at the level of the inter-twin membrane–placental junction is clearly seen. The dividing membrane is also thick due to the interposing chorion. **(B)** With advancing gestation, the thickness of the membrane as well as the prominence of the 'lambda' sign decrease.

- Thickness of the dividing membrane: In dichorionic placentation, the dividing membrane has four layers, two amnions externally and two layers of interposing chorion, which may be fused. This composition makes the membrane thicker in dichorionic-diamniotic placentation than in cases of monochorionic-diamniotic placentation, in which there are only two amnions without interposing chorion (Figure 3.5). The dividing membrane thickness can be measured by ultrasound under adequate magnification and image settings, ideally in a parallel view in relation to the ultrasound beam.[7] Although the dividing membrane is thinner in monochorionic-diamniotic placentation, the absence of a clearly defined cut-off thickness to differentiate between monochorionic versus dichorionic twins and lack of a standardised method to measure membrane thickness limit the usefulness of this technique. Although a cut-off thickness of 2 mm in the second and third trimesters has been proposed, measurements have a high inter- and intra-observer variability and the membrane thickness becomes difficult to assess as pregnancy progresses.[7] An additional sonographic feature is the number of layers of the dividing membrane.[7] Using high-resolution ultrasound, more than two membranes may be visible, but it is usually difficult to visualise the four layers of dichorionic placentation in clinical practice. Due to these limitations, this technique has not gained wide acceptance in the ultrasound community. Another simple sign, particularly useful in the third trimester, is the detection of splitting membranes, known as the 'split membrane' sign. This represents local accumulation of fluid within the membranes and is a characteristic of dichorionic placentation, as it has not been described in monochorionic-diamniotic twin pregnancies. It was noted as a third-trimester sign of dichorionic-diamniotic twins, although it occasionally can be detected in second-trimester twins (Figure 3.11).

Amnionicity

The amniotic cavity is the space filled with amniotic fluid that surrounds the embryo and fetus during intrauterine development. This cavity is enclosed by the amnion, a thin membrane measuring less than 0.5 mm. In multiple pregnancies, the term 'amnionicity' is used to refer to the number of amniotic cavities. This terminology comes from 'amnion' (Greek *amnos*, 'little lamb', 'vase in which the blood of a sacrifice was caught', 'membrane around a fetus'). In clinical practice, determination of amnionicity is only relevant to

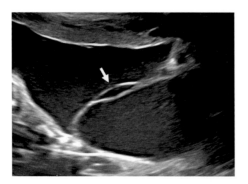

Figure 3.11 The 'split membrane' sign characteristic of a dichorionic-diamniotic placentation at 25 weeks (arrow).

monochorionic twin pregnancies, as all dichorionic twin pregnancies have two amniotic sacs and are therefore diamniotic.

Based on the number of amniotic cavities, monochorionic twin pregnancies are classified into two groups: diamniotic and monoamniotic. In monochorionic-diamniotic twins, each twin has its own amniotic cavity whereas monochorionic-monoamniotic twins share a single amniotic cavity. In the latter condition, entanglement of the umbilical cords invariably occurs as the fetuses freely move within the amniotic cavity and the umbilical cord placental insertion sites remain fixed. Continuous fetal movement may result in entwining of the umbilical cords and a subsequent cord accident. A unique form of monochorionic-monoamniotic twin pregnancy is the development of conjoined twins, in which the inner cell mass only partially splits after 12 days after conception, resulting in different degrees of fusion at the level of head (cephalopagus), chest (thoracopagus), abdomen (omphalopagus) or pelvis (ischiopagus).[2] The ultrasound diagnosis of conjoined twins relies on the context of fused body parts in the setting of a monochorionic-monoamniotic placentation. In the rostral type of conjoined twins, which accounts for around 50% of the cases, there is a single umbilical cord so cord entanglement is not possible. In the other types of conjoined twins, cord entanglement is possible but uncommon due to the restriction of movement of the two fetuses relative to each other.

Prenatal Determination of Amnionicity

Diamniotic twins: In monochorionic twins, amnionicity can be determined by direct identification of the inter-twin amniotic membrane, which appears sonographically at around the 8th week. This inter-twin membrane is characteristically thin throughout pregnancy and is formed by the apposition of the two amnions, one from each twin, and lacks interposing chorion. As the amniotic cavities increase in size over time, a progressively smaller chorionic cavity develops, which is sonographically visualised as an anechoic pyramid-shaped space (the 'black lambda' sign). Two yolk sacs located within the single chorionic cavity but outside the amniotic cavity can be visualised (Figure 3.12). Sometimes they are adjacent to each other and have a characteristic appearance known as the 'eight' or 'spectacles' sign (Figure 3.13). In the second and third trimesters, determination of diamnionicity is straightforward with visualisation of the inter-twin membrane separating the two fetuses in both dichorionic-diamniotic and monochorionic-diamniotic pregnancies, although the location of the membrane occasionally may be more difficult to identify with advancing gestation and in ases of severe oligohydramnios in one of the twins.

Monoamniotic twins: By definition, monochorionic-monoamniotic twins lack an inter-twin dividing membrane. This type of twinning occurs in less than 1% of monochorionic twin pregnancies.[2] As the dividing amniotic membrane is confidently visualised only after the 8th week, other sonographic landmarks have been suggested to determine amnionicity in very early gestation. There is evidence that counting the number of yolk sacs helps differentiate between monochorionic-diamniotic and monochorionic-monoamniotic twins when the dividing membrane is not visualised or difficult to ascertain. Bromley and Benacerraf[13] were the first to suggest the use of the number of yolk sacs to determine amnionicity before the 8th week. In their review of 22 monochorionic twin pregnancies between the 6th and 9th week, they noted that in 19 of the 20 (95%) diamniotic twin pregnancies, two yolk sacs were seen. The remaining case was first examined at 6 weeks

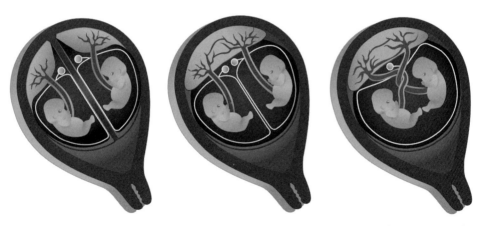

WSepulveda & CGutierrez 2020 ©

Figure 3.12 Schematic representation of the relation between yolk sac number and amnionicity in early pregnancy. In all dichorionic-diamniotic twin pregnancies, the yolk sacs are separated by chorionic tissue (left panel). In monochorionic-diamniotic twin pregnancies, two yolk sacs are present in the single chorionic cavity (middle panel). In monochorionic-monoamniotic twin pregnancies, only one yolk sac is usually identified (right panel). (A black and white version of this figure will appear in some formats. For the colour version, please refer to the plate section.)

when only one yolk sac was visualised; however, at re-examination at 8 weeks, two yolk sacs were clearly identified. In contrast, in the remaining two monoamniotic twin pregnancies examined, only one yolk sac was visualised (Figure 3.14). Although this observation was confirmed by the other authors, subsequent reports questioned the use of this technique; though mainly based on single case reports, two yolk sacs were documented in several pregnancies which ultimately proved to be monochorionic-monoamniotic. More recently, large series have shown compelling evidence that counting the number of yolk sacs is not a reliable technique for determining amnionicity in early monochorionic pregnancies. Fenton et al.[14] reviewed the number of yolk sacs in 38 monochorionic-monoamniotic twin pregnancies and found only one yolk sac in 26 (68%) and two yolk sacs in 12 (32%) of the cases. In the review of their own experience as well as the literature, a total of 22 cases of monochorionic-monoamniotic twin pregnancies with two yolk sacs were documented in early pregnancy. Therefore, additional sonographic follow-up examinations are required to provide a confident diagnosis of monoamnionicity.

From the late first trimester onwards, the dividing membrane can be clearly visualised sonographically between the fetuses in most cases. This thin structure is better identified using transvaginal ultrasound in the first trimester and by abdominal sonography in the second and third trimesters. In order to enhance visibility, it is advised that the ultrasound beam should insonate the membrane perpendicularly, ideally as close to 90 degrees as possible. In advancing monochorionic pregnancies, the visualisation of the dividing membrane should be taken as a definitive proof of diamnionicity. If the dividing membrane is not identified, every effort should be made to visualise the umbilical cords for entanglement. Although this can be identified with conventional two-dimensional ultrasound, colour Doppler imaging can provide

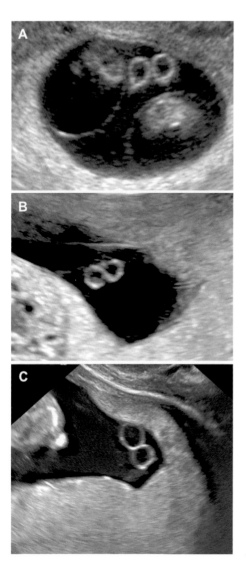

Figure 3.13 Amnionicity in first-trimester monochorionic-diamniotic twins. Two yolk sacs are seen in close proximity to each other within the single chorionic cavity (the 'spectacles' sign). **(A)** At 9 weeks. **(B)** At 11 weeks. **(C)** At 12 weeks.

compelling evidence of umbilical cord entanglement, especially later in pregnancy (Figure 3.15).

Pseudo-amnionicity: Spontaneous rupture of the dividing membranes in dichorionic-diamniotic or monochorionic-diamniotic twins is exceedingly rare. In contrast, iatrogenic amniotomy secondary to invasive procedures such as diagnostic or therapeutic amniocentesis and fetoscopic procedures is well documented in the literature.[2] In all of these cases, the history of an invasive procedure and the identification of membranes floating freely within the amniotic cavity make the diagnosis straightforward. Umbilical cord entanglement and amniotic band syndrome are well-known complications occurring in the context of pseudo-amnionicity.

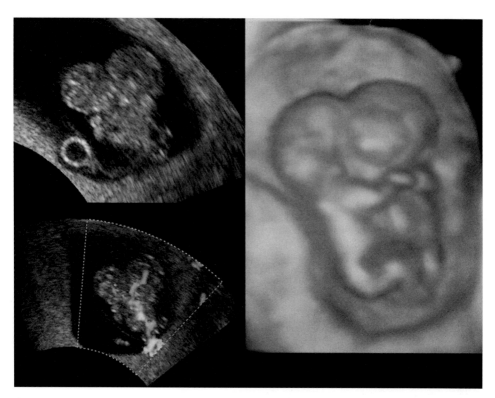

Figure 3.14 Amnionicity in early first-trimester monochorionic-monoamniotic twins. In this set of monochorionic-monoamniotic conjoined twins (thoracopagus type), there is only one yolk sac in the common chorionic cavity. (A black and white version of this figure will appear in some formats. For the colour version, please refer to the plate section.)

Triplets and Other Higher-Order Multiple Pregnancies

Higher-order multiple pregnancy is defined as a pregnancy with three or more fetuses. The number of fetuses is an independent prognostic factor for pregnancy outcome; the greater the number of fetuses, the higher the risk for the pregnancy. Spontaneous higher-order multiple pregnancies are rare. However, the transfer of multiple embryos in in vitro fertilisation patients resulted in an excessively high prevalence of higher-order multiple pregnancies until single embryo transfer became a more common standard of care in patients with infertility. Determination of chorionicity and amnionicity in higher-order multiple pregnancies has tremendous importance for the subsequent management of the pregnancy. If a set of monochorionic fetuses is present, the pregnancy risks are further increased from that based merely on the number of fetuses due to the unique risks associated with monochorionicity. When embryo reduction is being considered in this situation, the entire monochorionic set is often targeted to maximise the risk reduction conferred by the procedure particularly since reduction of only one monochorionic fetus must be avoided due to the associated risks for the surviving co-twin.[2,8]

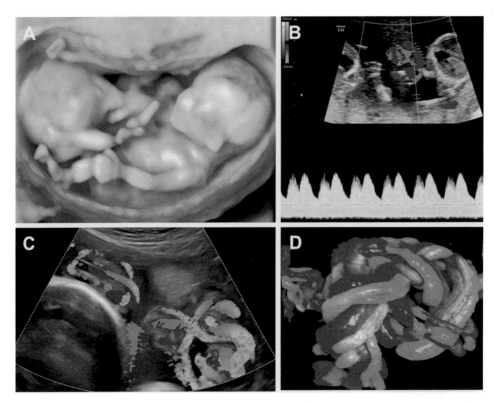

Figure 3.15 Monochorionic-monoamniotic twin pregnancy at 12 weeks 6 days. **(A)** Three-dimensional ultrasound shows two fetuses lying close together. The amniotic membrane was not identified. **(B)** Entanglement of the umbilical cords confirmed monoamnionicity. Spectral Doppler ultrasound demonstrates the two cardiac beats in the area of entanglement of the umbilical cords. **(C)** At 30 weeks, entanglement of the umbilical cords is evident as visualised with colour flow mapping. **D,** Three-dimensional HD live flow mapping demonstrates entanglement of the umbilical cords. (A black and white version of this figure will appear in some formats. For the colour version, please refer to the plate section.)

Determination of chorionicity and amnionicity in this setting is often performed early in pregnancy, at which time transvaginal and transabdominal imaging approaches are usually complementary. The first step is determining the number of fetuses. The second is establishing the placentation of each fetus in relation to the surrounding fetuses.[2,8] The same criteria used in twin pregnancies apply to each fetus from a higher-order multiple pregnancy, with careful evaluation to determine if a monochorionic set is present. As determining the number of placentas can be technically challenging, chorionicity is most commonly assessed based on the thickness of the dividing membrane in conjunction with the assessment of the inter-twin membrane–placental junction. In triplet pregnancies, assessment of the area where the amniotic sacs converge provides information on chorionicity.[15] This area, known as the 'Ypsilon' zone or 'Mercedes' sign (Figure 3.16), has been shown to be a reliable criterion to differentiate trichorionic from dichorionic and monochorionic triplet pregnancies. Nevertheless, it is important that all of these higher-order multiple pregnancies be managed at tertiary referral centres.

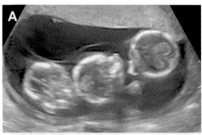

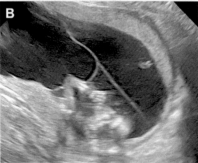

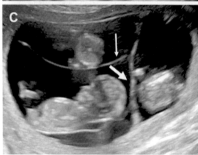

Figure 3.16 Assessment of the 'Ypsilon' zone to determine chorionicity and amnionicity in higher-order multiple pregnancies. **(A)** Three fetuses are seen at 14 weeks. There was a single placental mass and the dividing membranes were subjectively thin. **(B)** Evaluation at the area where the three amniotic cavities joined demonstrates a thin membrane with similar thickness, suggesting monochorionicity. **(C)** For comparison, a dichorionic-triamniotic triplet pregnancy at 12 weeks is presented. Note that one membrane is thicker (thick arrow) in comparison with the other (thin arrow), suggesting the presence of a monochorionic set.

Acknowledgments

This work was supported by an unrestricted research grant from the 'Sociedad Profesional de Medicina Fetal 'Fetalmed' Ltda., Chile.

Key Points

- Monozygotic twins are genetically identical but can be associated with dichorionic-diamniotic, monochorionic-diamniotic or monochorionic-monoamniotic placentation depending on the timing of embryonic splitting.
- Dizygotic twins are genetically different and are associated with only dichorionic-diamniotic placentation.
- The optimal time for accurate classification of multiple pregnancy is during the first trimester, ideally before the 11th week of gestation.
- Dichorionicity can be sonographically diagnosed in early pregnancy with the presence of two gestational sacs.
- The diagnosis of monochorionicity requires visualisation of multiple embryonic structures within a single gestational sac.

- Key features that should be assessed to determine chorionicity consist of: fetal sex, number of placentas, appearance of the inter-twin membrane–placental junction and thickness of the inter-twin dividing membrane.
- The 'lambda' or 'twin peak' sign is characteristic of dichorionic placentation and the 'T sign' is characteristic of monochorionic placentation.
- Monoamnionicity is rare and is often difficult to diagnose in the early first trimester due to the thinness of the amniotic membrane. If a dividing membrane cannot be confidently identified later in the pregnancy, evaluation for umbilical cord entanglement should be performed.

References

1. Moise KJ Jr, Johnson A. There is NO diagnosis of twins. Am J Obstet Gynecol 2010;**203**:1–2.

2. Blickstein I, Keith LG (eds.). Multiple Pregnancy: Epidemiology, Gestation & Perinatal Outcome. 2nd Edition. New York: Informa Healthcare, 2005.

3. Khalil A, Rodgers M, Baschat A, Bhide A, Gratacos E, Hecher K, et al. ISUOG Practice Guidelines: role of ultrasound in twin pregnancy. Ultrasound Obstet Gynecol 2016;**47**:247–63.

4. McNamara HC, Kane SC, Craig JM, Short RV, Umstad MP. A review of the mechanisms and evidence for typical and atypical twinning. Am J Obstet Gynecol 2016;**214**:172–91.

5. Norwitz ER, McNeill G, Kalyan A, Rivers E, Ahmed E, Meng L, et al. Validation of a single-nucleotide polymorphism-based non-invasive prenatal test in twin gestations: determination of zygosity, individual fetal sex, and fetal aneuploidy. J Clin Med 2019;**8**(7).pii:E937.

6. Gratacos E, Ortiz JU, Martinez JM. A systematic approach to the differential diagnosis and management of the complications of monochorionic twin pregnancies. Fetal Diagn Ther 2012;**32**:145–55.

7. Jha P, Morgan TA, Kennedy A. US evaluation of twin pregnancies: importance of chorionicity and amnionicity. RadioGraphics 2019;**39**:2146–66.

8. Monteagudo A, Timor-Tritsch IE, Sharma S. Early and simple determination of chorionic and amniotic type in multifetal gestations in the first fourteen weeks by high-frequency transvaginal ultrasonography. Am J Obstet Gynecol 1994;**170**:824–9.

9. Bessis R, Papiernik E. Echographic imagery of amniotic membranes in twin pregnancies. In Twin Research 3: Twin Biology and Multiple Pregnancy, Gedda L, Parisi P, Nance WE (eds.). New York: Alan Liss, 1981;183–7.

10. Finberg HJ. The 'twin peak' sign: reliable evidence of dichorionic twinning. J Ultrasound Med 1992;**11**:571–7.

11. Sepulveda W, Sebire NJ, Hughes K, Odibo A, Nicolaides KH. The lambda sign at 10–14 weeks of gestation as a predictor of chorionicity in twin pregnancies. Ultrasound Obstet Gynecol 1996;**7**:421–3.

12. Sepulveda W, Sebire NJ, Hughes K, Kalogeropoulos A, Nicolaides KH. Evolution of the lambda or twin-chorionic peak sign in dichorionic twin pregnancies. Obstet Gynecol 1997;**89**:439–41.

13. Bromley B, Benacerraf B. Using the number of yolk sacs to determine amnionicity in early first trimester monochorionic twins. J Ultrasound Med 1995;**14**:415–19.

14. Fenton C, Reidy K, Demyanenko M, Palma-Dias R, Cole S, Umstad MP. The significance of yolk sac number in monoamniotic twins. Fetal Diagn Ther 2019;**46**:193–9.

15. Sepulveda W, Sebire NJ, Odibo A, Psarra A, Nicolaides KH. Prenatal determination of chorionicity in triplet pregnancy by ultrasonographic examination of the ipsilon zone. Obstet Gynecol 1996;**88**:855–8.

Multifetal Pregnancy Reduction

Simi Gupta Talati and Andrei Rebarber

The Facts

The triplet and higher-order multiple birth rate was 101.6 per 100,000 births in 2017. This rate is not significantly different from 2016; however, 2016 and 2017 had the lowest triplet and higher-order multiple birth rates in more than two decades. On the other hand, the twin birth rate was 33.3 per 1,000 births in 2017, which is only slightly less than the highest reported rate of 33.9 per 1,000 births in 2014.[1]

Multiple gestations have been associated with a number of adverse pregnancy outcomes. Fetal mortality is increased due to a higher rate of stillbirth, and neonatal mortality is increased primarily due to a higher rate of preterm birth. Furthermore, multiple gestations have an increased risk of short-term and long-term neonatal and infant mortality switch to morbidity than singletons born at the same gestational age. Maternal morbidity is also increased with higher rates of hyperemesis gravidarum, gestational diabetes, anaemia, haemorrhage, caesarean section, post-partum depression and hypertension. Specifically, hypertension rates are 12.7% in twins and 20% in triplets as compared to 6.5% in singleton pregnancies and are associated with iatrogenic preterm delivery and abruption.[2]

Multifetal pregnancy reduction (MFPR) is one option to reduce the number of fetuses in a pregnancy. In this procedure, the fetus or fetuses chosen for reduction are determined based on technical considerations and the ease of accessibility for the procedure or by chorionicity in a triplet or higher-order multiple pregnancy with one or more monochorionic fetuses. Selective termination (ST) is the application of the same procedure as with MFPR but the fetus or fetuses chosen for reduction are based on an anomaly.

Multifetal pregnancy reduction has been shown to reduce the risk of preterm delivery and other adverse pregnancy outcomes in multiple gestations with low procedure-related loss rates. The most recent data show that procedure-related loss rates are highest with higher starting fetal numbers (11% at five or more starting fetuses compared to 2.1% with two starting fetuses) and higher with a finishing twin pregnancy (5.3%) compared with a finishing singleton pregnancy (3.8%). Furthermore, gestational age at delivery and birthweight are lower with a finishing twin pregnancy compared with a finishing singleton pregnancy.[3]

In pregnancies with separate chorionicities, the standard technique is to first map the location of each fetus and placenta and confirm which fetus or fetuses will be reduced (see Figure 4.1). In MFPR, the fetus located closest to the fundus or anterior abdominal wall is usually chosen for reduction due to ease of accessibility. The next step is to administer potassium chloride into the fetal heart or thorax using a spinal needle under real-time ultrasound guidance. We use 2–10 cc of 2 mEq/ml of potassium chloride with a 20-gauge

(a)

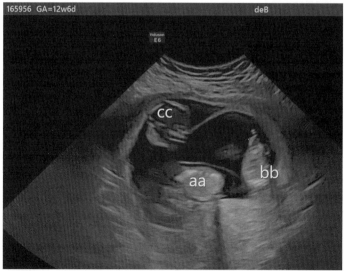

(b)

Figure 4.1 Mapping location and placentation prior to MFPR in a dichorionic-triamniotic triplet gestation

spinal needle. Asystole is usually confirmed within minutes. For additional fetuses, one may use the same needle puncture or a separate puncture depending on location.

The standard timing of the procedure is between 10 and 14 weeks gestation for MFPR and soon after diagnosis and decision-making in ST. Early embryo reduction via a transvaginal approach between 6 and 8 weeks gestation has been evaluated. However, recent data have shown a higher rate of procedure-related fetal loss (7.2% with embryo reduction versus 0.9% with fetal reduction at 11+ weeks, $p = 0.039$). This also translated to higher rates of overall fetal loss during the pregnancy and higher rates of miscarriage prior to 24 weeks with embryo reduction versus fetal reduction, without any decrease in the risk of preterm delivery or other adverse pregnancy outcomes.[4] Therefore, fetal reduction after 10 weeks gestation is recommended for MFPR. For selective reduction, studies have evaluated the risks and benefits of later gestational age at reduction. A large study showed a higher rate of pregnancy loss in patients undergoing ST after 18 weeks compared to less than 18 weeks (12% vs 0%, p = 0.05) and a higher rate of preterm birth with later gestational ages at ST.[5] Though the dividing gestational age threshold varies between studies, most studies show lower loss rates and improved pregnancy outcomes with earlier gestational ages at ST. One study evaluated outcomes in patients undergoing ST in the second versus the third trimester and found higher rates of extreme and early preterm delivery in patients undergoing ST in the second trimester compared to the third trimester (25% vs 0%, p = 0.02). They also found no difference in pregnancy loss rates between the two groups. While this study was small, and ethical and legal considerations may prevent ST at certain later gestational ages, this study does lend some data supporting the safety of ST at later gestational ages.[6]

Genetic screening or testing and first-trimester anatomy survey should be offered prior to MFPR in order to decrease the risk of reducing a genetic or congenital normal fetus or fetuses and continuing the pregnancy of a genetic or congenitally abnormal fetus. Chorionic villus sampling (CVS) prior to MFPR has not been shown to increase the pregnancy loss rate after MFPR and data suggest that it may actually decrease loss rates by improved selection of abnormal fetuses for reduction. One study showed a 3.1% rate of abnormal fluorescence in situ hybridisation (FISH) results in patients with a sonographically normal fetus prior to reduction.[7] For patients who do not desire invasive testing, screening can be offered through ultrasound for early anatomy, nuchal translucency, nasal bone and first-trimester biochemical screening, and/or non-invasive prenatal screening. Abnormal results may then prompt patients to pursue CVS prior to MFPR or to reduce the suspected abnormal fetus. The cross-sampling rate of CVS (contamination of villi from the other fetus) reported in the literature is usually based on cases where incorrect gender determination or XX/XY mosaicism is identified. Initial sampling error rates reported as high as 4–5% have decreased to almost none.[8] DNA fingerprinting can be used to determine zygosity when required in same-sex twins to determine if sampling error may have occurred. However, little published data have been described to that level of accuracy to identify the true rate of cross-sampling error in multichorionic gestations prior to fetal reduction, and this technique would not differentiate if sampling error occurred in monochorionic gestations or if monozygotic fetuses exist within multichorionic gestations.

Monochorionic Multiple Gestations

In pregnancies that share a placenta (monochorionic), potassium chloride injections into the fetal heart or thorax cannot be performed because of concern about transplacental passage of the potassium chloride to the other fetus(es)and because hemodynamic changes in the reduced fetus may cause neurological morbidity or mortality to the other fetus. Therefore, an alternative technique, primarily some form of umbilical cord occlusion, is utilised.

There are four main techniques for umbilical cord occlusion: suture ligation, laser coagulation, bipolar coagulation and radiofrequency ablation. In the original suture ligation procedure, a port is introduced into the uterine cavity and a vicryl suture is placed into the cavity through the port. The suture is then looped around the cord by ultrasound guidance and tied in a knot extra-corporeally, and a knot pusher is used to secure the knot. This is repeated in a second position along the cord to ensure complete cord occlusion.[9] In the technique of laser coagulation, again a small port is used for uterine entry, and an operative endoscope is used to visualise the appropriate cord. The umbilical vessels are then photocoagulated using a 600 microm quart Nd-YAG non-contact laser fibre (with a power of 20–40 W) through the operating channel of the endoscopy. Each pulse lasts 2–3 seconds and is repeated until coagulation is completed as determined by lack of blood flow using colour and pulsed Doppler ultrasound. If bipolar coagulation is being used, the umbilical cord is grasped with a 3 mm bipolar forceps introduced through a uterine port and coagulation is performed at a power setting of 30–50 watts for 30 seconds. Additional cord segments can be coagulated as a precaution and cessation of flow in the umbilical vessels is confirmed by colour Doppler. In the technique of radiofrequency ablation, a 17-gauge Starburst radiofrequency needle is inserted into the fetal abdomen adjacent to the area of the umbilical cord insertion and the prongs of the device are partially deployed. Radiofrequency energy is applied for 4 minutes at 95 watts to generate a target temperature of 100 degrees Celsius. The procedure is repeated for an additional one or two cycles until cessation of cord blood flow is confirmed using colour and power Doppler velocimetry.

There are pros and cons to the different procedures which may guide choice of procedure. Bipolar coagulation requires a larger-calibre operative sleeve and therefore may be more useful in mid second-trimester cases where there is enough amniotic fluid to accommodate the larger operative sleeve or where additional procedures may be required through the port. The benefit of bipolar coagulation is complete occlusion with first application. Radiofrequency or laser ablation has the benefit of a smaller-diameter device and therefore may be preferred in cases at earlier gestation, with low amniotic fluid or with a shorter umbilical cord. However, the occlusion is slower, which may alter flow patterns between the fetuses and increase the risk of fetal demise. There is also a concern about an increased risk of rupture of membranes from thermal damage from the device. Finally, suture ligation may be the best option at late gestational ages when the bipolar forceps may not fit around the umbilical cord.

In recent years, only bipolar coagulation and radiofrequency ablation have been compared in observational trials and a large systematic review and meta-analysis showed no difference in co-twin death rates, live birth rates, neonatal death rates or overall survival. There was a slight increase in preterm premature rupture of membranes with bipolar coagulation versus radiofrequency ablation (28.2% vs 17.7%, p = 0.01), but no difference in preterm delivery rates before 28 or 32 weeks of gestation. This study also showed that the outcome data with selective reduction in monochorionic twin pregnancies are worse than with dichorionic twin pregnancies with an overall survival rate – live birth rate minus neonatal death rate – of only 76.8% with radiofrequency ablation and 79.1% with bipolar coagulation. The risk of preterm delivery was also high with a mean gestational age at delivery of 34.7 weeks with radiofrequency ablation and 35.1 weeks with bipolar coagulation.[10] The second, older systematic review also showed lower survival rates in selective reduction in monochorionic pregnancies of 86% with radiofrequency ablation, 72% with bipolar coagulation, 72% with laser coagulation and 70% with cord ligation.[11] The third study looked at long-term neurodevelopmental impairment in children at least two years of age after selective reduction in monochorionic pregnancies and found a 6.8% risk of neurodevelopmental impairment.[12]

Most selective reduction procedures in monochorionic pregnancies occur in the second trimester soon after the diagnosis for need is made. One systematic review showed improved survival rates when the procedure was performed after 18 weeks (89% vs prior to 18 weeks 69%, p = 0.02). However, the second study looking at timing of intervention of twin-reversed arterial perfusion (TRAP) cases showed worse outcomes when cases were managed conservatively with serial ultrasound, and therefore some advocate for early intervention in the second trimester as soon as the diagnosis is made.[13]

In addition to the different techniques for cord occlusion, some authors recommend antibiotics prior to, during and post procedure. Some also use tocolytics such as nifedipine and/or indomethacin around the time of the procedure. Depending on the author and procedure, patients are either discharged home the same day or monitored in the hospital for 24–48 hours prior to discharge. All patients are followed up at regular at 1–2-week intervals and most receive either a detailed fetal neurosonogram or fetal MRI to evaluate for cerebral injury post procedure.

Multifetal pregnancy reduction is usually not recommended in monochorionic-monoamniotic twin pregnancies due to the residual risk of cord entanglement even with cord occlusion. However, there have been reports in cases of fetal anomalies and the most recent case report discussed a technique of bipolar cord occlusion followed by laser ablation to transect the cord in two cases with selective intrauterine fetal demise of one twin. Both cases were reported to have good outcomes.[14]

The Issues

Multifetal Pregnancy Reduction in Triplet and Twin Pregnancies

While pregnancy loss rates continue to be low after reduction of trichorionic-triamniotic (TT) and dichorionic-diamniotic (DD) pregnancies, the reduction in adverse pregnancy outcomes appears to be more modest. For example, a recent study comparing continued TT pregnancies to TT pregnancies reduced to DD pregnancies showed no difference in preterm delivery rates prior to 34 weeks, but did show an increase in birthweight and a decrease in caesarean sections with MFPR. This study also showed no difference in pregnancy loss rate prior to 24 weeks between ongoing TT pregnancies and MFPR to DD pregnancies.[15]

Another study comparing continued DD pregnancies with MFPR to a singleton pregnancy showed reduction in preterm delivery rates prior to 37 weeks and 34 weeks with MFPR, but no reduction in preterm delivery rates prior to 32 weeks. It also showed a decrease in birthweight less than 10% and 5%, pre-eclampsia and caesarean section with MFPR. This study showed no difference in unintended pregnancy loss rates between DD and MFPR to singleton pregnancies.[16] While the most dramatic survival benefits are seen with reductions from higher initial starting numbers of fetuses in higher-order multifetal pregnancies, limited data have been published to identify whether there is improved long-term outcomes in twins reduced to singletons given the advances in neonatal care of late preterm births.

In dichorionic-triamniotic (DT) triplet pregnancies, there are three options for a triplet pregnancy of mixed chorionicity: reduction to two fetuses by reducing one of the monochorionic pair, reduction to two fetuses by preserving the monochorionic pair, and reduction to one fetus by reducing both fetuses from the monochorionic pair. The reduction of the monochorionic-diamniotic (MD) pair or the fetus with a separate placenta increases the gestational age at delivery compared to expectant management of DT pregnancies. However, the pregnancy loss rate appears to be higher with reduction of the fetus with a separate placenta, but similar between reduction of the MD pair and ongoing DT pregnancies. Overall reduction of one or more fetuses significantly reduces the risk of severe prematurity with a marginal impact on the miscarriage rate.

Management of Pregnancies after Multifetal Pregnancy Reduction or Selection Termination

While more recent studies have focused on comparing pregnancy outcomes between ongoing multiple gestation pregnancies and pregnancies after reduction, older studies compared pregnancy outcomes in pregnancies after reduction and pregnancies that originated as a singleton pregnancy. In these older studies, adverse pregnancy outcomes after reduction were higher than in pregnancies that originated as singleton pregnancies. Specifically, these older studies showed high rates of preterm delivery and intrauterine growth restriction in pregnancies after reduction than in pregnancies that originated as a singleton pregnancy. Therefore, one would assume that pregnancies after reduction would require a higher level of surveillance than routine singleton pregnancies.

Few studies have reviewed surveillance strategies after fetal reduction. Our group assessed the validity of vaginal fetal fibronectin (fFN) as a screening test for spontaneous preterm delivery in asymptomatic patients who had undergone MFPR. In this cohort of 63 patients, 13 singleton gestations and 50 twin gestations, a median of 4 fFN assays were performed per patient. A total of 234 fFN tests were performed with 222 negative results and 12 positive results. The fFN test had similar validity to predict spontaneous preterm birth in these at-risk pregnancies as previously published cohorts.[17] Additionally, our group also evaluated the utility of serial cervical-length evaluation in asymptomatic twins with and without fetal reduction procedures to address the potential effect from the procedure on the measurements. The study group of 35 twins after MFPR was compared to 83 twin gestations who had not had the procedure, and the results noted that cervical length across gestation was not affected by the MFPR procedure.[18] However, there are no studies evaluating prospectively different management protocols after reduction. Our management suggestions are listed in what follows.

Management Options

Multifetal Pregnancy Reduction or Selective Termination in Pregnancies with Separate Chorionicities

Pre-pregnancy Counselling

- Patients are counselled about the risks and benefits of MFPR or ST based on starting number, ending number and gestational age at decision-making.
- Patients who are planning on undergoing MFPR are counselled about the options of genetic screening/testing and are offered non-invasive prenatal screening, nuchal translucency/nasal bone screening and/or CVS with FISH, karyotype and/or microarray. They are also offered first-trimester anatomy screening to assess for congenital anomalies.

- Patients are scheduled for MFPR as soon after genetic screening/testing results are returned or for ST as soon as the diagnosis of a fetal anomaly is made, but not before 10 weeks of gestation.

Multifetal Pregnancy Reduction or Selective Termination Protocol

- Patients undergo ultrasound mapping of each fetus and placenta. For patients undergoing genetic screening/testing, all attempts are made to have the same physician and sonographer who perform the mapping for genetic screening/testing also perform the reduction procedure in order to minimise the risk of error.
- Two to 10 cc of 2 mEq/ml of potassium chloride are transabdominally administered into the fetal heart or thorax with a 20-gauge spinal needle under ultrasound guidance. Asystole is confirmed. For additional fetuses, one may use the same needle puncture or a separate puncture depending on location of the other fetus(es).
- Rhogam is administered as needed for Rh-negative patients.

Post-reduction Pregnancy Management

- Maternal serum alpha feto-protein levels are not drawn for patients who have undergone reduction procedures as they may be falsely elevated.
- Patient instead undergoes an initial anatomy scan at 16–18 weeks to evaluate for congenital anomalies. They also undergo the routine anatomy scan at 20–22 weeks.
- Patients are followed with serial cervical length measurements to assess for risk of preterm delivery. Low-risk treatment options for short cervix such as vaginal progesterone for patients with a cervical length < 2.5 cm are recommended in appropriate patients, while treatment options such as cervical cerclage are offered on an as-needed, case-by-case basis, particularly in the setting of an extremely shortened or dilated cervix.
- Patients are followed with serial ultrasounds for fetal growth every 4 weeks after 20 weeks to detect intrauterine growth restriction. Additional monitoring for pregnancies diagnosed with intrauterine growth restriction such as antenatal testing with biophysical profiles or fetal Doppler evaluation is performed as needed.
- Routine antenatal testing with biophysical profiles is started weekly at 32–34 weeks of gestation or earlier if clinically indicated.
- Timing and mode of delivery are per usual obstetric indications.

Selective Termination in Monochorionic Pregnancies

- Patients undergo an initial anatomy scan at 16–18 weeks to evaluate for congenital anomalies. They also undergo a routine anatomy scan at 20–22 weeks.
- Patients are followed with serial cervical length measurements to assess the risk of preterm delivery. Low-risk treatment options for short cervix such as vaginal progesterone for patients with a cervical length < 2.5 cm are recommended in appropriate patients, while treatment options with higher risks such as cervical cerclage are offered as needed on a case-by-case basis, particularly in the setting of an extremely shortened cervix or a dilated external observational study prior to 24 weeks.
- Patients are followed with serial ultrasounds for fetal growth every 4 weeks after 20 weeks to detect intrauterine growth restriction. Additional monitoring for pregnancies

diagnosed with intrauterine growth restriction such as antenatal testing with biophysical profiles or fetal Doppler evaluation are performed as needed.
- Timing and mode of delivery are per usual obstetric indications.

Key Points

- Obstetric caregivers should be aware that multifetal pregnancies increase maternal and perinatal morbidity and mortality. The greater the number of fetus(es) the higher the risks to both mothers and infants.
- Non-directive patient counselling should be offered to all women with multiple gestations regarding the potential medical benefits of fetal reduction.
- Prior to fetal reductions, attempts should be made with either non-invasive or invasive testing to determine the genetic/structural normality of the fetus that will remain.
- Multifetal pregnancy reduction and selective termination are generally performed between 11 and 14 weeks or as soon as possible after diagnosis of an anomaly, and the loss rate of the pregnancy is based on the starting number as well as the number remaining.
- Biochemical screening for aneuploidy and/or spina bifida should not be performed after the procedure.
- Serial assessment of fetal growth should be considered in these pregnancies, particularly in remaining twin gestations.
- Consider second-trimester cervical length screening +/− fFN screening in both singleton and twin gestations.

References

1. Martin JA, Hamilton BE, Osterman MJK, Driscoll AK, Drake P. Births: final data for 2017. National Vital Statistics Reports 2018;**67**(8):1–50.

2. American College of Obstetricians and Gynecologists. Multifetal gestations: twin, triplet, and higher-order multifetal pregnancies. Practice Bulletin No. 169. Obstet Gynecol 2018;**128**: e131–e146.

3. Stone J, Ferrara L, Kamrath J, Getrajdam J, Berkowitz R, Moshier E et al. Contemporary outcomes with the latest 1000 cases of multifetal pregnancy reduction (MFPR). Am J Obstet Gynecol 2008;**199**:406.e1– 406.e4.

4. Kim MS, Choi DH, Kwon H, Ahn E, Cho HY, Baek MJ et al. Procedural and obstetrical outcomes after embryo reduction vs fetal reduction in multifetal pregnancy. Ultrasound Obstet Gynecol 2019;**53**:214–18.

5. Bigelow C, Factor S, Moshier E, Bianco A, Eddleman K, Stone J. Timing and outcomes after selective termination of anomalous fetuses in dichorionic twin pregnancies. Prenat Diagn 2014;**34**:1320–5.

6. Dural O, Yasa C, Kalelioglu I, Can S, Yilmaz G, Esmer AC et al. Comparison of perinatal outcomes of selective termination in dichorionic twin pregnancies performed at different gestational ages. J Matern Fetal Neonatal Med 2017;**30**(12):1388–92.

7. Rosner M, Pergament E, Andriole S, Gebb J, Dar P, Evans M. Detection of genetic abnormalities by using CVS and FISH prior to fetal reduction in sonographically normal appearing fetuses. Prenat Diagn 2013;**33**:940–4.

8. Evans MI, Andriole S, Evans SM. Screening and testing in multiples. Clin Lab Med 2016;**36**(2):289–303.

9. Wilmasundra RC. Selective reduction and termination of multiple pregnancies. Semin Fetal Neonat 2010;**15**:327–35.

10. Gaerty K, Greer R, Kumar S. Systematic review and metaanalysis of perinatal outcomes after radiofrequency ablation and bipolar cord occlusion in monochorionic pregnancies. Am J Obstet Gynecol 2017:637–43.

11. Rossi AC, D'Addario V. Umbilical cord occlusion for selective feticide in complicated monochorionic twins: a systematic review of literature. Am J Obstet Gynecol 2009:123–9.

12. Van Klink JMM, Koopman HM, Middeldorp JM, Klumper FJ, Rijken M, Oepkes D et al. Long-term neurodevelopmental outcomes after selective feticide in monochorionic pregnancies. BJOG 2015;122:1517–24.

13. Bebbington M. Selective reduction in complex monochorionic gestations. Am J Perinatol 2014;21:S51–S58.

14. Greimel P, Csapo B, Haeusler M, Lang U, Klaritsch P. A modified technique for cord transection in monochorionic monoamniotic twin pregnancies. Fetal Diagn Ther 2018;44:236–40.

15. Herlihy N, Naqvi M, Romero J, Gupta S, Monteagudo A, Rebarber A et al. Multifetal pregnancy reduction of trichorionic triplet gestations: what is the benefit? Am J Perinatol 2017;34:1417–23.

16. Viera L, Warren L, Pan S, Ferrar L, Stone J. Comparing pregnancy outcomes and loss rates in elective twin pregnancy reduction with ongoing twin gestations in a large contemporary cohort. Am J Obstet Gynecol 2019;221:253.e1–8.

17. Roman AS, Rebarber A, Lipkind H, Mulholland J, Minior V, Roshan D. Vaginal fetal fibronectin as a predictor of spontaneous preterm delivery after multifetal pregnancy reduction. Am J Obstet Gynecol 2004;190(1):142–6.

18. Rebarber A, Carreno CA, Lipkind H et al. Cervical length after multifetal pregnancy reduction in remaining twin gestations. Am J Obstet Gynecol 2001;185(5):1113–17.

Gestational Dating in Multiple Pregnancy

Pierre Macé, Houman Mahallati and Laurent J. Salomon

Introduction

In addition to determining chorionicity and amnionicity, screening for aneuploidies and structural defects, dating of the pregnancy is one of the important goals of ultrasound in twin pregnancies, especially when exams are done in the first trimester. The primary purpose of dating in twin pregnancies is not entirely the same as in singleton pregnancies in that the estimation of a due date is not as relevant in the context of multiple pregnancies. Most deliveries take place before 40 weeks of gestation, either spontaneously or due to a medical indication. The main objective of dating in multiple pregnancies is to make subsequent ultrasound examinations at later term more effective in the screening and management of complications either specific to twin pregnancies (twin–twin transfusion syndrome (TTTS) or selective fetal growth restriction (FGR)) or more frequent in these pregnancies (preterm birth, structural defects, aneuploidies). One of the recurrent questions is the choice of the fetus upon which to base dating, especially when there is a significant difference between the size of the two twins. This must be done in a manner that does not ignore potential complications and that at the same time does not generate unnecessary parental anxiety or result in further unnecessary investigations.

The Issues

When and How?

Routine dating of a singleton pregnancy from a measurement of the crown–rump length (CRL) at the time of first-trimester ultrasound has been shown to be superior to the use of menstrual dates or dating after 14 weeks of gestational age.[1][2] It is likely that the same should apply in twins, although there have been no specific studies demonstrating that it performs better than the last menstrual period. The question is therefore whether the CRL reference charts used in singleton pregnancies can also be used in twin pregnancies. In cases where the patient presents after 14 weeks of gestation or the CRL measurement is greater than 84 mm, one must use the biometric measurements producing the most accurate prediction of gestational age. Dating options in cases where pregnancies are conceived via assisted reproductive technologies (ART) are discussed later in this chapter.

Which Twin?

While it is likely that dating in the first trimester is desirable, there is less consensus on whether pregnancy should be dated on measurements taken on the smallest twin, the largest twin or the mean measurements of the two twins.[3] Theoretically, the choice of the smallest twin has the advantage of not creating unnecessary parental anxiety about possible growth restriction as early as the first trimester. The exception to this would be cases with significant and obviously pathological CRL discordances (see later in this chapter). There are three potential disadvantages to this strategy: (1) ignoring growth restriction in the smaller fetus; (2) the potential to incorrectly assume there is fetal macrosomia of the larger twin at a later term; and (3) the risk of neglecting a post-term twin pregnancy. These risks and the relative infrequency of large-for-gestational-age fetuses in twin pregnancies explain the common practice of dating the pregnancy based on the larger twin. In this situation, the choice is effectively that of increasing the sensitivity of screening for selective FGR whilst recognising the increased risk of a higher number of false positives and potentially unnecessary additional testing and increasing parental anxiety. The choice should therefore be based on the most accurate measurement in this context, but unfortunately the literature is inconsistent as to what constitutes the most accurate measurement, with several authors finding a higher performance of either the smallest CRL,[3,7] or the mean of the two measurements,[4] while the largest CRL often leads to the greatest difference with the assumed date of pregnancy by in-vitro fertilisation timing.

Putting this into perspective, given that CRL discordance in twin pregnancies is rare (less than 10% of twins have a discordance of more than 10%), the mean discrepancy between twins at the time of first-trimester ultrasound would be expected to be very low.[3,8]

In a prospective study including 182 twin pregnancies, Salomon et al.[3] showed that the mean difference in the CRL measurement between the two twins was 3.4 mm or 1.2 days. This was supported in a large retrospective study on 6,225 twin pregnancies which stated that the mean difference in CRL measurement was 3.2 mm in dichorionic pregnancies and 3.6 mm in monochorionic-diamniotic pregnancies.[8] In this sense, using the formula reported by Robinson et al., a 3 mm difference in CRL measurement is at most equivalent to a difference of 2 days of gestational age.[9] As mentioned later, this difference may simply reflect different growth patterns and/or measurement errors of two normal fetuses and is well below the measurement error reported for CRL assessment. It is therefore unlikely to have a significant impact on subsequent pregnancy follow-up.

The situation is different in the presence of a major discrepancy between CRL measurements. Several different cut-offs of significant CRL discrepancy have been proposed, which is itself a concern as the association between CRL discordance and adverse outcomes is highly dependent on the threshold adopted. It is therefore important to set a threshold to define a significant discrepancy that could impact the pregnancy outcome. The ≥10mm or 15% CRL discordance are the most commonly used thresholds to represent the higher centiles of discordance, and the 95th percentile for CRL discrepancy seems to be around 10 mm, which is a 14% difference in CRL measurement or 3.6 days of gestational age.[3] Again, according to Robinson et al., a 10 mm difference is equivalent to a difference of between 4 and 6 days depending on the gestation at the time of measurement.[9]

Above these limits, the dating of the pregnancy should be based on the larger twin's CRL, as this major discrepancy probably indicates a very early-onset growth restriction of the smallest twin, which may have the same significance as in a singleton pregnancy and reveal a chromosomal defect or structural abnormalities.[3] However, it is to be noted that the role of CRL discordance in screening for aneuploidy is probably limited with the introduction of non-invasive prenatal testing. A significant CRL discordance has also been reported as an early predictor of adverse pregnancy outcomes such as significant birthweight discrepancy[10], selective intrauterine growth restriction (IUGR), fetal loss before 20 or 24 weeks of gestation, preterm birth,[8,11] fetal loss after 24 weeks of gestation[11] or TTTS in monochorionic twins [8,12–14] – with a moderate strength of association and too poor prediction accuracy to form a clinically relevant screening test for these adverse outcomes.[8,11]

The Management Option

When and How?

The dating of twin pregnancies should ideally be based on that of singletons and should be performed when the CRL measurement is between 45 and 84 mm (i.e. 11+0 to 13+6 weeks of gestation), using the same singleton reference chart used at the time of the routine first-trimester examination.[4,5]

Dias et al.[4] compared the dating of twin and singleton pregnancies (controls) conceived following ART by measuring the CRL (Robinson charts[9]) and compared CRL-based dates with the known date of conception. They showed that the variation in CRL between singletons and twins was unlikely to be clinically relevant, with a maximum variation of about 2 mm or 1 day, well within the first-trimester ultrasound accuracy range for dating pregnancy, and probably consistent with normal physiological variation. If the woman presents after 14 weeks of gestational age and with a CRL measurement above 84 mm, the dating of pregnancy should be based on measurement of the head circumference,[2,5] which appears to produce the most reliable prediction.[15]

As is the case for singleton pregnancies, twin pregnancies conceived via ART should be dated using the oocyte retrieval date or the embryonic age from fertilisation.[5] In the case of pregnancies conceived either spontaneously or via ART, significant discrepancy between the two twins (>10 mm, >15%) should lead to consideration of additional investigations of the smallest twin, which is the twin at higher risk of aneuploidy or FGR, and closer follow-up of the pregnancy should be instituted. This is despite the poor screening performance for adverse pregnancy outcomes as stated earlier in this chapter. An additional earlier scan at 14 weeks for monochorionic pregnancies and 16 weeks of gestational age for dichorionic pregnancies should still be offered. With regards to the risk of aneuploidy, future research should investigate the relevance of major CRL discrepancy in the era of cfDNA testing.

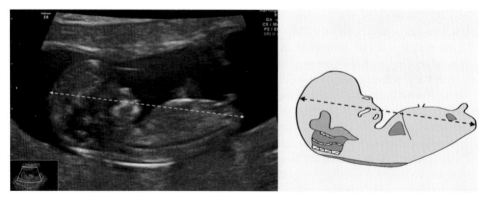

Figure 5.1 Crown–rump length measurement, left: ultrasound view, right: schematic view

Which Twin?

In the vast majority of twin pregnancies for which the discordance is less than 15% (i.e. in practice less than 7–12 mm), the question of which twin to use for dating remains debatable.

While the smaller twin, which appears closer to the actual age in ART-conceived pregnancies, could be used for dating, this will decrease the FGR detection rate later in pregnancy.[3,7] The use of the average CRL will reduce the random error of the measurements. Finally, the use of the larger twin allows for a simple and consistent practice since it applies even in the case of a major discrepancy related to aneuploidy or structural defects of the smaller one and increases the sensitivity of subsequent selective FGR screening. This recommendation has also recently been stated in the International Society of Ultrasound in Obstetrics and Gynecology (ISUOG) guidelines on the role of ultrasound in twin pregnancies and is likely to ensure, through its simplicity, a much-needed standardisation of practices.[5] To add emphasis, such a recommendation can be applied in all cases regardless of the discrepancy in CRL between the twins. If the woman presents after 14 weeks of gestational age, the larger head circumference should be used for dating pregnancy. The following flow chart summarises the management options for the dating of twin pregnancies.

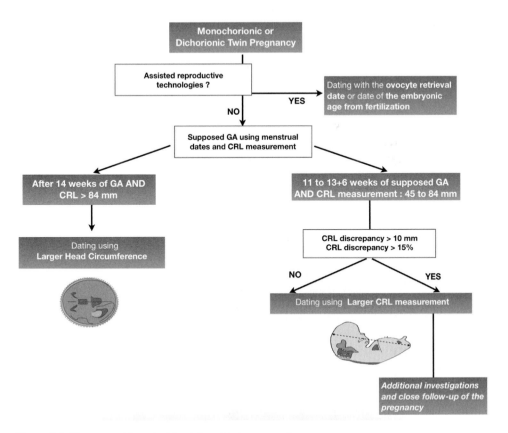

Figure 5.2 Management flow chart for dating of twin pregnancies

Key Points

- Dating of the pregnancy is one of the main objectives of first-trimester ultrasound in twin pregnancies.
- Unlike singleton pregnancies where dating establishes term, due to frequent earlier delivery dates, the main objective of dating twin pregnancies is to improve the screening and management of twin pregnancy complications, especially selective IUGR.
- Twin pregnancies conceived via ART should be dated using the oocyte retrieval date or the embryonic age from fertilisation.
- The dating of twin pregnancies should be based on CRL measurements between 45 and 84 mm (i.e. 11+0 to 13+6 weeks of gestation) using the same reference charts used for singleton pregnancies.
- The mean discrepancy between twins at the time of the first-trimester ultrasound appears to be clinically irrelevant and is unlikely to have a significant impact on subsequent pregnancy follow-up.
- Dating of twin pregnancies using the largest CRL measurement, as advised by the ISUOG guidelines, is the simplest and the most common practice and allows high sensitivity for the screening of selective IUGR.
- If the CRL measurement discrepancy is >10 mm or >15%, additional investigations should be considered for the smaller twin, which is at higher risk of aneuploidy or FGR despite the poor prediction accuracy of CRL discrepancy for adverse pregnancy outcomes.
- After 14 weeks of gestational age or if the CRL measurement is above 84 mm, the larger head circumference should be used for dating pregnancy.

References

1. Whitworth M, Bricker L, Mullan C. Ultrasound for fetal assessment in early pregnancy. Cochrane Pregnancy and Childbirth Group, editor. Cochrane Database of Systematic Reviews [Internet]. 2015 Jul 14 [cited 2019 Apr 11]. http://doi.wiley.com/10.1002/14651858.CD007058.pub3

2. ISUOG Practice Guidelines: performance of first-trimester fetal ultrasound scan. Ultrasound in Obstetrics & Gynecology 2013 Jan;41(1):102–13.

3. Salomon LJ, Cavicchioni O, Bernard JP, Duyme M, Ville Y. Growth discrepancy in twins in the first trimester of pregnancy. Ultrasound in Obstetrics & Gynecology 2005;26(5):512–26.

4. Dias T, Mahsud-Dornan S, Thilaganathan B, Papageorghiou A, Bhide A. First-trimester ultrasound dating of twin pregnancy: are singleton charts reliable? BJOG 2010;117(8):979–84.

5. Khalil A, Rodgers M, Baschat A, Bhide A, Gratacos E, Hecher K et al. ISUOG Practice Guidelines: role of ultrasound in twin pregnancy. Ultrasound in Obstetrics & Gynecology 2016;47(2):247–63.

6. Sebire NJ, D'Ercole C, Soares W, Nayar R, Nicolaides KH. Intertwin disparity in fetal size in monochorionic and dichorionic pregnancies. Obstet Gynecol 1998 Jan;91(1):82–5.

7. Chaudhuri K, Su L-L, Wong P-C, Chan Y-H, Choolani MA, Chia D et al. Determination of gestational age in twin pregnancy: which fetal crown–rump length should be used? Gestational dating in twins. Journal of Obstetrics and Gynaecology Research 2013 Apr;39(4):761–5.

8. Litwinska E, Syngelaki A, Cimpoca B, Sapantzoglou I, Nicolaides KH. Intertwin discordance in fetal size at 11–13 weeks' gestation and pregnancy outcome. Ultrasound in Obstetrics & Gynecology

2020 Feb;**55**(2):189–97. https://obgyn-onlinelibrary-wiley-com.lama.univ-amu.fr/doi/10.1002/uog.21923

9. Robinson HP, Fleming JEE. A critical evaluation of sonar 'crown–rump length' measurements. Br J Obstet Gynaecol 1975 Sep;**82**(9):702–10.

10. Kalish RB, Chasen ST, Gupta M, Sharma G, Perni SC, Chervenak FA. First trimester prediction of growth discordance in twin gestations. Am J Obstet Gynecol 2003 Sep;**189**(3):706–9.

11. D'Antonio F, Khalil A, Pagani G, Papageorghiou AT, Bhide A, Thilaganathan B. Crown–rump length discordance and adverse perinatal outcome in twin pregnancies: systematic review and meta-analysis. Ultrasound in Obstetrics & Gynecology 2014;**44**(2):138–46.

12. Mackie FL, Hall MJ, Morris RK, Kilby MD. Early prognostic factors of outcomes in monochorionic twin pregnancy: systematic review and meta-analysis. American Journal of Obstetrics and Gynecology 2018 Nov;**219**(5):436–46.

13. Stagnati V, Zanardini C, Fichera A, Pagani G, Quintero RA, Bellocco R et al. Early prediction of twin-to-twin transfusion syndrome: systematic review and meta-analysis. Ultrasound in Obstetrics & Gynecology 2017 May;**49**(5):573–82.

14. Memmo A, Dias T, Mahsud-Dornan S, Papageorghiou AT, Bhide A, Thilaganathan B. Prediction of selective fetal growth restriction and twin-to-twin transfusion syndrome in monochorionic twins.BJOG 2012;**119**(4):417–21.

15. Papageorghiou AT, Kemp B, Stones W, Ohuma EO, Kennedy SH, Purwar M et al. Ultrasound-based gestational-age estimation in late pregnancy. Ultrasound Obstet Gynecol 2016 Dec 1;**48**(6):719–26.

Screening for Fetal Aneuploidy in Multiple Pregnancy

Maria del Mar Gil and Kypros Nicolaides

The Facts

Aneuploidies, particularly trisomies 21, 18 and 13, are common and major causes of perinatal death and childhood handicap and their prenatal detection has been one of the main goals of fetal medicine. Diagnosis of fetal aneuploidies necessitates invasive testing by amniocentesis or chorionic villus sampling (CVS) and karyotyping of amniotic fluid and chorionic tissue, respectively. However, these procedures are associated with an increased risk of miscarriage and therefore these tests are carried out only in pregnancies considered at high risk for aneuploidies. Consequently, strategies have focused on the development of effective methods of screening to define the group in need of such invasive testing.

The primary aim of screening was always prenatal detection of trisomy 21; however, a beneficial consequence of such screening was the detection of trisomies 18 and 13, Turner syndrome, triploidy and some other rare chromosomal defects.[1] In the past 50 years, screening for aneuploidies in singleton pregnancies has evolved from maternal age in the 1970s with detection rate (DR) for Down syndrome of 30% and false positive rate (FPR) of 5%, to second-trimester serum biochemical testing in the 1980s with DR of 50–70% at FPR of 5%, to the first-trimester combined test with maternal age, fetal nuchal translucency (NT) and maternal serum pregnancy-associated plasma protein A (PAPP-A) and free β-human chorionic gonadotrophin (β-hCG) in the 1990s, with DR of 90% at FPR of 5%. Finally, in the past 10 years, several externally blinded validation and implementation studies have shown that it is possible through analysis of cell-free (cf) DNA in maternal blood to detect 99.7%, 97.9% and 99.0% of cases of trisomy 21, trisomy 18 and trisomy 13, respectively, with FPR of about 0.4%, 0.4% and 0.4%, respectively.[2]

Overall, dizygotic twin pregnancies are at higher risk for aneuploidy than singleton pregnancies because either of the two fetuses could be affected and also because women with such pregnancies are usually older than women with singleton pregnancies. Consequently, the proportion of these pregnancies that are positive by the traditional methods of screening is considerably higher than in singleton pregnancies. However, prenatal screening and diagnosis for aneuploidy in multiple pregnancies is limited by significant clinical, technical and ethical issues.

The Issues

In multiple pregnancies, compared with singleton pregnancies, prenatal diagnosis is complicated because, first, the techniques of invasive testing may provide uncertain results or may be associated with higher risks of miscarriage; second, the fetuses may be discordant for the abnormality; third, the different methods of screening described for singletons need specific corrections and their performance may be lower; fourth, the number of affected cases studied in multiple pregnancies is much lower than in singleton pregnancies; therefore, estimates of test performance will always be less precise.

Monozygotic pregnancies are genetically identical in the vast majority of cases (with very rare exceptions due to post-zygotic changes) and therefore all fetuses are either affected or unaffected, whereas dizygotic (or higher order) pregnancies are genetically different and therefore most likely discordant for the aneuploidy, with one fetus affected and the other(s) not. When screening monozygotic pregnancies, an overall risk assessment is provided for the entire pregnancy, while pregnancies of higher zygosity order will be provided a specific risk for each fetus, being the risk of aneuploidy for each fetus more or less independent of the risk for the other (although NT measurements in both fetuses may be somehow correlated). However, zygosity can only be determined by DNA fingerprinting, which requires amniocentesis, CVS or cordocentesis. Thus, chorionicity, which can be indirectly determined by ultrasound, is used as a proxy for zygosity in prenatal diagnosis: all monochorionic twins are monozygotic and about 85% of dichorionic twins are dizygotic. Conversely, all dizygotic twins are dichorionic whereas two-thirds of monozygotic twins are monochorionic and one-third are dichorionic, depending on the timing of embryo splitting.

Monochorionic twins carry a higher risk of structural abnormalities, but the risk of aneuploidy appears similar to the risk in singletons. On the other hand, in dizygotic pregnancies, the maternal age-related risk for chromosomal abnormalities for each twin is the same as in singleton pregnancies and therefore the chance that at least one fetus is affected by a chromosomal defect is about twice as high as in singleton pregnancies.

In multiple pregnancies, effective screening for trisomies can be provided by a combination of maternal age and fetal NT thickness. However, in monochorionic pregnancies, the false positive rate of NT screening is higher than in singletons due to an early manifestation of a twin–twin transfusion syndrome seen as discordant NT thickness among fetuses.[3]

Serum biochemical marker concentrations used for risk assessment in the first or second trimester in twin pregnancies reflect the presence of two fetuses rather than one and are also different according to chorionicity – that is, around gestational weeks 11–13, maternal serum concentrations in twins are approximately double than those found in singletons.[4-6] For this reason, risk assessment for twin pregnancies by the first-trimester combined test or by the second-trimester triple or quadruple test needs adjustment by chorionicity and it is not possible in multiple pregnancies of higher order. Additionally, biochemical markers are not fetus-specific, and therefore the abnormality from one fetus may be masked by the normal fetus and vice versa.

In cfDNA testing, the ability to detect a small increase in the amount of a given chromosome in maternal plasma in a trisomic compared to a disomic pregnancy is directly related to the proportion of the fetal to maternal origin of the cfDNA. This proportion of cfDNA from the fetus in the mother's bloodstream is known as fetal fraction. When the fetal fraction is low, it is more difficult to discriminate between aneuploid and euploid pregnancies. In twin pregnancies, cfDNA testing is more complex than in singleton pregnancies because the two fetuses could be either monozygotic, which are therefore genetically identical, or dizygotic, in which case only one fetus is likely to have the aneuploidy when present. When performing analysis of cfDNA in maternal blood in dizygotic twins, each fetus contributes different amounts of cfDNA into the maternal circulation, which could vary by nearly twofold.[7] It is therefore possible that in a dizygotic twin pregnancy discordant for aneuploidy, the fetal fraction of the affected fetus is below the minimal threshold (normally about 4%) required for successful testing. This could lead to an erroneous result of low risk for aneuploidy because a high contribution from the disomic co-twin could result in a satisfactory total fetal fraction (Figure 6.1). This phenomenon would happen more frequently in multiple pregnancies of increasing order. To avoid this potential error, two strategies have been proposed: first, to determine the fetal fraction for each twin and to use the lowest of the two for risk estimation, and, second, to increase the fetal fraction threshold for reporting a result – that is, from 4% to 8%. However, these approaches will inevitably lead to a higher proportion of tests that will not yield a result. Although the number of affected cases evaluated is significantly lower than that for singletons, performance of cfDNA testing for trisomy 21 in twin pregnancies is similar to that in singletons.[7] However, there are insufficient data to accurately report the performance of the test for conditions other than trisomy 21 or for multiple pregnancies of order three or higher.

The Management Options

A summary of screening performance for trisomy 21 of each screening method in twin pregnancies is provided in Table 6.1.

Screening by Maternal Age

When defining a risk cut-off for screening of aneuploidies, we must always state when that probability refers to. Since the rate of fetal death between 12 weeks of gestation and term is about 30% for trisomy 21, 80% for trisomies 18 and 13 and only 1–2% for euploid fetuses, the risk for trisomies decreases with gestation and the risk cut-off will vary depending on when the risk assessment is performed.[8] For example, in screening for aneuploidies by maternal age, the estimated risks for fetal trisomies 21, 18 and 13 for a woman aged 20 years at 12 weeks of gestation are about 1 in 1,000, 1 in 2,500 and 1 in 8,000, respectively, whereas the risks of such woman delivering an affected baby at term are 1 in 1,500, 1 in 18,000 and 1 in 42,000, respectively. Conversely, the respective risks for these aneuploidies for a 35-year-old woman at 12 weeks of gestation are about 1 in 250, 1 in 600 and 1 in 1,800, and the risks of delivering an affected baby at term are 1 in 350, 1 in 4,000 and 1 in 10,000. Monosomy X (45,X) has a prevalence of about 1 in 1,500 at 12 weeks and 1 in 4,000 at 40 weeks and is not related to maternal age. Other sex chromosome aneuploidies (47,XXX, 47,XXY and 47,

Table 6.1 Performance of different methods of screening for trisomy 21

Method of screening	Detection rate	False positive rate
Maternal age	40	65
Maternal age + fetal NT	75–80	8
First-trimester combined test	90	6 (DC), 9 (MC)
Quadruple test	45	5
Cell free DNA test	> 99	0.05

NT: nuchal translucency; DC: dichorionic; MC: monochorionic

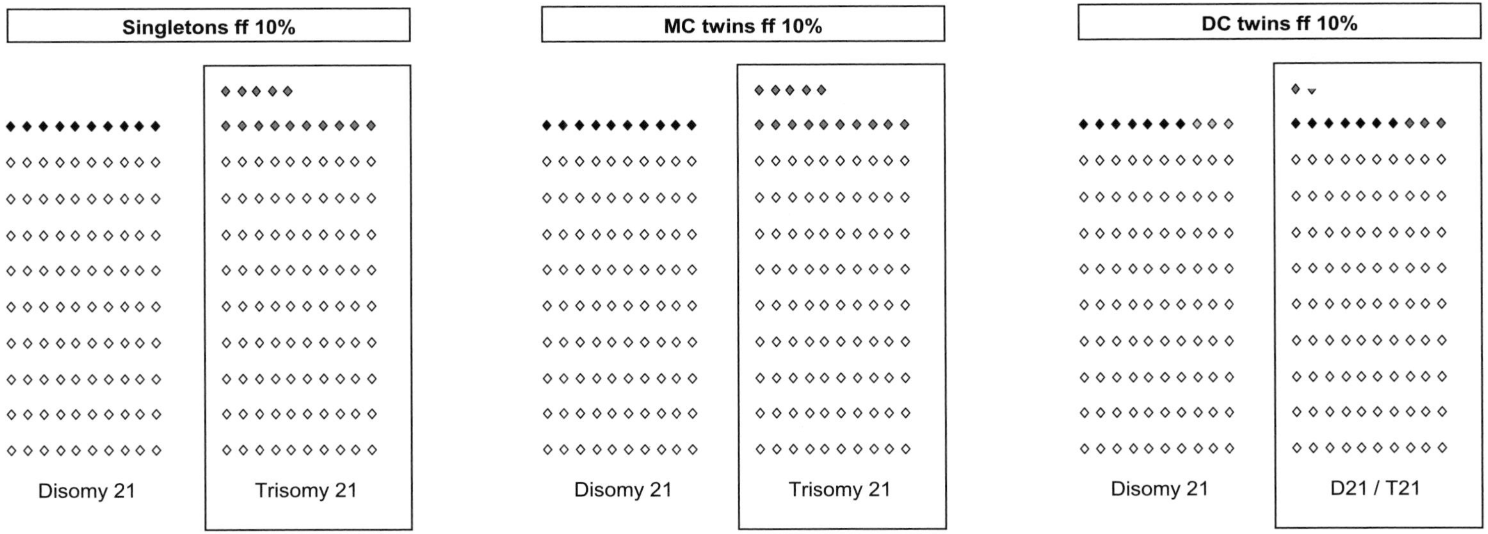

Figure 6.1

XYY) have the same rate of fetal death as euploid fetuses and therefore their overall prevalence (about 1 in 500) does not decrease with gestation and also it does not significantly change with maternal age. Finally, triploidy is unrelated to maternal age and has a prevalence of about 1 in 2,000 but, because most of the affected fetuses die by 20 weeks, it is rarely seen in live births.

Unlike with singletons, there is little direct information on the prior maternal age-specific risk in twins and almost non-existent information in multiple pregnancies of higher order. If the risk of trisomy 21 for each fetus was completely independent of the risk of the other(s), the risk that at least one fetus is affected in a twin pregnancy would be double than in a singleton pregnancy. Actually, the risk is somewhat less than double (about 1.6) for two reasons: first, monozygotic pregnancies are concordant for the aneuploidy, and second, because NT measurements in euploid twins are somehow correlated even after accounting for the sonographer.[9]

In monochorionic pregnancies where both fetuses are assumed to be genetically identical, the prior risk for aneuploidies for the whole pregnancy according to maternal age is the same as in singleton pregnancies. In dichorionic twins, it has been estimated by modelling charts that the traditional threshold of 35 years used to define the high-risk group by maternal age alone (risk cut-off: 1 in 250 at 12 weeks of gestation) in singleton pregnancies corresponds to 31–33-year-olds in a dichorionic twin pregnancy (Table 6.2). The same rationale applies to multiple pregnancies of higher order.

However, screening for aneuploidies based on maternal age alone in multiple pregnancies should be discouraged for several reasons: first, lowering the cut-off to define the high-risk group in addition to a higher proportion of elderly women in this group of patients would inevitably lead to a disproportionally increased screened positive rate of about 65%. Second, there is a higher miscarriage rate related to invasive diagnostic procedures in these pregnancies, and therefore the aim should be to reduce the screen positive rate. Third, the observed incidence of trisomy 21 in twin pregnancies is lower than that predicted by theoretical models, and therefore it is likely that these figures are overestimating the risk.[10]

Screening by Nuchal Translucency

Chorionic villus sampling for fetal karyotyping is the preferred method for prenatal diagnosis in singleton pregnancies due to the advantages of early diagnosis and early selective termination of pregnancy as an option. However, although the risk of miscarriage following CVS in twin pregnancies is not higher than that of amniocentesis, in about 5% of cases, it may be unclear whether the same placenta has been sampled and hence it may be argued that the best method for fetal karyotyping is amniocentesis. However, it must be kept in mind that cytogenetic results from amniocentesis may not be available until 18–20 weeks, when the risk of miscarriage of performing a selective feticide is about three times higher than if it is performed before 16 weeks. Therefore, there must be a proper and early risk assessment to help select the most appropriate invasive diagnostic procedure according to the likelihood of ending requiring a selective termination of pregnancy. In this respect, screening by fetal nuchal translucency in the first trimester provided a major step in the management of fetal aneuploidies in multiple pregnancies.

In multiple pregnancies, effective screening for chromosomal abnormalities is provided by a combination of maternal age and fetal NT thickness. The optimal time for measuring NT thickness is between 11+0 and 13+6 weeks of gestation, when the fetal crown–rump

Table 6.2 Risk for trisomy 21 in singleton pregnancies at 12 weeks of gestation and risk estimates of the same risk for both, monochorionic and dichorionic twin pregnancies

Maternal age (years)	Risk for trisomy 21 in singletons and MC twins (1 in X)	Risk for trisomy 21 in DC twins (1 in X)
20	1,068	534
25	946	483
30	626	313
31	544	272
32	460	230
33	380	190
34	312	156
35	250	125
36	200	100
37	150	75
38	118	59
39	90	45
40	68	34
41	50	25
42	38	19
43	30	15
44	20	10
45	16	8

DC: dichorionic; MC: monochorionic

length ranges from 45 to 84 mm. Fetal NT thickness increases with crown–rump length and a measurement above the 95th centile detects about 75–80% of trisomy 21 fetuses in both singleton and multiple pregnancies.[3,8] Furthermore, NT thickness is independent of maternal age; therefore, data from these two parameters can be combined, increasing DR of trisomy 21 to 80–85% at an FPR of 5% in singletons, while the same DR can be achieved in twins at the expense of a higher FPR of about 8%, likely as a consequence of fetal heart failure of the recipient in monochorionic pregnancies complicated by early twin–twin transfusion syndrome.[3,6,8] Because neither serum biomarkers nor cfDNA testing can be used in multiple pregnancies of order three or higher, screening by a combination of fetal NT thickness and maternal age is the preferred method for screening of trisomy 21 in these pregnancies.

Screening by First-Trimester Combined Test

Performance of screening by fetal NT thickness and maternal age in the first trimester can be improved by the addition of maternal serum biochemistry when appropriate adjustments for chorionicity are performed. At 11+0 to 13+6 weeks, the levels of maternal serum-free β-hCG and PAPP-A in dichorionic pregnancies are twice as high as in singleton pregnancies.[4-6] In monochorionic twins, these levels are also higher than in singletons but lower than in dichorionic twins.[4-6] The use of serum biomarkers has not been validated in multiple pregnancies of order three or higher.

The addition of likelihood ratios for PAPP-A and free β-hCG to risk assessment by maternal age and fetal NT in dichorionic twins increases the DR for fetal trisomy 21 up to 90% and decreases the FPR from approximately 8% to 6%, which is similar than the screening performance of the first-trimester combined test in singletons.[6,11] However, there appears to be no improvement in the DR of fetal aneuploidy in monochorionic twins, which is about 85–90% for trisomy 21, nor in the FPR, which remains around 9%, by the addition of biochemical markers.[6]

In monochorionic twins, risks for trisomy 21 are calculated for each fetus using maternal age, fetal NT thickness and crown–rump length and serum levels of free β-hCG and PAPP-A corrected by chorionicity. Then the average of the two risks is calculated to estimate the overall pregnancy risk. However, in dichorionic twins, risks for trisomy 21 are calculated in the same way but provided for each fetus separately. It can be assumed that the two fetuses are independent or, alternatively, the correlation in NT measurements between fetuses can be taken into account for the risk calculation.[8,9] This measure may not have a significant impact on the overall performance of screening, but it does have a substantial impact on the estimated patient-specific risk.[9]

Screening by Second-Trimester Serum Biomarkers

Several second-trimester serum biomarkers have been incorporated to improve DR of screening for trisomy 21 by maternal age alone from 14 weeks of gestation onwards. In singleton pregnancies, at a fixed FPR of 5%, the DR by combining maternal age with serum alpha fetoprotein and free β-hCG (double test) is about 60–65%. With the addition of unconjugated estriol (triple test), it is about 65–70%, and with the addition of inhibin A (quadruple test), it is about 70–75%. However, in twin pregnancies, the maximum DR that can be achieved by this method is only about 45–50% at the same FPR of 5%.[12]

One limitation of screening for trisomy 21 by serum biomarkers alone in twins is that the pregnancy is classified as high risk as a whole without any indication of which fetus may be the affected one, unlike ultrasound markers, which are fetus-specific. This method is not validated for pregnancies of order three or higher, and for twin pregnancies, it would only be recommended when other screening methods with higher performance are not available.

Screening by Cell-Free DNA Testing

Analysis of cfDNA testing in maternal blood for screening of aneuploidies should not be performed before 10 weeks of gestation to ensure accurate results, without an upper limit for testing. Several clinical validation and implementation studies have been published, and this method is currently recommended either as first-line screening or as contingent screening following the results from a previously performed screening method.

Performance of cfDNA testing for trisomy 21 in twin pregnancies is similar to that reported in singleton pregnancies, showing a DR of about 98% and an FPR of 0.05%.[7] Although the number of cases reported in the literature is still insufficient to properly evaluate performance of cfDNA screening for trisomy 18, DR and FPR are about 90% and 0.03%, respectively.[7] The use of cfDNA testing for screening of other aneuploidies or genetic conditions is currently not validated and therefore not recommended.

Despite its good performance, cfDNA testing remains as a screening test, which means that a high-risk result requires confirmation by invasive testing and that a negative result, although reassuring, does not mean that the pregnancy is certainly not affected.

The two main concerns when screening for trisomy 21 by cfDNA testing in twin pregnancies relate to, first, the limited available data and, second, to the increased rate of tests that do not yield a result (no-result rate) in dichorionic twins as compared to singletons (5% versus 1% after second testing).[13] One of the main reasons for this increased no-result rate in dichorionic twins is directly related to twinning and the necessity of being very conservative with the minimal fetal fraction required in order to ensure accurate results. However, another risk factor for an increased no-result rate that has been repeatedly associated with a lower fetal fraction and therefore to an increased no-result rate is the use of assisted reproductive techniques for pregnancy conception, something which is far more frequent in twin than in singleton pregnancies.[13] Other risk factors for not obtaining a result after testing are increasing maternal weight, nulliparity, certain ethnic origins, like Afro-Caribbean or South Asian, and factors related to a smaller placental size, like earlier gestational age or low serum levels of free β-hCG and PAPP-A.[13] Likewise, aneuploidies related to a small placenta, such as trisomies 18 and 13 and digynic triploidy but not trisomy 21, have a lower fetal fraction, and therefore they are also associated with an increased no-result rate. Therefore, when a result is not obtained from cfDNA testing, careful ultrasound assessment of the fetal anatomy must be carried out in order to rule out the presence of any structural defects related to any of the aforementioned conditions; if those are excluded, repeating the test is a sensible management option, and a result will be obtained in the second draw in about 50% of cases.[13] In those cases where a result is not reported after second testing, other risk factors or screening tests must be considered to help decide if an invasive diagnostic testing is advisable (Figure 6.2). Therefore, pretest counselling should not only include DR and FPR but also the no-result rate since it is a component of the test screening performance.

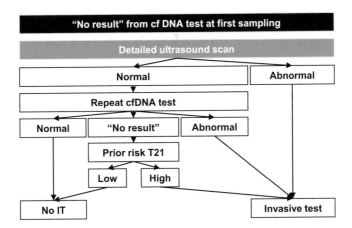

Figure 6.2 Management algorithm if cfDNA test yields 'no-result'

Although it has been tested in triplets, cfDNA screening has not been validated for pregnancies of order three or higher. As for serum biomarkers, it has the disadvantage of not being fetus-specific, and therefore, the results are provided for the whole pregnancy without any information on which can be the affected fetus. Consequently, it is recommended that cfDNA testing is always accompanied by a comprehensive ultrasound assessment.

Screening of Aneuploidies in the Presence of a Vanishing Twin

The presence of a vanishing twin may complicate screening using maternal serum biomarkers or cfDNA testing since placental products from the interrupted pregnancy are present in the maternal bloodstream for several weeks.

Although it was generally recommended not to use serum biomarkers when there is a measurable fetal pole,[14] it has been recently reported that, unlike PAPP-A levels, which are always increased in vanishing twin pregnancies even if only an empty sac is visible, free β-hCG levels are not significantly different from those in normal singleton pregnancies, regardless of when the fetal demise occurred.[15] This knowledge may allow performing first-trimester screening by combining maternal age, fetal NT thickness and free β-hCG in these pregnancies, increasing DR from 80% to 85% as compared to screening by maternal age and NT alone, both at 5% FPR.[15]

The cfDNA testing should not be performed in vanishing twin pregnancies because of flooding of cfDNA into the maternal plasma from the necrotic cytotrophoblasts, which may persist for at least 15 weeks after fetal demise. This persisting cfDNA from the vanishing twin in the maternal circulation may reduce DR and increase false positive and no-result rates.

Key Points

- For monochorionic pregnancies, an overall risk assessment is provided for the entire pregnancy, while for dichorionic (or higher chorionicity order) a specific risk is provided for each fetus.
- In monochorionic pregnancies, the risk of aneuploidy appears similar to the risk in singleton pregnancies; in dizygotic pregnancies, the chance that at least one fetus is affected by a chromosomal defect is about twice as high as in singleton pregnancies.
- Screening by a combination of maternal age and fetal NT thickness in multiple pregnancies shows a similar DR to that in singleton pregnancies, of about 80–85%, but at a higher FPR with higher number of fetuses. This is the recommended method for multiple pregnancies of order three or higher.
- First-trimester combined tests in twins show a similar detection rate to singletons of about 90%, but at a higher FPR, of 6% for dichorionic twins and 9% for monochorionic twins. It is not possible to screen multiple pregnancies of order three or higher by this method.
- Screening for trisomy 21 in twins by the second-trimester quadruple test will only achieve a DR of about 45% at a 5% false positive rate. It is not possible to screen multiple pregnancies of order three or higher by this method.
- Analysis of cfDNA in maternal blood for screening of trisomy 21 in twin pregnancies achieves similar performance to singleton pregnancies, showing a DR of 98% at FPR of 0.05%. Data are limited for other aneuploidies and genetic conditions as well as for multiple pregnancies of order three or higher.

- In the presence of a vanishing twin with a measurable fetal pole it is recommended to screen by maternal age and fetal NT thickness (+/− free β-hCG) since contamination of maternal blood by placental products from the interrupted pregnancy may affect serum biomarkers levels and cfDNA analysis.

References

1. Santorum M, Wright D, Syngelaki A, Karagioti N, Nicolaides KH. Accuracy of first-trimester combined test in screening for trisomies 21, 18 and 13. Ultrasound Obstet Gynecol 2017;49:714–20.

2. Gil MM, Accurti V, Santacruz B, Plana MN, Nicolaides KH. Analysis of cell-free DNA in maternal blood in screening for aneuploidies: updated meta-analysis. Ultrasound Obstet Gynecol 2017;50:302–14.

3. Sebire NJ, Snijders RJ, Hughes K, Sepulveda W, Nicolaides KH. Screening for trisomy 21 in twin pregnancies by maternal age and fetal nuchal translucency thickness at 10–14 weeks of gestation. Br J Obstet Gynaecol 1996;103:999–1003.

4. Spencer K. Screening for trisomy 21 in twin pregnancies in the first trimester using free beta-hCG and PAPP-A combined with fetal nuchal translucency thickness. Prenat Diagn 2000;20:91–5.

5. Spencer K, Kagan KO, Nicolaides KH. Screening for trisomy 21 in twin pregnancies in the first trimester: an update of the impact of chorionicity on maternal serum markers. Prenat Diagn 2008;28:49–52.

6. Madsen HN, Ball S, Wright D et al. A reassessment of biochemical marker distributions in trisomy 21-affected and unaffected twin pregnancies in the first trimester. Ultrasound Obstet Gynecol 2011;37:38–47.

7. Gil MM, Galeva S, Jani J et al. Screening for trisomies by cfDNA testing of maternal blood in twin pregnancy: update of the Fetal Medicine Foundation results and meta-analysis. Ultrasound Obstet Gynecol 2019;53:734–42.

8. Nicolaides KH. Screening for fetal aneuploidies at 11 to 13 weeks. Prenat Diagn 2011;31:7–15.

9. Wright D, Syngelaki A, Staboulidou I, Cruz J, Nicolaides KH. Screening for trisomies in dichorionic twins by measurement of fetal nuchal translucency thickness according to the mixture model. Prenat Diagn 2011;31:16–21.

10. Audibert F, Gagnon A, Genetics Committee of the Society of Obstetricians and Gynaecologists of Canada, Prenatal Diagnosis Committee of the Canadian College of Medical Geneticists. Prenatal screening for and diagnosis of aneuploidy in twin pregnancies. J Obstet Gynaecol Can 2011;33:754–67.

11. Prats P, Rodríguez I, Comas C, Puerto B. Systematic review of screening for trisomy 21 in twin pregnancies in first trimester combining nuchal translucency and biochemical markers: a meta-analysis. Prenat Diagn 2014;34:1077–83.

12. Cuckle H. Down's syndrome screening in twins. J Med Screen. 1998;5:3–4.

13. Galeva S, Gil MM, Konstantinidou L, Akolekar R, Nicolaides KH. First-trimester screening for trisomies by cfDNA testing of maternal blood in singleton and twin pregnancies: factors affecting test failure. Ultrasound Obstet Gynecol 2019;53:804–9.

14. Khalil A, Rodgers M, Baschat A et al. ISUOG Practice Guidelines: role of ultrasound in twin pregnancy. Ultrasound Obstet Gynecol. 2016 Feb;47(2):247–63. doi: 10.1002/uog.15821. Erratum in Ultrasound Obstet Gynecol. 2018 Jul;52(1):140. PMID: 26577371.

15. Chaveeva P, Wright A, Syngelaki A, Konstantinidou L, Wright D, Nicolaides KH. First-trimester screening for trisomies in pregnancies with vanishing twin.Ultrasound Obstet Gynecol. 2020 Mar;55(3):326–31. doi: 10.1002/uog.21922. Epub 2020 Feb 13. PMID: 31710734.

Screening for Fetal Abnormality in Multiple Pregnancy

Carolina Bibbo, Julian N. Robinson and Beryl Benacerraf

The Facts

Chorionicity and the Risk of Fetal Abnormality

Determination of chorio-amnionicity in the early first trimester is of great importance to establish the amount of risk that can be associated with the pregnancy. Monochorionic twin pregnancies have an increased incidence of perinatal morbidity and mortality given the shared placental–fetal circulation. Such complications can be due to the occurrence of twin–twin transfusion syndrome (TTTS) and selective intrauterine growth restriction (sIUGR) or a mixture of the two (both of these conditions are dealt with in detail in Chapter 13).[1] Chorionicity and amnionicity are most accurately determined by ultrasound in the first trimester after 7 weeks with a sensitivity of more than 98%.[1] The typical findings on ultrasound are the 'lambda sign' for dichorionic-diamniotic twins and the 'T-sign' for monochorionic-diamniotic twins (Figures 7.1, 7.2). Monochorionic-monoamniotic twins are characterised by the absence of the inter-twin membrane (Figure 7.3).

Although chorionicity can be easily determined by ultrasound, chorionicity does not accurately determine zygosity (dichorionic twins can be monozygous). Knowing the zygosity is important to determine the risk of aneuploidy for the pregnancy. Zygosity needs to be included in genetic counselling, the management of genetic screening and diagnostic testing options. Knowing the chorionicity is important for the management of these pregnancies that are at risk for TTTS and sIUGR. Chorionicity determines the protocol for routine antenatal care and ultrasound surveillance that will be followed throughout the pregnancy (ultrasound surveillance every 2–3 weeks for monochorionic twins and monthly

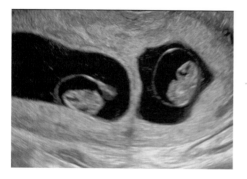

Figure 7.1 This image represents a dichorionic-diamniotic twin pregnancy at 8 weeks. The inter-twin membrane with the 'twin peak' or 'lambda sign' is characteristic of the triangular projection of tissue from a fused dichorionic placenta.

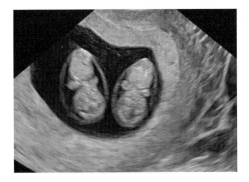

Figure 7.2 This image represents monochorionic-diamniotic twins at 9 weeks.

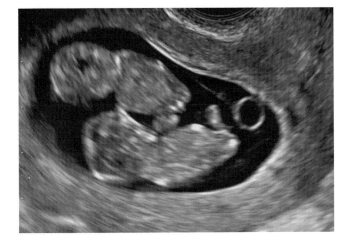

Figure 7.3 This image represents monochorionic-monoamniotic twins at 11 weeks. The inter-twin membrane is absent.

for dichorionic twins). Chorionicity, amnionicity and zygosity are dealt with in detail in Chapter 3.

Dizygotic twin pregnancies carry double the risk of aneuploidy as a maternal age-matched singleton pregnancy (with the pregnancy likely being discordant for aneuploidy). Twin conceptions can also result in a single, normal-appearing fetus adjacent to a partial or complete molar twin (Figure 7.4).

Structural anomalies are more common in monozygotic twins, at least double that of singletons. The chance of a malformation in at least one fetus is four times as high as in a singleton pregnancy (8%). This risk is highest in monoamniotic twins (17%).[1] There is conjecture that the mechanical process of the embryo splitting may precipitate structural abnormalities. Dizygotic twins have the same incidence of malformations as singletons, but the overall risk of a malformation in at least one fetus is twice as high as in a singleton pregnancy (4%).[2]

Despite being genetically identical, monozygotic twins can be discordant for structural abnormality. Only 20% of malformations are concordant in monozygotic twins.[2] Congenital heart disease is more prevalent in monochorionic twins, a proportion of which is caused in response to the abnormal physiology of TTTS.[3] Among the most

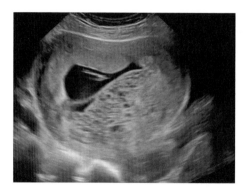

Figure 7.4 This image represents a twin conception with a normal fetus and a coexistent molar pregnancy at 9 weeks.

common structural malformations in twin pregnancies are cardiac anomalies, neural tube and brain malformations and gastrointestinal and abdominal wall defects.

A common error in clinical practice is to miss multiple structural abnormalities once one abnormality has been diagnosed. The distraction of finding an abnormality can affect the clinical performance of the rest of the study. However, detecting one abnormality should trigger increased suspicion for another anatomic defect as an underlying genetic syndrome may be present.

Some of the malformations seen in monozygotic twins are inherent to the twining process itself, such as acardiac twinning and conjoined twins. These malformations can be easily diagnosed in the first trimester. It has been our experience that the twin-reversed arterial perfusion (TRAP) sequence, also known as an acardiac twin, can be misdiagnosed as a structural abnormality or as a co-twin fetal demise in the first-trimester scan (Figures 7.5, 7.6). In these situations, colour Doppler showing reversed perfusion within the acardiac twin or the use of transvaginal ultrasound to enhance anatomic detail can aid in the diagnosis. Conjoined twins can also be diagnosed in the first-trimester scan. The typical findings are proximity of fetal poles and lack of independent movement of body/limbs from each twin. Sometimes the fusion of the organs can be apparent even in the first trimester (Figures 7.7, 7.8).

For all first-trimester ultrasound performed in this setting, the operator should have a low threshold for utilising both transabdominal and transvaginal ultrasound. In modern practice, the use of transvaginal ultrasound is routine due to higher-frequency transducers and closer proximity to the fetal parts. Doppler can be useful but should be used with caution and for specific indications due to the higher power exposure of this modality.

Discrepancy in Inter-twin Crump–Rump Length Measurement

The observation of size discordance in the first trimester is important. When there is discordance in the crump–rump length (CRL) measurement in twins, the dating should be established by the larger. The discordance in CRL is calculated as the difference between the larger CRL and the smaller CRL, divided by the larger CRL and multiplied by 100.

The prevalence of discordance in inter-twin CRL is not accurately known. The body of literature pertaining to this subject is heterogeneous not only in the definition of the discordance thresholds, but also in the inclusion criteria of the study populations (aneuploid fetuses, anomalous fetuses, monochorionic twins). Most published reports define inter-twin CRL discordance when the discordance in CRL is ≥10%.[4] This 10% discordance

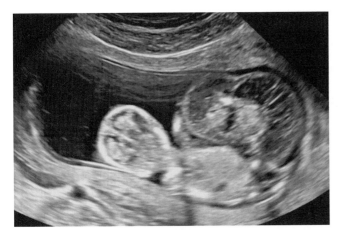

Figures 7.5 and 7.6 These images represent a monochorionic-diamniotic twin pregnancy at 12 weeks affected by twin-reversed arterial perfusion (TRAP sequence), also known as acardiac twin.

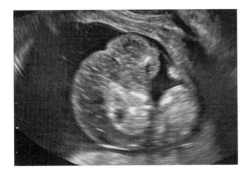

represents the 90th or 95th percentile distribution in most studies. The degree of CRL discrepancy is not related to chorionicity or the mode of conception.[5] Monochorionic twins are at a much higher risk of fetal size discrepancy, loss and other complications.[6]

The studies that have focused on the outcomes of twins with inter-twin CRL discordance in a dichorionic twin population (excluding monochorionic twins) have conflicting findings. Kalish et al. and Salomon et al. in the early 2000s showed that dichorionic twins with inter-twin CRL discordance > 90th percentile (>10%) were more likely to have a twin with either a chromosomal or anatomic anomaly.[5,7] Kalish et al.'s work emphasised the poor predictive value of this finding showing that when the inter-twin CRL discordance was >10%, the sensitivity to predict birth discordance (>20%) was 18.8% with a specificity of 92.1%.[7] Fareeduddin et al. have published that in euploid dichorionic twins that are structurally normal, first-trimester inter-twin CRL discordance is associated with adverse pregnancy outcomes, including preterm birth, preterm premature rupture of the membranes (PPROM) and lower birthweights.[6] Harper et al. have reported that dichorionic twin pregnancies affected by CRL discordance are more likely to result in the loss of one of the twins prior to 20 weeks (10.5 vs 1.3%; RR 7.8 (95% CI 3–20.5)). Furthermore, their study showed that the risk of structural abnormality was 60% higher than in twins with concordant CRL. However, if the pregnancy did not result in a loss of one twin or one of the twins

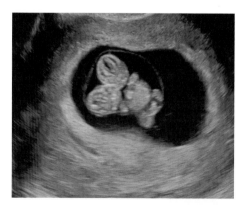

Figures 7.7 and 7.8 These images represent conjoined monochorionic-monoamniotic at 9 weeks. Colour Doppler is used to clarify the anatomy and identification of the conjoined twins which are thoracopagus (fusion from thorax to umbilicus). (A black and white version of this figure will appear in some formats. For the colour version, please refer to the plate section.)

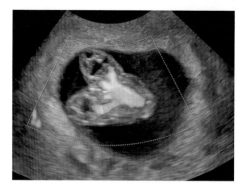

having an anomaly, the pregnancy was not associated with a higher risk of stillbirth, intrauterine growth restriction or preterm delivery prior to 34 weeks.[8]

D'Antonio and his collaborators demonstrated that once structural malformations and aneuploidy have been excluded, CRL discordance is weakly associated with poor adverse perinatal outcome, and as such, it is a poor predictor of these events in both dichorionic and monochorionic twins.[9] A recently published systematic review of 17 studies confirmed this finding. This review showed that inter-twin CRL discordance has been associated with a higher risk of adverse perinatal outcomes including fetal loss, weight discordance, fetal anomalies and preterm delivery. However, despite this association, such discordance had a low positive predictive value and its use in clinical practice is limited.[4] These authors suggest that such a finding should not change clinical management.

In conclusion, discordance in inter-twin CRL measurement raises concern to the obstetrician. Studies including only dichorionic twins or both dichorionic and monochorionic have found an association with fetal loss and fetal anomaly. As fetuses with chromosomal abnormalities have been found to have a smaller CRL than expected, CRL discordance might prompt investigation for aneuploidy. Despite the potential association with poor pregnancy outcome, the CRL discordance has a poor predictive value of such events. However, if there is a large discrepancy in the size of the gestational sacs that accompanies the CRL discrepancy, the prognosis is guarded (Figure 7.9). In our opinion, first-trimester CRL discordance warrants concern for aneuploidy and structural abnormality and should trigger genetic counselling and further ultrasound surveillance. No

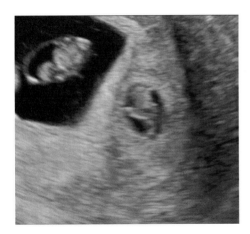

Figure 7.9 This image represents dichorionic-diamniotic twins at 7 weeks with a large discrepancy in the size of the gestational sacs (small gestational sac size of the smaller twin) that accompanies the CRL discrepancy.

long-term predictions regarding pregnancy outcome should be made due to such findings without further pertinent information.

Nuchal Translucency Measurement Discordance

The nuchal translucency (NT) thickness can be measured between 10 and 13 weeks to screen for aneuploidy and fetal structural abnormality. As in singleton pregnancies, a thickened nuchal translucency or cystic hygroma is equally concerning for fetal aneuploidy and fetal abnormality in twin pregnancies. In twin pregnancies, sonographic genetic screening with nuchal translucency has an increased importance since serum screening is less accurate.

The interpretation of maternal serum genetic screening is challenging in dichorionic twin pregnancies (the majority dizygotic) as both twins contribute to the concentration of these markers and the overall results do not specify which twin is affected. The measurement of the nuchal translucency thickness can certainly improve the aneuploidy detection rate and better identify the affected twin in these pregnancies. The test sensitivity in dichorionic twins of first-trimester maternal serum markers and nuchal translucency measurement is 86% (95% CI 73–94) and the test sensitivity in monochorionic twins is 87% (95% CI 53–98).[10]

It is important to mention that early in the first trimester, underlying hemodynamic changes in TTTS can result in an increased NT thickness in the recipient twin.[11] Therefore the false positive rate of NT screening is higher in monochorionic twins than in dichorionic twins, as the pathogenesis can reflect early severe TTTS rather than aneuploidy.

Kagan et al. studied inter-twin discordance in NT and its predictive value in severe TTTS. Their study excluded pregnancies diagnosed with chromosomal or major structural abnormalities. They found that 25% of monochorionic twins had an inter-twin discordance in NT of ≥20%. When there was such a finding, the risk of complications (death of one or both twins < 18 weeks or severe TTTS requiring laser intervention) was >30%. If the discordance was <20%, then the risk of these complications was <10%.[11]

More recently, Stagnati et al. published a systematic review with different conclusions. They found that the ability of inter-twin NT and CRL discrepancy to predict TTTS was low. Both findings were associated with an increased likelihood of developing severe TTTS;

however, their predictive accuracy was insufficient to recommend any changes in clinical management at the time of diagnosis.[12]

In conclusion, for monochorionic twin pregnancies, significant discrepancy in NT measurement in the first trimester raises concern for the development of severe TTTS. This finding warrants close ultrasound surveillance as it is customary for this type of twin gestation; therefore, no modifications should be made in antenatal management. In both dichorionic and monochorionic twin pregnancies, a thickened NT or a cystic hygroma is associated with aneuploidy and/or a structural fetal anomaly. These patients should be offered genetic counselling with the option of diagnostic testing and early anatomic surveys.

The Issues

Labelling Twins

There is little information regarding reproducible methods for labelling multifetal gestations during antenatal ultrasound. It is important to follow a consistent and reliable method for longitudinal follow-up of fetal growth and well-being. Such an approach is essential when there is an abnormality that warrants invasive prenatal testing prior to selective fetal reduction.

Dias et al. have described a simple method of labelling twins. Twin 1 is the fetus contained in the gestational sac which is closer to the maternal cervix. If the inter-twin membrane runs vertically along the longitudinal axis of the uterus, then the twins are oriented as either left or right. If the inter-twin membrane runs more horizontally, then the twins are oriented as top or bottom (Figure 7.10). In the case of dichorionic twins, more details should be given regarding the location of the placenta or fetal sacs to aid in the accurate labelling and identification of each twin.[13]

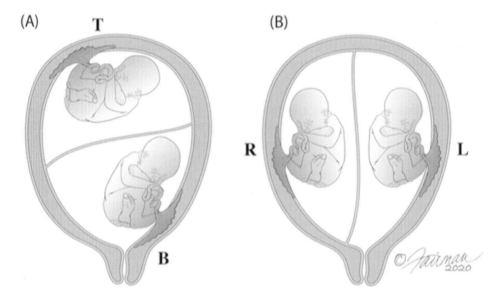

Figure 7.10 This illustration is a diagram of a dichorionic-diamniotic twin gestation in the late first trimester. The twin orientation is relative to the longitudinal axis of the uterus and the inter-twin membrane. Figure 7.10a shows twins with a vertical orientation, top (T) and bottom (B). Figure 7.10b shows twins with a lateral orientation, right (R) and left (L).

(A)   (B)

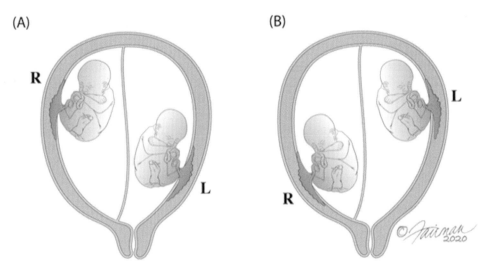

Figure 7.11 This illustration is a diagram of a dichorionic diamniotic twin gestation in the second trimester. This diagram shows how the twins' position in relationship to the cervix can change throughout gestation. At any point, either twin can be presenting (schematic represents left/right orientation). Figure 7.11a shows twin 1 presenting and Figure 7.11b shows twin 2 presenting. The gestational sac orientation remains unchanged throughout the pregnancy given the fixed inter-twin membrane base and thus, the labelling of the twins as 1 and 2 that was performed in the late first trimester should not change.

The gestational sac's position in relation to the maternal cervix does not change during the pregnancy. However, the position of either fetus in relationship to the cervix can vary (Figure 7.11). Hence the orientation of each twin with each other based on the location of the inter-twin membrane is helpful considering the inter-twin membrane is fixed.[13]

The labelling should occur in the late first trimester, and it should stay consistent throughout all antenatal ultrasounds. Even if twin 2 becomes the presenting twin, it should still be labelled as twin 2. In such a case, a comment should be made that twin 1 is non-presenting and twin 2 is presenting. The labelling of the twins should not be changed across gestation depending on the position of each fetus.

Antenatal sonographic identification of twin 1 and twin 2 is not necessarily the same as the labelling done by paediatricians at birth. Paediatricians identify twin 1 as the first born and twin 2 as the second born. However, this may not be consistent with the antenatal sonographic labelling that occurred during pregnancy. This is key in cases of discordant fetal anomalies that require immediate neonatal intervention. In cases where there are no fetal anomalies, the possibility of this 'perinatal switch' carries no significant clinical importance.

Dias et al. showed that twin 2 is delivered first in 25% of cases delivered by caesarean section, as twin 2 might be more accessible depending on the uterine position. The perinatal switch occurred in only 5% of cases during vaginal deliveries, likely due to twin 2 being delivered through a fold in the inter-twin membrane.[13]

In our practice, for higher-order multiples such as triplets, triplet 1 is labelled as the one whose gestational sac is closest to the cervix and then the remainder of the triplets are labelled in a clockwise fashion.

Role of Fetal Anatomic Scan: Timing and Mode

The traditional role of the first-trimester ultrasound is to establish the dating of the pregnancy and the determination of chorionicity and amnionicity. The first-trimester ultrasound is also utilised to assess the risk of aneuploidy and potential risk of fetal structural abnormality (in the presence of thickened NT and cystic hygroma). For monochorionic gestations, the first-trimester ultrasound is utilised to screen for TRAP sequence or conjoined twins which would require tailored management. Furthermore, the first-trimester ultrasound is an opportunity to screen for the presence of any major anomalies (some lethal) as this allows consideration of selective fetal reduction within the first trimester if warranted (avoiding having to wait until the mid-second trimester when the risks associated with the procedure are higher). However, when carrying out selective reduction early, the patient should be aware that anomalies cannot be completely excluded from the surviving fetus until later in gestation due to the limitations of a first-trimester anatomy survey.

In the second trimester, the International Society of Ultrasound in Obstetrics & Gynecology (ISUOG) recommends a complete fetal anatomic survey between 18 and 22 weeks of gestation for both monochorionic and dichorionic twins that are uncomplicated.[14] The overall rate of malformation for twins is higher than for a singleton. The incidence of malformation is around 4% in dichorionic twins, 7% in monochorionic-diamniotic twins and 17% in monochorionic-monoamniotic twins.[1]

Monochorionic twins are at a higher risk of congenital heart disease. These may represent true malformations or malformations acquired during the prenatal period because of the cardiovascular changes due to TTTS. The North American Fetal Therapy Network (NafTNET) recommends a fetal echocardiogram for all uncomplicated monochorionic gestations around the time of the anatomical survey.[1] This recommendation is not part of the clinical practice of all centres as it is rare to miss the diagnosis of a structural cardiac defect with a normal fetal survey (four chamber views, outflow tracts, sagittal views) performed by a maternal fetal medicine specialist. Furthermore, a fetal echocardiogram might not be easily accessible in all centres. In cases of TTTS, a fetal echocardiogram may be warranted to better assess cardiac dysfunction in the recipient twin.

The American College of Obstetricians and Gynecologists (ACOG) and the American Institute of Ultrasound in Medicine (AIUM) published their guidelines regarding ultrasound in pregnancy in 2016 and these were reaffirmed in 2018. Their recommendations regarding timing of ultrasounds are not different from those published by the ISUOG. If the pregnancy is otherwise low risk, with a negative family history and low-risk first-trimester genetic screening, it is reasonable to perform an anatomical survey between 18 and 22 weeks. If the pregnancy is at a higher risk based on family history, abnormal nuchal translucency thickness or a concern for anomalies during first-trimester ultrasound, an anatomic survey at 16 weeks or even earlier with the use of transvaginal ultrasound may be considered. Patients should understand the limitations of early ultrasound mainly in terms of neurological anatomy and the potential need to return in a few weeks to obtain views that may have been suboptimal in the initial survey. It is of importance for patients at high risk of fetal anomalies not to wait until 22 weeks to perform the fetal survey to ensure a better chance of earlier diagnosis and prompt pregnancy management.

Performing an anatomical ultrasound in a twin gestation can be challenging. Not only does it take longer, but it may also be difficult to see all the required fetal structures for both twins during a single study. Patients should be counselled that they often need to return a second time to complete the fetal anatomic survey.

For challenging patients who are obese, certain techniques can be helpful. The goal is to minimise the distance between the transducer and the uterus. These techniques include a full maternal bladder, the use of the umbilicus as an acoustic window, scanning above the pannus in a sitting position, using a maternal lateral position and scanning from the flank or groin, or a transvaginal scan.

In the past decades, there has been a trend towards earlier prenatal diagnosis. The role of first-trimester ultrasound to assess fetal anatomy has been studied specifically in patients who are obese. Most fetuses can be surveyed by ultrasound within 13 to 14 weeks as well as 18–22 weeks. Of note, not all anatomic structures are fully developed for an anatomy study to be completed by the end of the first or early in the second trimester. Structures such as the septum cavum pellucidum and the cerebellar vermis are usually neurologic. In the absence of an indication such as obesity, a first-trimester transvaginal ultrasound is not superior to the routine second-trimester ultrasound and it should not replace it. However, many specialists advocate for the use of first-trimester transvaginal ultrasound in patients with a body mass index > 35–40 as it can improve the rate of completion of the fetal anatomic survey.

Due to these nuances as discussed in this chapter, twin pregnancies with a diagnosis of a fetal anomaly should be referred to a maternal fetal medicine specialist to plan pregnancy management. A multidisciplinary approach including a team with experience in ultrasound, genetic counselling, invasive fetal genetic testing and paediatric specialists to discuss neonatal prognosis is recommended.[1]

Management of Twin Pregnancy Affected by a Fetal Anomaly

The management of a multifetal pregnancy affected by a fetal anomaly is complex. Depending on the degree of anomaly, whether there is also a chromosomal abnormality, the patient might opt to continue the pregnancy expectantly, proceed with selective fetal reduction or terminate the entire pregnancy (this topic is discussed in greater detail in Chapter 4).

The rationale for proceeding with selective fetal reduction is to improve the outcome of the unaffected fetus. The anomalous fetus may develop complications during the pregnancy (e.g. polyhydramnios and severe growth restriction) that may put the entire pregnancy at risk for either spontaneous or indicated preterm delivery. Even an uncomplicated twin pregnancy with no fetal anomaly is at a higher risk of preterm delivery than a singleton pregnancy. Some parents may prefer to have a reduction in the first or early second trimester than to carry an anomalous fetus to full term. The regulations regarding selective fetal reduction may vary, so it is important to be aware of the local law regarding termination of pregnancy.

When performing diagnostic testing in the first trimester (chorionic villus sampling) or in the second trimester (amniocentesis), a detailed description of the position of the gestational sacs and placentas should take place. This 'mapping' of the pregnancy prior to diagnostic testing and potential subsequent selective fetal reduction is very important to minimise the possibility of targeting the wrong fetus. If the selective fetal reduction is due to a structural abnormality, then the target fetus should be easily distinguishable. However, 'fetal mapping' becomes important when there is an absence of an obvious structural abnormality in the aneuploid fetus.

Fetal mapping can be considered similar to making a diagram of the multifetal pregnancy. One needs to take into consideration the location of the gestational sacs and the placentas. Of note, the presence of a full bladder can change the position of the fetuses; therefore, a notation should be made regarding the bladder fullness on the scan. Fetal sex is an obvious identifying feature. Another potential marker that can be used for identification of a fetus is biometry. If the biometry of one fetus is significantly smaller than the other one, this relationship should stay the same if the selective reduction is to be carried out a few days later than the diagnostic ultrasound. The possibility of both intra- and inter-observer variation should always be considered, making it desirable to have the same team of clinicians carry out the diagnostic study and the selective fetal reduction if these are not performed on the same occasion. Other sonographic findings can help identify a fetus such as an echogenic focus or bowel. However, one needs to be mindful of the gain settings and the machinery utilised for the original study as these findings may not be replicated reliably. The description and procedure for selective fetal reduction is discussed in detail in Chapter 4 and is not repeated here.

Key Points

- Zygosity will determine the aneuploidy and structural malformation risk for the pregnancy.
- Structural abnormalities are more common in monozygotic twins, with monochorionic-monoamniotic twins carrying the highest risk.
- Even though inter-twin CRL discordance in the first trimester has been associated with poor pregnancy outcome, it has a poor predictive value and should not be used as a prognostic tool.
- Increased NT or cystic hygroma increases the likelihood of aneuploidy or fetal anomaly.
- The labelling of twins should take place in the first trimester and should not change throughout gestation despite the position of the fetuses in relationship to the cervix. Twin 1 should be labelled as the twin whose gestational sac is closer to the maternal cervix.
- For uncomplicated twin pregnancies, fetal anatomic ultrasound is recommended around 18 to 22 weeks for both monochorionic and dichorionic twin gestations.
- In high-risk patients with concern for structural anomaly in the first trimester, a complete fetal anatomic ultrasound should be performed earlier in gestation at around 16 weeks.
- The management of a multifetal pregnancy affected by a fetal anomaly is complex and it requires a multidisciplinary team approach that encompasses maternal fetal medicine specialists, genetic counsellors and paediatric specialists.
- Prenatal diagnosis via CVS or amniocentesis is warranted in most cases. In clinical cases when selective fetal reduction is planned, careful 'mapping of the pregnancy' should be performed at the time of diagnostic testing to ensure that the correct fetus is targeted at the time of fetal reduction.

References

1. Emery SP et al. The North American Fetal Therapy Network Consensus Statement: prenatal management of uncomplicated monochorionic gestations. Obstet Gynecol 2015;**125**(5):1236–43.

2. Glinianaia SV, Rankin J, Wright C. Congenital anomalies in twins: a register-based study. Hum Reprod 2008;**23**(6):1306–11.

3. Bahtiyar MO et al. The North American Fetal Therapy Network consensus statement: prenatal surveillance of uncomplicated monochorionic gestations. Obstet Gynecol 2015;**125**(1):118–23.

4. D'Antonio F et al. Crown–rump length discordance and adverse perinatal outcome in twin pregnancies: systematic review and meta-analysis. Ultrasound Obstet Gynecol 2014;**44**(2):138–46.

5. Salomon LJ et al. Growth discrepancy in twins in the first trimester of pregnancy. Ultrasound Obstet Gynecol 2005;**26**(5):512–16.

6. Fareeduddin R et al. Discordance of first-trimester crown–rump length is a predictor of adverse outcomes in structurally normal euploid dichorionic twins. J Ultrasound Med 2010;**29**(10):1439–43.

7. Kalish RB et al. First trimester prediction of growth discordance in twin gestations. Am J Obstet Gynecol 2003;**189**(3):706–9.

8. Harper LM et al. First-trimester growth discordance and adverse pregnancy outcome in dichorionic twins. Ultrasound Obstet Gynecol 2013;**41**(6):627–31.

9. D'Antonio F et al. Crown–rump length discordance and adverse perinatal outcome in twins: analysis of the Southwest Thames Obstetric Research Collaborative (STORK) multiple pregnancy cohort. Ultrasound Obstet Gynecol 2013;**41**(6):621–6.

10. Prats P et al. Systematic review of screening for trisomy 21 in twin pregnancies in first trimester combining nuchal translucency and biochemical markers: a meta-analysis. Prenat Diagn 2014;**34**(11):1077–83.

11. Kagan KO et al. Discordance in nuchal translucency thickness in the prediction of severe twin-to-twin transfusion syndrome. Ultrasound Obstet Gynecol 2007;**29**(5):527–32.

12. Stagnati V et al. Early prediction of twin-to-twin transfusion syndrome: systematic review and meta-analysis. Ultrasound Obstet Gynecol 2017;**49**(5):573–82.

13. Dias T et al. Systematic labeling of twin pregnancies on ultrasound. Ultrasound Obstet Gynecol 2011;**38**(2):130–3.

14. Khalil A et al. ISUOG Practice Guidelines: role of ultrasound in twin pregnancy. Ultrasound Obstet Gynecol 2016;**47**(2):247–63.

Screening and Diagnosis of Complications of Shared Placentation

Caitlin D. Baptiste and Lynn Simpson

	Screening	Diagnosis	Management
Twin-to-twin transfusion syndrome	Ultrasounds q2 weeks starting at 16 weeks assessing: MVP of each sac Identification of fluid-filled bladder in each twin +/− Doppler flow of the umbilical artery if there is discordance in MVP or growth	Quintero staging system: Polyhydramnios (MVP > 8 cm) in one twin and oligohydramnios (MVP < 2 cm) in the other twin Fluid-filled bladder not visible in the donor twin for 60 minutes Doppler abnormalities Hydrops fetalis in one or both twins Death of one or both twins	Stage I: Consider expectant management with ultrasound surveillance at least once per week. Stages II, III, IV: Referral to fetal centre for laser treatment if between 16 and 25 6/7 weeks. Otherwise, consider amnioreduction. Stage V: Counsel on 10% risk of death and 10–30% risk of neurologic complications for co-twin. Consider expectant management.
Selective intrauterine growth restriction	Perform fetal growth assessments q3–4 weeks starting at 18 weeks	Estimated EFW of either twin is <10% and/or inter-twin growth discordance is >20% Staging system (based on umbilical artery Doppler's of IUGR twin:	Type I: Expectant management with serial surveillance. Consider delivery between 34 and 37 weeks. Types II/III: Discuss options for selective termination via cord occlusion if prior to

(cont.)

	Screening	Diagnosis	Management
		Positive end-diastolic flow Persistent absent or reversed end-diastolic flow Intermittent absent or reversed end-diastolic flow	viability. After viability, if expectant management is pursued, at least weekly ultrasound are recommended, or inpatient admission may be considered. Delivery between 32 and 34 weeks may be considered for REDF or AEDF, respectively.
Twin anaemia polycythaemia syndrome	Perform MCA Doppler studies q2 weeks starting at 20 weeks	Either: (1) MCA-PSV ≥ 1.5 MoM in one twin and ≤1.0–0.8 MoM in the other twin (2) An inter-twin MCA-PSV discordance ≥ 1.0 MoM	Weekly ultrasound surveillance at diagnosis Optimal timing and type of treatment remain unclear
Twin-reversed arterial perfusion syndrome	Screen during first-trimester ultrasound where monochorionicity is suspected and one twin appears anomalous or there is large CRL discordance	Doppler studies confirm retrograde arterial flow from the normal pump twin to the anomalous acardiac twin	Depending on gestational age at diagnosis, consider selective reduction (cord occlusion, interstitial laser or radiofrequency ablation) for anomalous twin or expectant management with increased ultrasound surveillance assessing for hydrops in pump twin.
Discordant anomalies	All monochorionic twin pregnancies should obtain detailed fetal anatomy between 18 and 22 weeks and a fetal echocardiogram.		Depending on gestational age at diagnosis, consider selective termination via cord occlusion of anomalous twin. Refer to appropriate medical and surgical paediatric specialists.

The Facts

Twins comprise 3–4% of all live births and their chorionicity greatly affects the rate of complications. In a monozygotic pregnancy, when the embryo splits ≥ 4 days after fertilisation, shared placentation, or monochorionicity, occurs. Monochorionic-diamniotic (MCDA) twins occur when an embryo splits 4–8 days after fertilisation and monochorionic-monoamniotic (MCMA) twins occur when splitting occurs ≥ 8 days after fertilisation. If division occurs ≥ 13 days after fertilisation, the twins will be conjoined. In the absence of assisted reproductive technology, 70% of twins are dichorionic. Although less than a third of twin pregnancies are monochorionic, these pregnancies account for 75% of the complications in twins.[1]

The estimated date of delivery for twin pregnancies should be confirmed when the crown–rump length (CRL) measures between 45 and 84 mm (around 11 0/7 to 13 6/7 weeks gestation). If there is a discrepancy in the CRL, the larger of the two should be used to estimate gestational age.[2] Ultrasound after 7 0/7 but before 13 6/7 weeks is the most effective way to determine chorionicity and amnionicity. Establish chorionicity by (1) assessing the membrane thickness at the site of insertion of the amniotic membrane into the placenta, (2) identifying the T sign (monochorionic) or lambda sign (dichorionic) or (3) counting the number of placental masses.[2] Please see Chapter 3 for more on zygosity, chorionicity and amnionicity.

Labelling twin fetuses allows for reliable and consistent identification of both twins. Use several characterising features to describe each twin, including location within the maternal uterus (superior, inferior, right, left), placental location (if dichorionic), placental cord insertion site, gender or discordant anomalies.

Monochorionic pregnancies may be complicated by twin–twin transfusion syndrome (TTTS), selective intrauterine growth restriction (sIUGR), twin anaemia polycythaemia syndrome (TAPS), twin-reversed arterial perfusion syndrome (TRAP) and discordant congenital anomalies. In the setting of monoamnionicity, cord entanglement may occur. All monochorionic pregnancies are at increased risk of co-twin death, which has potential implications for the surviving twin.

It remains difficult to predict in the first trimester which MCDA pregnancies will develop TTTS and how severe the condition will be. Currently, no single screening test exists to identify which MC pregnancies will develop complications and therefore all MC pregnancies are subject to costly and time-intensive antenatal surveillance, which has impact on both the patient and health care resources.[3]

Despite the plethora of complications monochorionic twins present, the prognosis improves with adequate surveillance and access to fetal therapy. In a recent cohort of 3,621 twin pregnancies in Denmark, 15% were monochorionic, of which 92.3% of MCDA and 66.7% of MCMA pregnancies resulted in at least one live born infant compared to 98.2% of dichorionic twins.[4] It is important to remember that the frequency and location of testing (inpatient versus outpatient) also influences the survival rate of these pregnancies with a shared placenta.

The Issues

All monochorionic twins have shared circulation through vascular anastomoses in the placenta. There are three types of anastomoses: arterio-arterial (A-A), veno-venous (V-V) and arterio-venous (A-V). Blood flow in A-V anastomoses is unidirectional and can lead to

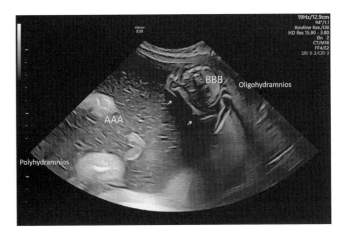

Figure 8.1 Monochorionic-diamniotic twin pregnancy with oligohydramnios-polyhydramnios sequence diagnostic of stage I TTTS. The separating membrane is seen draping around the stuck twin (arrows).

discordant blood flow between the two fetuses. If uncompensated, this unidirectional flow may lead to an imbalance of volume between the twins (Figure 8.1). The number and location of these anastomoses leads to the various complications seen in monochorionic twins. Pregnancies affected by growth discordance or sIUGR commonly have a sharing imbalance, high rates of velamentous cord insertions and large A-A anastomoses. Pregnancies affected by TTTS commonly have low numbers of A-A anastomoses whereas pregnancies complicated by TAPS have only a few, small, A-V anastomoses and few A-A anastomoses. These complications in order of prevalence, starting with the most common, are reviewed in what follows.

Twin–Twin Transfusion Syndrome

Twin–twin transfusion syndrome affects 10–15% of MCDA twins and usually occurs between 15 and 26 weeks of gestation. Although it can occur in any monozygotic pregnancy, it is exceptionally rarely seen in dichorionic-diamniotic (DCDA) twins and not often observed in MCMA twins. Twin–twin transfusion syndrome accounts for up to 17% of perinatal mortality in all twins and up to half of perinatal deaths in MCDA twins. The diagnosis is made when one twin in an MCDA twin pregnancy has oligohydramnios (defined as a maximum vertical pocket (MVP) < 2 cm) and the other twin has polyhydramnios (MVP > 8 cm).

The most common staging system by Quintero includes five stages based on sonographic findings (Table 8.1). This simple and replicable diagnostic staging system allows for standardisation of the diagnosis, improves communication between referring providers and fetal centres and helps identify cases most likely to benefit from treatment. However, it does not accurately predict outcomes or perinatal survival for an individual pregnancy. Twin–twin transfusion syndrome often does not progress in a predictable manner and robust natural history data are lacking. Most natural history data predate the standardised Quintero staging and therefore outcomes in these studies are not stratified by stage.[5] For example, stage I disease may evolve into stage IV or V disease without clearly progressing through stages II and III. Studies looking at the natural progression of staged disease report that 85% of stage I disease resolves or remains stable and only 15% progress to a higher

Table 8.1 Quintero staging system for twin–twin transfusion syndrome

Stage	Findings on ultrasound
I	Polyhydramnios (MVP > 8 cm) in one (recipient) twin Oligohydramnios (MVP < 2 cm) in other (donor) twin
II	Fluid-filled bladder not visible in donor twin
III	Doppler abnormalities: Umbilical artery Doppler shows absent or reversed end-diastolic flow Ductus venous with reversed flow in a-wave Umbilical vein pulsations in either twin
IV	Hydrops fetalis in one or both twins
V	Death of one or both twins

stage.[5] On the contrary, stage III/IV disease presenting before 26 weeks of gestation, if left untreated, has a perinatal loss rate of 70–100%.

Screening for Twin–Twin Transfusion Syndrome in the First Trimester

Although one cannot accurately predict disease in the first trimester, findings on ultrasound between 11 and 14 weeks may predict adverse outcomes. These include discordant nuchal translucency (NT) measurements and discordant CRLs.[1] A systematic review and meta-analysis of early prognostic factors in monochorionic twin pregnancies found a significant association between NT > 95% in one or both fetuses and the development of TTTS. However, the positive predictive value of one or both fetuses having an NT > 95% was only 22%. The same review noted a significant association between CRL discordance ≥ 10% and the later development of TTTS but again, the positive predictive value was only 28%. Collectively, these first-trimester ultrasound findings have been reported to have a false negative rate of 52%.[6] Although enlarged and/or discordant NT and discordant CRL demonstrate poor individual prognostic ability for the development of TTTS, the International Society for Ultrasound in Obstetrics and Gynecology recommends referral to a fetal medicine expert for all twin pregnancies where the CRL discordance is ≥10% or the NT discordance is ≥20%.[2,3]

Screening for Twin–Twin Transfusion Syndrome in the Second Trimester

Regular ultrasound in the second trimester is the mainstay of screening for TTTS. Although there are no randomised controlled trials on the optimal frequency of ultrasound surveillance in MCDA pregnancies, current recommendations suggest ultrasound every two weeks starting at 16 weeks of gestation. Ultrasound surveillance in the second trimester should include:

(1) MVP of each sac.

(2) identification of a fluid-filled bladder in each fetus.

(3) Doppler flow in the umbilical artery if there is discordance in fluid or growth.[5]

Screening for Twin–Twin Transfusion Syndrome with Fetal Echocardiogram

The role of routine fetal echocardiography in the assessment of TTTS remains unclear. Since the development of the initial Quintero staging of TTTS, much has been learned about the cardiovascular effects of TTTS on fetuses. Even in early stages of TTTS, changes in myocardial function are present in the recipient twin. Although several groups have evaluated changes in fetal cardiac function as a potential modifier of the current staging system, none of these proposed systems has been widely adopted. Currently, data are insufficient to change the current staging of TTTS based on findings on fetal echocardiography.

Diagnosis of Twin–Twin Transfusion Syndrome

When TTTS is diagnosed or suspected, prompt consultation with a fetal treatment centre is paramount. When indicated, laser therapy improves outcomes to a double survivor rate of 60–70% and a single survivor rate of 80–90%.[2] Despite the favourable obstetric prognosis after treatment, pregnancies complicated by TTTS remain at increased risk of neurodevelopmental disability. Although neurologic outcomes after laser therapy are improved compared to untreated TTTS cases, 9% of surviving children of TTTS pregnancies treated with laser have major neurodevelopmental delays at 6 years of age.[2] Please see Chapter 13 for further management of TTTS.

Selective Intrauterine Growth Restriction

Discordant growth, complicated by sIUGR of one fetus, affects 10–15% of monochorionic pregnancies. Discordant growth is commonly due to both vascular anastomoses and unequally shared placental territories. The smaller twin in pregnancies complicated by growth discordance commonly has a velamentous or marginal cord insertion and placental pathologic evaluation usually shows unequal placental sharing (Figure 8.2).[7] This discrepant placental share may be modified, for better or worse, by placental anastomoses. The natural history of the discordant growth in MCDA twins depends on both the discordance in placental territories and the pattern of vascular anastomoses between their circulations. Therefore, when TTTS simultaneously complicates these pregnancies and laser therapy is performed, the elimination of these anastomoses can disrupt their protective effect and lead to poor outcomes for the smaller twin.

Various diagnostic criteria exist for growth abnormalities in MCDA twins. Selective intrauterine growth restriction in MCDA twins may be diagnosed if the estimated fetal weight (EFW) of either twin is <10th percentile for the gestational age. When this definition is used, the prevalence of sIUGR in MCDA twins is 10–20%. If IUGR is defined as an abdominal circumference < 5th percentile irrespective of the overall EFW, the incidence of sIUGR in MCDA twins is 10–25%.[8] Still, others define discordant growth as fetal abdominal circumference discordance > 20–25% regardless of whether either twin meets criteria for IUGR and others use a combined EFW < 10th percentile and an inter-twin discordance of >20% to define sIUGR.

Both placental insufficiency and inter-twin vascular anastomoses affect the umbilical artery Doppler waveforms in MC twins. A classification system for sIUGR has been created based on Doppler assessment of the umbilical artery of the smaller twin (Table 8.2).[9]

The smaller twin in Type I sIUGR has positive end-diastolic flow in the umbilical artery and these pregnancies have a favourable prognosis. These cases are managed similarly to

Table 8.2 Classification of selective intrauterine growth restriction

Type	Umbilical artery Doppler findings of growth-restricted fetus
I	Positive end-diastolic flow
II	Persistent absent/reversed end-diastolic flow
III	Intermittent absent/reversed end-diastolic flow

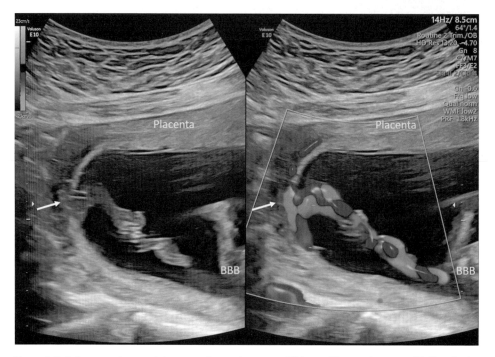

Figure 8.2 Split-screen ultrasound demonstrating a velamentous PCI (arrows) by two-dimensional (left) and colour flow (right) imaging with the anterior placenta several centimetres from the cord insertion. (A black and white version of this figure will appear in some formats. For the colour version, please refer to the plate section.)

that of singletons with IUGR with antenatal testing and indicated early delivery. Please see Chapter 16 for more on management of fetal growth pathology in multiple pregnancy. Adverse outcomes are somewhat unpredictable in these cases, but the intrauterine fetal demise rate of the smaller twin remains low at 2–4%.

The prognosis and management for Type II sIUGR, with *persistently* absent or reversed end-diastolic flow in the umbilical artery of the smaller twin, depends on the gestational age at diagnosis (Figure 8.3). These pregnancies are commonly affected by unequal placental sharing; the placental territory for the growth-restricted fetus is usually small and the number of vascular anastomoses fewer than with Type I sIUGR. Overall, 70–90% of Type II sIUGR cases will show signs of deterioration on fetal testing by 30 weeks of gestation. In a Japanese study in which selective termination was not available, the natural history showed

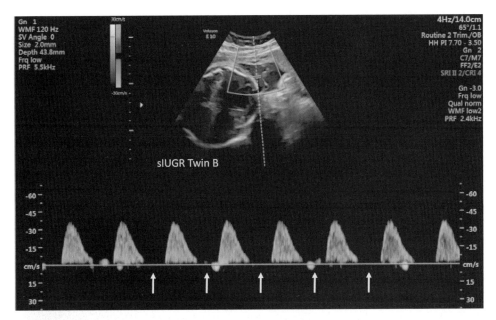

Figure 8.3 Doppler velocimetry of an MCDA twin with sIUGR demonstrating persistent absent end-diastolic flow (arrows). (A black and white version of this figure will appear in some formats. For the colour version, please refer to the plate section.)

a 37% intact survival rate for the smaller twin and a 55% intact survival rate for the larger twin, with a mean gestational age at delivery of 28 weeks.[10]

In the setting of Type II sIUGR, if the pregnancy is viable, consider hospital admission to increase fetal monitoring and perform Doppler interrogation of the ductus venosus to help predict imminent fetal deterioration. If persistently abnormal Doppler findings develop prior to viability, consider selective termination via cord occlusion. A series evaluating 90 cases of Type II and III sIUGR treated with cord occlusion showed a 93% survival rate of the remaining twin with a mean gestational age at delivery of 36.4 weeks.[11]

In pregnancies complicated by Type III sIUGR, the Doppler studies of the umbilical artery show *intermittently* absent or reversed end-diastolic flow that indicates the existence of large placental A-A anastomoses. The degree of placental territory discordance may be greatest in this type of sIUGR, but the placental vascular anastomoses help compensate for the territorial discordance. Given its variable nature, it is easy to miss this Doppler finding; it is generally more prominent and easily seen near the placental cord insertion. Due to the large anastomoses, there is a higher risk of acute feto-fetal transfusion and neurologic injury to the normally grown twin even if both are born alive. Although the overall prognosis of Type III is better than Type II sIUGR, the unpredictable clinical evolution of these cases makes them difficult to manage. If expectant management is undertaken at viability, at least weekly ultrasounds are recommended.[12]

One of the main risks of sIUGR and discordant twin growth is intrauterine demise of the smaller fetus. As with all cases of single fetal demise in a monochorionic pregnancy, there is risk to the remaining twin (see Chapter 12 on single fetal demise). Even when both twins survive, sIUGR may be associated with neurologic impairment of one or both twins.[12] This may in part be due to increased rates of prematurity but also due to the shared vasculature in utero. Please see Chapter 16 for further management of growth abnormalities in multiple pregnancies.

Twin Anaemia Polycythaemia Sequence

Twin anaemia polycythaemia sequence is a complication of monochorionic pregnancies when one twin, the donor, develops anaemia and the other twin, the recipient, becomes polycythaemic. The incidence of TAPS affects 2–5% of uncomplicated monochorionic pregnancies and 3–16% of cases post laser therapy for TTTS. Different governing bodies have different recommendations for screening and diagnosing TAPS. The International Society of Ultrasound in Obstetrics and Gynecology recommends screening for TAPS in monochorionic pregnancies starting at 20 weeks of gestation and obtaining an ultrasound every two weeks to assess the middle cerebral artery peak systolic velocity (MCA-PSV) by Doppler velocimetry. However, there is a lack of evidence that monitoring for TAPS with MCA-PSV at any gestational age, including >26 weeks, improves outcomes. Therefore, several groups, including the Society for Maternal Fetal Medicine, do not recommend performing routine screening for TAPS in otherwise uncomplicated monochorionic twin pregnancies.[6,13]

A recent Delphi process was conducted among international experts to determine the key diagnostic features and optimal monitoring approach for TAPS.[14] Based on their consensus, monitoring for the development of TAPS should occur every two weeks, although the gestational age at which to start screening remains unclear. If TAPS is diagnosed, obtain ultrasound assessment weekly. Evaluation on ultrasound should include MCA-PSV as well as evaluating for evidence of fetal hydrops and cardiac compromise.

Expert opinion considers a diagnosis of TAPS if either of the following are detected: (1) MCA-PSV ≥ 1.5 MoM in one twin and ≤ 0.8 MoM in the other twin or (2) an inter-twin MCA-PSV discordance ≥ 1.0 MoM (Figure 8.4). Other studies suggest a diagnosis of TAPS if the MCA-PSV is >1.5 MoM in the recipient and <1.0 MoM in the donor twin. While less commonly used, a staging system for TAPS has been proposed (Table 8.3).[13] It remains unclear how and when to treat TAPS. Options for treatment include fetoscopic laser therapy and/or percutaneous fetal blood transfusion of the anaemic twin and possible exchange transfusion of the polycythaemic twin. Postnatally, a haemoglobin difference ≥ 8 g/dL and an inter-twin reticulocyte ratio ≥ 1.7 confirm the diagnosis. Please see Chapter 14 for further management of TAPS.

Twin-Reversed Arterial Perfusion Sequence

Twin-reversed arterial perfusion sequence occurs in 0.3% of all monozygotic gestations.[15] Although the TRAP sequence can occur in both MCDA and MCMA twins, it is more common in MCMA twins due to the universal presence of A-A anastomoses in MCMA twins. Diagnosing TRAP requires a high index of suspicion, particularly in cases where one twin has abnormal or absent cardiac anatomy early in gestation. The TRAP sequence occurs when an acardiac mass is perfused by an anatomically normal pump twin (Figure 8.5). Although the acardiac twin can easily be misdiagnosed as an anomalous or demised twin, Doppler studies reveal *retrograde arterial flow from the pump twin to the acardiac twin*. This perfusion can occur through A-A anastomoses as well as through a common cord insertion site. The parasitic-like demands of the acardiac twin can lead to complications for the pump twin, including congestive heart failure and hydrops fetalis due to increased cardiac demand.

Table 8.3 Proposed classification for antenatal diagnosis TAPS*

Antenatal Classification: Ultrasound Findings	
Stage 1	MCA-PSV donor > 1.5 MoM MCA PSV recipient < 1.0 MoM No signs of fetal compromise
Stage 2	MCA-PSV donor > 1.7 MoM MCA PSV recipient < 0.8 MoM No signs of fetal compromise
Stage 3	MCA findings as above with any of the following: Abnormal umbilical artery Doppler studies (absent or reversed end-diastolic flow) Pulsatile flow in the umbilical vein Increased pulsatility index or reversed flow in the ductus venosus
Stage 4	Hydrops in donor twin
Stage 5	Intrauterine demise of one or both twins preceded by diagnosis of TAPS

* Based on Slaghekke et al. Twin anaemia-polycythaemia sequence: diagnostic criteria, classification, perinatal management and outcome. Fetal Diagnosis and Therapy 2010: 27: 181–90.

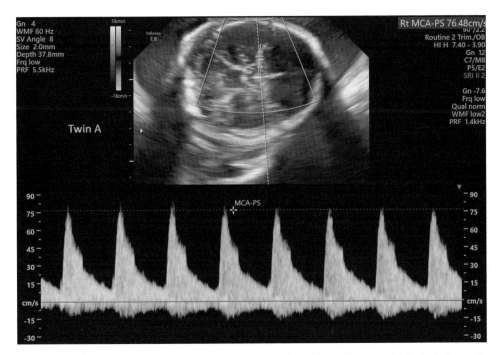

Figure 8.4 Elevated MCA-PSV in an MCDA twin pregnancy complicated by TAPS at 29 weeks after laser therapy for stage III TTTS at 21 weeks of gestation. (A black and white version of this figure will appear in some formats. For the colour version, please refer to the plate section.)

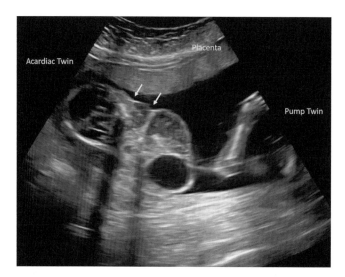

Figure 8.5 The amorphous acardiac twin of this MCDA pregnancy complicated by TRAP appeared stuck (arrows) but continued to grow in the second trimester, resulting in cardiac failure in the pump twin which was treated with cord occlusion of the acardiac twin.

If a single demise is diagnosed in the first trimester, perform Doppler assessments to exclude reversed perfusion of the demised twin. For ongoing pregnancies affected by the TRAP sequence, one or more of the following poor prognostic factors raise the risk for pump twin mortality:[16] evidence of congestive heart failure or hydrops fetalis, abnormal Doppler studies in the umbilical artery of the pump twin, EFW acardiac to EFW pump > 0.7, polyhydramnios or monoamniotic pregnancy.[16] Without early detection and therapy, mortality rates for the pump twin range from 50% to 70%. Concern for the TRAP sequence should prompt an early referral to a fetal therapy centre to discuss the options of termination of the entire pregnancy, selective reduction (cord occlusion, interstitial laser or radiofrequency ablation) or conservative management with serial surveillance. The anomalies of the acardiac twin are incompatible with life, so the focus should be on improving the survival of the pump twin. Early detection, close follow-up and selective cord occlusion of a large or rapidly growing acardiac mass can increase survival for the pump twin to 80–90%. Please see Chapter 15 for further management of the TRAP sequence.

Single Fetal Demise

Due to the inter-twin vascular anastomoses within the single placenta and the acute drop in vascular resistance that occurs when one twin dies, the risk of severe neurologic handicap in the remaining twin is 10–30% with a 10% risk of death.[5] Please see Chapter 12 for more details on management of single fetal demise in MC pregnancies.

Screening and Diagnosis of Complications of Monochorionic-Monoamniotic Twins

Monochorionic-monoamniotic twins make up 1–2% of all monozygotic twin pregnancies and occur when an embryo splits ≥ 8 days after fertilisation. Monochorionic-monoamniotic twins share both a chorion and amnion and lack a dividing membrane.

The absence of a dividing membrane early in pregnancy should be considered an MCMA pregnancy until a dividing membrane is visualised, which may not be possible until about 12 weeks. It is important not to incorrectly diagnose MCMA in what is actually an MCDA pregnancy complicated by TTTS where the donor twin is 'stuck' underneath a draped dividing membrane. In a monoamniotic twin pregnancy, both twins should move throughout the uterus and neither twin should appear stuck in the same location throughout the exam.

Monoamnionicity can be confirmed by the presence of cord entanglement on obstetric ultrasound, particularly when colour flow imaging is utilised (Figure 8.6). Cord entanglement is detected prenatally in almost all cases of MCMA twins and is responsible for the perinatal mortality rate of 70%. Recommendations for monitoring for cord entanglement and its impact on the monoamniotic twins vary. Any advice for twin surveillance, including whether monitoring should take place as an inpatient or outpatient, must balance the reduced fetal morbidity and mortality against the inconvenience and possible psychological and financial strain on the mother and her family, costs to the health care system and the possibility of iatrogenic prematurity or other adverse events.

Although the same complications that plague MCDA twins may occur in MCMA twins, the frequency varies. For example, the incidence of TTTS in MCMA pregnancies is 2–3% compared to the 10–15% seen in MCDA twins. This is likely due to the nearly universal presence of A-A anastomoses seen in MCMA twins, which are protective against TTTS and significant growth discordance.

Similar to MCDA twins, ultrasound assessment of MCMA twins may begin at 16 weeks, with assessment every two weeks pending the findings. Many providers consider admission

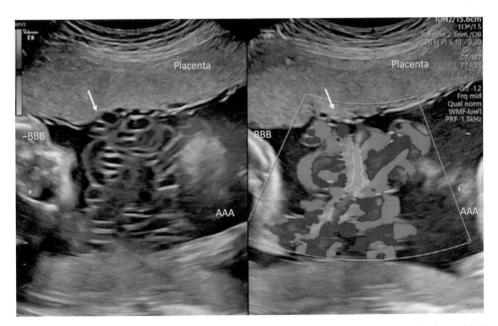

Figure 8.6 Split-screen ultrasound demonstrating umbilical cord entanglement (arrows) by two-dimensional (left) and colour flow (right) imaging in monoamniotic twins. (A black and white version of this figure will appear in some formats. For the colour version, please refer to the plate section.)

with increased monitoring between 24 and 28 weeks with delivery at 32–34 weeks. Great debate exists on whether and when to admit patients with MCMA twins to the hospital for increased surveillance of the twins. A recent retrospective analysis – the MONOMONO study – reported on 195 MCMA pregnancies at 22 participating sites in the United States and Europe and found no significant differences in outcomes between inpatient and outpatient monitoring. In this study, the peak fetal death rate was at 29 weeks with no fetal or neonatal deaths after 32 weeks, regardless of the location of testing.[17] Please see Chapter 17 for further discussion on management of MCMA twins.

Structural Anomalies

Compared to singletons, the rate of major congenital anomalies is fourfold higher in monozygotic twins and threefold higher than that of dizygotic twins. Of monozygotic twins, those with monochorionic-monoamniotic placentation have the highest rate of congenital anomalies. The rates of discordant anomalies are also very high and thus careful attention must be paid to evaluating each fetus individually for anomalies. Given the increased rate of congenital anomalies and heart defects, all monozygotic pregnancies should undergo a detailed anatomical survey and fetal echocardiogram. While an assessment for major anomalies may occur during the first trimester, a follow-up anatomical survey at 18–22 weeks should be performed given its higher detection rate for major malformations (50% vs 70%). Please see Chapters 7 and 11 for further discussion on screening for fetal abnormalities in multiples and management of discordant twin anomalies, respectively.

Preterm Birth Risk Assessment

All twin pregnancies are at risk of preterm birth. As a screening tool for preterm birth, cervical length assessment is recommended during the fetal anatomy scan but may be obtained more frequently during the second trimester. Asymptomatic women found to have a cervical length < 25 mm in mid trimester are at an increased risk of spontaneous preterm birth. A cervical length < 20 mm between 20 and 24 weeks is a reasonable predictor of preterm birth before 32–34 weeks.[2] Unfortunately, there is no effective strategy to prevent preterm birth in multiple gestations, so the impact of detecting a short cervix in a patient with twins is uncertain. Please see Chapters 19 and 20 for more discussion of preterm birth in multiple gestations.

The Management

An organised and standardised approach to the management of monochorionic twins improves outcomes. Checklists from the Society for Maternal Fetal Medicine and the American College of Obstetrics and Gynecology help optimally care for monochorionic twin pregnancies.

By 14 weeks, confirm the estimated date of delivery (EDD), chorionicity and amnionicity. During the first few prenatal visits, counsel the patient on the increased maternal risks of twin pregnancies such as hypertensive disorders of pregnancy, gestational diabetes and postpartum haemorrhage. Neonatal risks including TTTS, discordant growth, sIUGR, preterm birth and the potential sequelae to a surviving co-twin in the event of a single twin demise should also be discussed early in care. Review options for genetic screening and diagnosis during the initial prenatal visit.

Begin serial ultrasound monitoring of all monochorionic pregnancies at 16 weeks of gestation. Ultrasound assessment should include measuring the MVP of each sac and visualisation of a fluid-filled bladder for each twin. Obtain ultrasounds every two weeks until 26 weeks and then every two to three weeks until delivery. Assess fetal growth every three to four weeks starting at 16 weeks and continue until delivery. Obtain Doppler studies if either twin is growth restricted or growth or fluid discordance is noted. Perform a detailed anatomical survey and a fetal echocardiogram at 18–22 weeks. If there is concern for TTTS or discordant growth with selective IUGR, consider early consultation with a fetal therapy centre. If possible, perform screening ultrasounds and serial surveillance of monochorionic twins early in the workweek to allow time for referral and travel to a fetal therapy centre to help avoid delays in care when complications are encountered.

The Society for Maternal Fetal Medicine recommends delivery of uncomplicated monochorionic diamniotic pregnancies by 37 6/7 weeks and delivery of uncomplicated monochorionic monoamniotic pregnancies by caesarean section between 32 and 34 weeks of gestation. See Chapter 23 for more discussion on delivery timing in multiple pregnancies.

Key Points

- Establish EDD, amnionicity and chorionicity in the first trimester.
- Start serial ultrasound surveillance at 16 weeks and repeat every two weeks until 26 weeks with an assessment of MVP in each sac, presence of fetal bladders and Doppler studies if TTTS and/or sIUGR are diagnosed.
- In the second trimester, obtain a detailed fetal anatomical survey and fetal echocardiogram of both twins.
- Obtain baseline cervical length in the second trimester to assess risk for preterm birth.
- Assess twin growth every three to four weeks.
- Refer to fetal therapy centre if there is concern for TRAP, TTTS, sIUGR or TAPS.
- Deliver MCDA twins between 34 and 37 weeks.
- Deliver MCMA twins between 32 and 34 weeks by caesarean section.

Management of Monochorionic-Diamniotic Twin Pregnancies

By 14 weeks
- Establish EDD, amnionicity and chorionicity between 7 and 13 6/7 weeks
- Discuss risks of monochorionic pregnancy
- Assess for major congenital anomalies during first trimester ultrasound
- Obtain genetic screening and/or diagnosis

16 weeks
- Start obtaining ultraosounds every 2 weeks assessing:
- Maximum vertical pocket of each twin
- Fluid filled bladder identified for each twin
- Consider Doppler assessment of the umbilical artery and middle cerebral artery

18–22 weeks
- Obtain detailed anatomical survey and measure fetal growth
- Obtain fetal echocardiogram
- Measure cervical length to assess risk for preterm birth
- Continue twice weekly ultrasound assessment

22–28 weeks
- Continue twice weekly ultrasound assessment
- Obtain fetal growth every 3–4 weeks

28–37 weeks
- Continue ultrasound assessment every 2–3 weeks
- Contiue fetal growth scans every 3–4 weeks
- Deliver between 34–37 weeks

References

1. Sebire NJ, D'Ercole C, Hughes K, Carvalho M, Nicolaides KH. Increased nuchal translucency thickness at 10–14 weeks of gestation as a predictor of severe twin to twin transfusion syndrome. Ultrasound Obstet Gynecol 1997 Aug;**10**(20):86–9.

2. Khalil A et al. ISUOG practice guidelines: role of ultrasound in twin pregnancy. Ultrasound Obstet Gynecol 2016;**47**:247–63.

3. Mackie FL, Hall MJ, Morris RK, Kilby MD. Early prognostic factors of outcomes in monochorionic twin pregnancy: a systematic review and meta analysis. Am J Obstet Gynecol 2018 Nov;**2019**(5):436–46.

4. Kristiansen MK, Joensen BS, Ekelund CK, Petersen OB, Sandager P. Perinatal outcome after first-trimester risk assessment in monochorionic and dichorionic twin pregnancies: a population-based register study. BJOG 2015 Sep;**122**(10):1362–9.

5. Simpson LL. Twin–twin transfusion syndrome. Am J Obstet Gynecol 2013 Jan; **208**(1):3–18.

6. Kagan KO, Gazzoni A, Sepulveda-Gonzalez G, Sotiriadis A, Nicolaides KH. Discordance in nuchal translucency thickness in prediction of severe twin-to-twin transfusion syndrome.

Ultrasound Obstet Gynecol 2007. May;29(5):527–32.

7. Da Paepe ME, Shapiro S, Young L, Luks FL. Placental characteristics in selective birth weight discordance in diamniotic-monochorionic twin gestations. Placenta 2010. May;31(5):380–6.

8. Buca D, Pagani G, Rizzo G et al. Outcome of monochorionic twin pregnancy with selective intrauterine growth restriction according to umbilical artery Doppler flow pattern of smaller twin: systematic review and meta-analysis. Ultrasound Obstet Gynecol 2017 Nov;50(5):559–68.

9. Gratacós E, Lewi L, Muñoz B et al. A classification system for sIUGR in MC pregnancies according to UA Doppler flow in the smaller twin. Ultrasound Obstet Gynecol 2007 Jul;30(1):28–34.

10. Ishii K, Murakoshi T, Takahashi Y et al. Perinatal outcome of monochorionic twins with selective intrauterine growth restriction and different types of umbilical artery Doppler under expectant management. Fetal Diag Ther 2009;26 (3):157–61.

11. Parra-Cordero M, Bennasar M, Martínez JM, Eixarch E, Torres X, Gratacós E. Cord occlusion in monochorionic twins with early selective intrauterine growth restriction and abnormal umbilical artery Doppler: a consecutive series of 90 cases. Fetal Diagn Ther 2016;39(3):186–91.

12. Bennasar M, Eixarch E, Martinez JM, Gratacos E. Selective intrauterine growth restriction in monochorionic diamniotic twin pregnancies. Seminars in Fetal and Neonatal Medicine 2017;22:376–82.

13. Slaghekke F, Kist WJ, Oepkes D et al. Twin anemia-polycythemia sequence: diagnostic criteria, classification, perinatal management and outcome. Fetal Diagn Ther 2010;27:181–90.

14. Khalil A, Gordijn S, Ganzevoort W et al. Consensus diagnostic criteria and monitoring of twin anemia polycythemia sequence: a Delphi procedure. Ultrasound Obstet Gynecol 2019 Oct 12.

15. Bornstein E, Monteaguode A, Dong R, Schwartz N, Timor-Tristch IE. Detection of twin reversed arterial perfusion sequence at the time of first-trimester screening. The added value of 3-dimensional volume and color Doppler sonography. J Ultrasound Med 2008:1105–9.

16. Moore TR, Gale S, Benirschke K. Perinatal outcome of forty-nine pregnancies complicated by acardiac twinning. Am J Obstet Gynecol 1990;163:907.

17. MONOMONO Working Group. Inpatient vs outpatient management and timing of delivery of uncomplicated monochorionic monoamniotic twin pregnancy: the MONOMONO study. Ultrasound Obstet Gynecol 2019 Feb;53(2):175–83.

Invasive Prenatal Diagnosis in Multiple Pregnancy

Ranjit Akolekar

The Facts

Introduction

Chorionic villus sampling (CVS) and amniocentesis are commonly performed invasive procedures for prenatal invasive diagnosis. Prior to any invasive procedure in pregnancy, there should be a discussion with women regarding the potential risks associated with the procedure. There are various indications for carrying out invasive procedures in pregnancy. The main one remains the confirmation or exclusion of fetal aneuploidies following abnormal screening test results. Screening for fetal aneuploidies has evolved considerably in the past few decades from being based primarily on maternal age in the 1970s to the widespread implementation of routine first-trimester combined screening based on the assessment of fetal nuchal translucency thickness and maternal serum biochemistry.

Screening in twins is based on similar principles and carried out in a similar way as screening in singletons. An important aspect assessing the risk of aneuploidies as well as undertaking invasive procedures is knowledge of the chorionicity of a multiple pregnancy as the risk of complications is associated with chorionicity rather than zygosity. At the first-trimester scan at 11–13 weeks' gestation, demonstration of a triangular echogenic placental chorionic tissue between the amniotic sacs at the junction with the placenta (λ-sign) is diagnostic of a dichorionic pregnancy, whereas absence of this echogenic chorionic tissue with the amniotic membranes joining the placenta (T-sign) is suggestive of a monochorionic pregnancy. In a dichorionic pregnancy, the risk of fetal aneuploidies is assessed independently for each of the fetuses. In monochorionic pregnancies, however, the risk is based on an average of likelihood ratios derived from assessment of maternal characteristics, nuchal translucency (NT) in both twins and maternal biochemistry. Detection rates (DR) and false positive rates (FPR) of the combined screening for fetal aneuploidies between 11 and 13 weeks in twin pregnancies are comparable with singleton pregnancies with DR of 90% and FPR of about 6%. In monochorionic twin pregnancies, the false positive rate is higher compared to dichorionic pregnancies as the increased NT may be present in a higher proportion of chromosomally normal fetuses as a consequence of early presentation of twin–twin transfusion syndrome or due to higher incidence of fetal cardiac defects. The prevalence of multiple pregnancies is higher in mothers with advanced maternal age and those conceived by assisted reproductive techniques. Chromosomal abnormalities and structural defects are more common in multiple pregnancies, monochorionic pregnancies in particular. Therefore, accurate prenatal diagnosis is of crucial importance in management of these high-risk pregnancies.

Invasive Diagnostic Procedures

Chorionic Villus Sampling (CVS)

Several cohort and case-control studies, systematic reviews and meta-analyses demonstrate that CVS in singleton pregnancies is safe with a procedure-related risk of pregnancy loss of 0.3–0.5%. The advantages of CVS in twins are similar to those in singleton pregnancies, but in multiple pregnancies, it has additional benefits as well. First, CVS allows for a definitive prenatal diagnosis at an earlier gestation and therefore provides reassurance if the results are normal, but if the results are abnormal, it facilitates earlier decision-making regarding termination of pregnancy. Second, early cytogenetic testing with CVS allows selective fetal reduction of the affected fetus with a potentially lower risk of complications. It is also likely to have a reduced psychological impact on parents if the selective fetal terminations are performed early in pregnancy.

Amniocentesis

Amniocentesis is a safe and accurate method for prenatal diagnosis in singletons. Similar to CVS, there is extensive evidence from cohort studies, systematic reviews and meta-analysis in singleton pregnancies suggesting that the procedure-related risk of miscarriage is not significantly different from controls and is 0.1–0.2%. The advantage of amniocentesis compared to CVS is that the results are based on culture and analysis of amniocytes and therefore there is no chance of placental mosaicism as is noted in some pregnancies that undergo a CVS. The potential disadvantage of amniocentesis is that it can only safely be carried out at or after 15 weeks of gestation, and therefore the results of prenatal diagnosis are available to parents at a later gestation, which results in a management plan being made at a more advanced gestation compared to CVS. Scholars have carried out studies of amniocentesis in twins prior to 15 weeks' gestation, but similar to singleton pregnancies, early amniocentesis is associated with increased rate of fetal loss, failed procedures, multiple needle insertions, failed culture and fetal talipes equinovarus when compared to samplings carried out at gestation after 15 weeks. Early amniocentesis is therefore not recommended.

Fetal Blood Sampling (FBS)

Fetal blood sampling (FBS) has been previously suggested for rapid karyotyping in twin pregnancies. With the widely accessible quantitative fluorescent polymerase chain reaction (QF-PCR) analysis with the results available within potentially 24–48 working hours, indications for FBS are limited. A study by Antsaklis et al. reported the results of FBS carried out in 84 twin pregnancies, mainly for prenatal diagnosis of hemoglobinopathies with an overall 8.2% procedure-related fetal loss up to 2 weeks post procedure. This is around four times higher than the risk of pregnancy loss associated with FBS in singleton pregnancy. Fetal blood sampling is still of clinical importance in multiple pregnancies, but this should be reserved for pregnancies with fetal anaemia, thrombocytopenia, fetal infection and fetal hydrops.

The Issues

Technical Considerations

Chorionic Villus Sampling

The main issues concerning CVS in multiple pregnancies include the technical challenges of sampling and higher procedure-related risks and sampling errors compared to singleton pregnancies. Due to technical challenges associated with obtaining adequate samples in multiple pregnancies whilst ensuring low procedure-related loss rates, it is advisable that these procedures should only be carried out by experienced fetal medicine operators to ensure that accurate 'mapping' of the fetuses and placentae is done and correct ultrasound-guided placement of the instruments into each specific placenta is carried out. An important concern in multifetal CVS is sampling error and cross-contamination, mainly in cases when there are difficulties in identifying the placental margins by ultrasound or in pregnancies with fused dichorionic placentae. As with ultrasound assessment of fetal anatomy and the risk of chromosomal abnormalities, it is important to ensure that chorionicity, location of the amniotic sacs in relation to the cervix and the uterine fundus, their related placentas and the location of the cord insertions is accurately checked and documented prior to undertaking invasive testing. This is especially important as not only it will allow accurate sampling for prenatal diagnosis, but it is also important if a selective termination of pregnancy is required.

Different techniques have been described for CVS in twin pregnancies, including transabdominal, transcervical or even a combined approach, especially in pregnancies with both anterior high and posterior low placentae. Transabdominal CVS can be performed with a special CVS needle which can be used for a single-puncture procedure or, alternatively, a double-needle approach can be used. If the latter is used, it is prudent to use different needles to ensure there is no contamination, especially when sampling dichorionic placentae. It is always good practice to sample the affected fetus that has either a structural defect or is at high risk of chromosomal abnormality first and then proceed to sample the placenta of the other fetus. Transcervical CVS can be performed using aspiration catheter or biopsy forceps. As in the transabdominal approach, it is advisable to use a different instrument for each placenta. Systematic review of the literature has showed no superior CVS technique – that is, transabdominal, transcervical, a single-needle system, a double-needled system or a single uterine entry compared to double uterine entry are associated with similar risks and safety profiles.

Amniocentesis

Similar to CVS procedures, the issues relating to amniocentesis are technical challenges of undertaking the procedure, higher procedure-related risks and sampling errors compared to singleton pregnancies. Therefore, amniocentesis in multifetal pregnancies should be undertaken by experienced operators as with other procedures. Amniocentesis in twin pregnancies requires accurate sampling of different amniotic sacs, and it is therefore important to identify the inter-fetal amniotic membrane to ensure sampling is done on either side of the membrane or across it from different sacs.

Essentially two different techniques are described for carrying out amniocentesis in multiple pregnancies. The first technique which is commonly used is two different needles inserted separately and sequentially into each amniotic cavity under ultrasound guidance. After the insertion of the first needle, about 20 mL of fluid is aspirated for cytogenetic evaluation and the needle is withdrawn. Then the second needle is inserted from a different or the same entry point and the second amniotic sac is sampled. In order to reduce the risk of resampling the same amniotic sac from a different angle, it is reasonable to choose two different entry points as far from each other as possible. The second technique, which avoids the potential for sampling error, is the use of a single-needle technique. An optimal view of the different amniotic sacs with an intervening amniotic membrane should be visualised and the needle is inserted into the first sac which is proximal to the insertion site. After aspiration of the amniotic fluid from the first sac, the stilette is reintroduced into the needle, which is then advanced into the second sac across the amniotic membrane into the distal sac. An initial 1 mL of fluid is aspirated and discarded (to lower the risk of contamination from the first sac) and then 20 mL is collected from the distal sac. Some operators suggest the use of dye as a marker in one of the amniotic cavities to ensure accurate sampling; but in current practice, it is rarely used as it is feasible to carry out the procedure by ensuring sampling across different sides of the amniotic membrane.

Procedure-Related Pregnancy Loss

A systematic review in 2013 reported that procedure-related pregnancy loss in twin pregnancies following CVS was about 1.0% higher than the background risk in controls. Similarly, in pregnancies undergoing amniocentesis, the procedure-related risk of miscarriage in twins was 1.1% higher compared to twins that did not undergo invasive testing. The authors did not find any statistically significant differences in pregnancy loss, regardless of the technique.

A recently published systematic review and meta-analysis by Mascio et al. also demonstrated that the procedure-related risk of pregnancy loss in twins following invasive procedures is not significantly different compared to control twin pregnancies that did not have an invasive procedure. In twin pregnancies undergoing CVS, the background risk of fetal loss was 2.0% compared with 1.8% in controls with a prevalence of procedure-related fetal loss of 0.5% (95%CI 0.0–2.2), which is similar to data from singleton pregnancies. Similarly, in twins undergoing amniocentesis, the incidence of fetal loss was 2.4% (95% CI 1.4–3.6) compared with 2.4% (95% CI 0.9–4.6) for twin pregnancies not undergoing amniocentesis. In addition to the total rate of fetal loss, the authors examined the fetal loss rate prior to 24 weeks and within 4 weeks of the procedure and found no significant difference in overall fetal loss in those that had an amniocentesis or CVS compared to those that did not. In twin pregnancies undergoing amniocentesis, there was no significant difference in the risk of fetal loss < 24 weeks of gestation (p = 0.11) or within 4 weeks of the procedure (p = 0.80) compared to those that did not have an invasive procedure. They reported similar results for fetal loss < 24 weeks in twin pregnancies undergoing CVS with no statistically significant difference in rate of fetal loss. Regarding different techniques, results from systematic reviews showed no statistically significant difference in fetal loss between the single uterine entry techniques versus the double uterine entry technique.

Special Considerations

Delayed Cytogenetic Testing

In some pregnancies, such as those that are discordant for fetal defects or chromosomal abnormalities, the management option of delayed cytogenetic testing in the third trimester can be discussed. In these cases, the choice between management options depends on weighing the pros and cons of the risk assessment of chromosomal abnormalities and the risks of procedure-related loss, particularly of the unaffected fetus. The decision to discuss delayed invasive testing option should take into account the implications of prenatal diagnostic testing on further management options in the pregnancy such as the potential for termination of pregnancy at that gestational age as the gestational limit for termination will vary depending on guidelines in different countries. A potential advantage of delayed or late cytogenetic testing is the reduction in risk of miscarriage or morbidity and morbidity secondary to extreme prematurity in case of preterm delivery of the unaffected co-twin. The disadvantage of delayed or late testing in the third trimester is the possibility of preterm delivery before invasive testing can be undertaken and, in such circumstances, the impact of delivery of a fetus with a structural or chromosomal abnormality on the perinatal outcome.

Testing in Monochorionic Pregnancies

One of the questions regarding cytogenetic testing in monochorionic pregnancies is whether invasive testing should be done for one or both of the monochorionic fetuses. Essentially, all monochorionic pregnancies are monozygotic, therefore by implication they have identical genotypes. There are, however, reports of monochorionic twins that are discordant for chromosomal abnormalities, and these are called heterokaryotypic pregnancies. The exact prevalence of these heterokaryotypic pregnancies is not known, but they are reportedly caused by mosaicism, skewed X inactivation, differential gene imprinting and micro deletions. Examples of such monozygotic twins with discordant karyotypes include mosaicism for Turner syndrome, Down syndrome, Patau syndrome, trisomy 1 and 22q11 deletion syndrome.

Caution should be exercised in twin pregnancies when the results of the QF-PCR suggest monozygotic pregnancy due to identical genotype. This is expected in a monochorionic pregnancy, but in cases of a dichorionic pregnancy with a similar gender, an identical genotype could represent a monozygotic pregnancy, but it could also be due to sampling error because of sampling the same placenta. The latter should be borne in mind and this possibility should be discussed with the parents. A further management option in this situation is an amniocentesis ensuring that sampling is from separate sacs.

Higher-Order Pregnancies

Data are limited regarding the risks of invasive procedures in higher-order multiple pregnancies. Similar to twin pregnancies, these are technically challenging procedures and should be carried out in tertiary fetal medicine units by experienced operators.

The Management Options

Chorionic villus sampling and amniocentesis are both relatively safe procedures for invasive prenatal diagnosis in twin pregnancies, and women and their families can be reassured that the overall rate of fetal loss is low. Although the overall rate of fetal loss in monochorionic twin pregnancies is higher compared to dichorionic twin pregnancies, the procedure-related risk of fetal loss, especially prior to 24 weeks or within 4 weeks of the procedure, is not significantly different in both when compared to those not undergoing invasive procedures. Although there is a paucity of data comparing different techniques such as single-needle versus double-needle insertion for carrying out procedures, there is evidence that use of a double-needle technique is not associated with higher risks of fetal loss and therefore can be used safely for carrying out these procedures. As in the case of singleton pregnancies, CVS should be carried out after 11 weeks of gestation and amniocentesis can be carried out after 15 weeks of gestation. It is critical that chorionicity of the pregnancy is determined prior to undertaking assessment of fetal anatomy and combined screening, but also to ensure that invasive procedures are carried out safely. Invasive procedures in twin pregnancies are technically challenging and they should be undertaken by experienced operators in specialist fetal medicine centres.

Key Points

- The prevalence of multiple pregnancies is increasing worldwide due to the use of assisted reproductive techniques
- Combined screening for aneuploidies has a high detection rate of chromosomal abnormalities as in singleton pregnancies.
- Assessment of chorionicity is not just an essential prerequisite for undertaking a comprehensive assessment of fetal anatomy and combined screening for chromosomal abnormalities, but is an equally important assessment prior to undertaking invasive prenatal diagnosis.
- Pre-procedure planning with detailed ultrasound survey including assessment of chorionicity, location of placentae, amniotic sacs and labelling of twins is essential as it reduces the risk of sampling error.
- Chorionic villus sampling should not be carried out prior to 11 weeks of gestation and amniocentesis should not be carried out prior to 15 weeks of gestation.
- Women and their families should be reassured that the risk of procedure-related fetal loss before 24 weeks of gestation and within 4 weeks of the invasive procedure in twin pregnancies undergoing CVS and amniocentesis is low and not significantly different compared to the background rate of fetal loss in pregnancies not undergoing invasive procedures.
- There is no evidence of the superiority of any specific technique for performing invasive procedures, and although there is a lack of robust evidence comparing these techniques, both double-needle and single-needle entry appear to be safe.
- Invasive prenatal diagnostic procedures should be carried out by experienced operators in specialist fetal medicine centres.

References

1. Agarwal K, Alfirevic Z. Pregnancy loss after chorionic villus sampling and genetic amniocentesis in twin pregnancies: a systematic review. Ultrasound Obstet Gynecol 2012;**40**:128–34.

2. Antsaklis A, Daskalakis G, Souka AP, Kavalakis Y, Michalas S. Fetal blood sampling in twin pregnancies. Ultrasound Obstet Gynecol 2003;**22**:377–9.

3. Di Mascio D, Khalil A, Rizzo G, Buca D, Liberati M, Martellucci C, Falcco ME, Manzoli L, D'Antonio F. Risk of fetal loss following amniocentesis or chorionic villous sampling in twin pregnancies: a systematic review and meta-analysis. Ultrasound Obstet Gynecol 2020;**56**:647–55.

4. Krispin E, Wertheimer A, Trigerman S, Ben-Haroush A, Meizner I, Wiznitzer A, Bardin R. Single or double needle insertion in twin's

amniocentesis: does the technique influence the risk of complications? Eur J Obstet Gynecol Reprod Biol 2019;3:100051.

5. Sebire NJ, Noble PL, Odibo A, Malligiannis P, Nicolaides KH. Single uterine entry for genetic amniocentesis in twin pregnancies. Ultrasound Obstet Gynecol 1996;7:26–31.

6. Spencer K, Nicolaides KH. Screening for trisomy 21 in twins using first trimester ultrasound and maternal serum biochemistry in a one-stop clinic: a review of three years' experience BJOG 2003;**110**:276–80.

7. Vink J, Wapner R, D'Alton ME. Prenatal diagnosis in twin gestations. Semin Perinatol 2012;**36**:169–74.

8. Weisz B, Rodeck CH. Invasive diagnostic procedures in twin pregnancies. Prenat Diagn 2005;**25**:751–8.

Chapter 1

Conjoined Twinning
Diagnosis and Management

Alice King and Michael A. Belfort

The Facts

Conjoined twins are a rare anomaly where identical twins are born physically connected. The incidence is reported to be 1 in 50,000–200,000 births, and conjoined twins occur in approximately 1% of monozygotic twins.[1] There is a significant prevalence of female gender (75% or greater). The inheritance is sporadic and there is no increased incidence of conjoined twinning in subsequent pregnancies.

Although the exact survival rate is unknown, there is a very high perinatal mortality rate. Approximately 40–60% of prenatally diagnosed conjoined twins undergo in utero fetal demise. Following delivery, a persistently high mortality rate continues with 30% dying within the first 24 hours of life. The risk of death of one or both of the twins is dependent on their anatomy and physiology.[2]

The embryology of conjoined twins is thought to be a result of abnormal monozygotic twinning with two prevailing theories: an abnormality in either fission or fusion. Normal monozygotic twins are the result of fission, in which a single fertilised ovum splits into two identical diploid cells that develop into two identical embryos. Depending on the stage at which the split occurs, the extent of shared amnion and chorion between the fetuses varies. When the split occurs later (days 14–18) at the primitive streak stage, one embryonic axis splits into two parallel axes and this is thought to greatly increase the risk of forming conjoined twins, with abnormal or incomplete division of the single axis into two. An alternate (although largely discarded) theory proposes that there is complete division with subsequent rejoining at vulnerable locations through fusion of the axes. Conjoined twins tend to be joined at a few specific anatomic locations. This fusion theory helps to better explain atypical conjoined twinning, such as chimeric, asymmetrically conjoined and fetus-in-fetu. This chapter focuses on symmetric twins.

Conjoined twins are joined in ventral, lateral or dorsal unions at homologous anatomic locations (i.e. chest to chest and pelvis to pelvis).[3] They are most commonly classified according to the site of anatomic attachment followed by the suffix -pagus, derived from the Greek term for fixed. This standardised anatomic classification was championed by Spencer in 1996 in order to improve consistency in the nomenclature and in reports in the literature.[4]

Ventral Unions

Cephalopagus

Cephalopagus twins fused from the top of the head to the umbilicus represent 11% of conjoined twins. There may be a common cranium with either one composite face or two faces on opposite sides of the conjoined head. The thorax and upper abdomen show fusion of liver, heart and the upper gastrointestinal system down to Meckel's diverticulum. The lower abdomen and pelvis are not involved and each twin will have two arms and two legs. These twins tend to be non-viable.

Thoracopagus

Thoracopagus twins represent 20–40% of conjoined twins and are joined from the chest to the umbilicus. There is always involvement of the heart; however, the degree of involvement varies from a single shared organ to the presence of a single interatrial vessel. Liver parenchyma is always fused in thoracopagus twins, but the biliary system is shared in only 25% and the upper digestive tract in 50%. The pelvis is not typically involved and each twin will have two arms and two legs.

Omphalopagus

Omphalopagus twins occur in 18–33% of conjoined twins and are similar to thoraco-pagus twins with union primarily around the umbilicus with possible extension superiorly to the lower thorax. However, there is never involvement of the heart. The liver parenchyma is shared in 80% of omphalopagus twins. They typically have separate upper digestive tracts, although approximately one-third will share terminal ileum and proximal colon. Each twin typically has a separate pelvis with two arms and two legs.

Ischiopagus

Ischiopagus twins occur at a reported incidence of 6–11% and involve joining from the umbilicus to the pelvis. There is typically a single, large, conjoined pelvis with two sacra and one or two symphysis pubi. There is always involvement of the external genitalia and anus. These twins are mostly commonly joined end to end, but may also be joined face to face. Each twin always has two arms and two legs.

Lateral Union

Parapagus

Parapagus twins represent 28% of conjoined twins and are primarily joined ventral-laterally from the umbilicus, lower abdomen and pelvis. These twins always share a conjoined pelvis with one symphysis pubis. They may have one or two sacra, depending on the extent of ventrolateral rotation. The degree of fusion may extend superiorly and involve the thorax. The variable degree of union leads to a wide range in phenotype, from two separate thoraces with more inferior fusion of the abdomen and pelvis (dithoracic), to a single trunk with two separate heads (dicephalic), to a shared trunk and head with two faces (diprosopic). In diprosopic parapagus twins, the faces typically present on the same side of the head. Parapagus twins may have two, three or four arms and two or three legs.

Dorsal Union

Craniopagus

Craniopagus twins are rare and represent 2% of conjoined twins. They are characterised by the union of any portion of the skull except the face and foramen magnum. Each twin always has two arms and two legs. These twins may share cranium, meninges and brain. Additional classification systems have been developed to further characterise these twins in an effort to give a more comprehensive description of their union. These classifications are based on different variables, including the deepest structure shared (Winston classification), the angle between the shared dural venous sinus and longitudinal axes (Stone and Goodrich classification) or the size of union and extracranial versus intracranial involvement (O'Connell classification). Ultimately, multiple subclassifications are often used together to fully describe these twins, leading to difficulty in obtaining a clear understanding of the literature.

Pygopagus

Pygopagus twins have been reported to represent 18–28% of conjoined twins. They are joined along the back with involvement of the sacrococcygeal and perineal regions. There is typically a single anus with two rectums. A variable amount of spinal cord may be shared between the twins. Each twin has two arms and two legs.

Rachipagus

Rachipagus twins are very rare with fusion along the back above the sacrum. There may be involvement of the occiput and/or the vertebral column.

The Issues

Prenatal Imaging

Early and accurate prenatal diagnosis of conjoined twins is important in order to facilitate clinical care and provide thorough prenatal counselling. Prenatal diagnosis of conjoined twins was initially described in 1976. With the advent of high-resolution transvaginal ultrasound, the diagnosis has been made at an increasingly early gestational age. The majority of conjoined twins are diagnosed around 11–14 weeks of gestation at the time of first-trimester screening. However, initial diagnosis may be suspected as early as 7–8 weeks of gestation. At an earlier gestational age, there is a higher risk of false-positive diagnosis due to less fetal movement of the twins, which may result in overlapping body parts. Fetal movement slowly increases after 8 weeks of gestation and may demonstrate distinctly separate twins to rule out conjoining. Therefore, if conjoined twins are suspected at a very early stage of pregnancy, a repeat ultrasound is highly recommended prior to final decision-making in order to confirm the diagnosis, as well as to better delineate the anatomy of the suspected conjoined twins.[6]

Early sonography will demonstrate one yolk sac alongside two embryos consistent with monoamniotic-monochorionic twins. Sonographic findings suspicious for conjoined twinning will usually show fixed fetal position with the lack of a separating membrane between the twins and the inability to separate the fetal bodies when following skin contours.[7] In most cases, further evaluation will demonstrate fixed relative positions of the fetal heads with possible scoliosis and neck hyperextension, as well as atypical limb positioning. Oftentimes, the umbilical cord will present with more than three vessels. Care should be taken when assessing suspected conjoined twins since in cases where there is a small zone of fusion the twins may rotate through as much as 180 degrees, giving an impression of vertex and breech presentations which can be confusing. Another potential error occurs when there are such high degrees of fusion that the twins are difficult to distinguish and a singleton is diagnosed. Close serial follow-up is required throughout pregnancy to monitor for polyhydramnios as well as hydrops.

A referral to a dedicated fetal centre with experience in diagnosis and management of conjoined twins is recommended for further evaluation when conjoined twins is suspected. Special attention should be focused on the fusion site to delineate the vascular connections in the liver and heart with colour Doppler to diagnose common arterial and intra-cardiac connections.

On initial evaluation, the twins are assigned designations, such as twin A and twin B. This naming convention is maintained throughout later imaging studies and permits more clear and succinct communication. Typically, evaluation begins with two-dimensional ultrasonography which allows for categorisation of the type of union, such as ventral, dorsal or lateral. All limbs should also be identified and labelled. As noted earlier, Doppler techniques are applied to help evaluate shared vasculature. Additional adjuncts include transvaginal scans as needed, as well as the use of a high-resolution linear probe for increased detail. During each ultrasound evaluation, it is also important to assess the uterine environment, including placental location, umbilical cord position and the number of vessels within the umbilical cord, as well as an estimate of the amniotic fluid volume and the status of the cervix.

Fetal magnetic resonance imaging (MRI) is used alongside sonography for more detailed evaluation of shared anatomy. Different sequences are obtained in order to best visualise different aspects of the twins' anatomy. T2-weighted single-shot fast spin echo (SSFSE) can be very helpful in visualising vasculature, while T1-weighted gradient echo (GRE) can help delineate bowel where meconium will typically appear T1-hyperintense. Additional sequences which may be helpful include echoplanar imaging (EPI) for bone and cartilage, as well as diffusion-weighted imaging (DWI) for brain and kidneys. A second-trimester MRI can be very helpful, as most major anomalies may be detected prenatally to help guide counselling and postnatal care.

Fetal echocardiography is an essential component of prenatal evaluation. Cardiac involvement has a profound effect on outcomes. Prenatal echocardiogram has been suggested to be superior to postnatal scans, as the amniotic fluid can act as a buffer for the scans. Postnatally, echocardiography may be limited depending on where the twins are physically connected. There may be very limited pericardial windows, particularly for thoracopagus twins. Some series have compared the severity of disease predicted by prenatal echocardiography to autopsy results and have suggested that prenatal echo tends to underestimate the severity of disease. The clinical implications of these findings suggest that prenatal prediction of poor outcomes and mortality in conjoined twins are often very accurate.[7]

After initial evaluation and confirmation of the diagnosis of conjoined twins, if appropriate, termination of the pregnancy should be discussed and offered. In the event of termination being chosen, a destructive procedure may be required, and this frequently requires special expertise to safely accomplish. If possible, it is in the best interests of the mother to have a vaginal delivery and to avoid a hysterotomy.

In ongoing pregnancies, it is important to continue to follow closely throughout the remainder of gestation. During serial ultrasounds, each twin should be assessed individually, as conjoined twins may show differing growth rates and body compositions. Conjoined twins have been shown to have discrepant sizes, with the hypothesis that the smaller twin is supplying nutrients to the larger twin. Additionally, other complications including polyhydramnios (up to 75% of cases) or hydrops may be detected and warrant intervention such as amnioreduction or delivery if the viability of one or both twins may be affected.

The most common complication of monoamniotic twin pregnancy – that is, cord strangulation due to entanglement – is less likely to occur in conjoined twins because of the fixed positions of the babies. Close monitoring is still indicated because of the polyhydramnios and the potential for the extremities to become entangled in the cords.

Intra-partum Management

Timing of the delivery is important and a scheduled caesarean section is the preferred method for viable babies. Given the amount of pre-delivery organisation required to set up for delivery and initial resuscitation of the babies, it is not advisable to allow the patient to labour. A scheduled caesarean section with the entire team fresh and ready provides the optimum environment for the best outcome. Gestational age at delivery is dependent on prior obstetric history, current pregnancy circumstances and available resources. This should be individualised. There is no need for deliberate very preterm delivery unless obstetrically indicated since the larger the babies are at birth, the better they will do. Given that the majority of conjoined twin pregnancies have polyhydramnios there is a risk of preterm contractions, preterm premature rupture of the membranes (PPROM) and preterm delivery. Because of the abnormal shape of the uterine contents, PPROM is associated with a very real risk of umbilical cord prolapse, and careful consideration should be employed when considering prolongation of the pregnancy.

At the time of caesarean section care, we recommend a midline abdominal incision which allows for extension if required. Care should also be taken with the uterine incision because of the large fetal mass and potential difficulty in getting this mass delivered (especially when the babies are conjoined in such a way as to prevent easy manipulation and flexion). A bulky and inflexible fetal mass with multiple intertwined extremities can be very confusing and pre-hysterotomy ultrasound examination is advised to establish the lie and presentation of the twins in order to plan their orderly exit from the uterus. Given the extensive manipulation frequently required to effect the delivery there is an increased risk of inadvertently extending the hysterotomy into the uterine arteries with subsequent massive blood loss. We generally advise a lower-segment vertical hysterotomy (DeLee incision) which can be extended into the upper segment (classical hysterotomy) if required to give additional space. Attention should be given to managing uterine atony aggressively (and pre-emptively), and this should be anticipated given the frequently attendant polyhydramnios and overextended uterine cavity. An experienced anaesthesiology and surgical team familiar with the various medical and surgical approaches to reversing and controlling uterine atony and haemorrhage should be present. Adequate blood supplies and attention to blood loss, with early packed red cell transfusion and blood product replacement, cannot be overstressed. There is a very real risk of post-partum haemorrhage.

Postnatal Imaging

Following delivery, postnatal imaging is needed in the process of neonatal resuscitation and stabilisation, as well as to evaluate the anatomy to plan for further care and possible surgical separation.

Plain radiographs are needed to help confirm placement of endotracheal tubes, venous and arterial lines, as well as to evaluate the hearts and lungs. X-rays are also used to help assess bowel gas patterns. Depending on the twins' anatomic configuration, strategies to obtain and interpret radiographs are needed. Ventral union conjoined twins will need to be placed on their side, resulting in lateral views, while lateral union conjoined twins are usually positioned on their backs, resulting in anterior–posterior views.

Perinatal ultrasonography is very helpful in the evaluation of conjoined twins. This modality can be performed at the bedside and is used to evaluate a broad array of systems from cranial structures to abdominal solid organs. It is particularly helpful for vascular structures. For example, in cases of shared liver parenchyma, the hepatic vasculature will be evaluated with greyscale, colour Doppler and pulse-wave techniques. For vessels that bridge shared portions of the liver, waveforms can be examined for possible sharing. Additionally, vessels can be accurately traced back to each twin to delineate areas of involvement.

Fluoroscopy is used to help distinguish shared gastrointestinal and genitourinary tracts in conjoined twins. If prenatal imaging is suggestive of urinary tract anomalies, a voiding cystoureterogram (VCUG) should be performed postnatally. In addition to obtaining a roadmap or an outline of the shared anatomy, it will also help assess any vesicoureteral reflux. In cases of ambiguous external genitalia, a combination of retrograde fluoroscopic studies to delineate anatomy is helpful. Along with VCUG, fistula or anomalous communications and connections can be evaluated with the help of a contrast enema or genitogram. These are usually obtained via retrograde injection into the rectum or vagina respectively and may be performed with or without sedation. Often, a cystoscopy may be performed to augment the evaluation of the genitourinary system and to check for abnormal connections between the bladder, vagina and gastrointestinal system.

Further evaluation with cross-sectional computed tomography (CT) or MRI may be obtained to better understand the unique anatomy of each set of conjoined twins. Both CT and MRI are typically performed under anaesthesia in order to eliminate motion-related artifacts which can significantly degrade image quality. With the use of an angiography protocol, both CT angiography and MR angiography can help provide understanding of the sharing of organs and vessels. CT angiography (CTA) is superior to MR angiography for spatial resolution and has faster imaging acquisition, which helps obviate the need for breath-holding. The major disadvantage of CTA over magnetic resonance is the exposure to excess ionising radiation, an issue which is compounded if multiple CTAs are needed.

Due to the complexity of conjoined twin anatomy and the large degree of cross-circulation noted between many conjoined twins, multidisciplinary discussions to develop optimal radiographic strategies for contrast imaging are needed to formulate the best plan for each case. Computerised tomogram angiography has largely replaced the use of traditional angiography. In order to gain a complete understanding of their anatomy, separate scans with contrast injected into each baby may be needed. Selecting different gating will help optimise the visualisation of different systems. Computerised tomogram angiography of the thorax with electrocardiographic (ECG) gating can effectively delineate cardiac anatomy, even if the heart rates vary between the twins. This imaging is critical for surgical planning and may identify fused or shared chambers, which may render successful separation impossible. Computerised tomogram angiography of the chest will also exclude other vascular anomalies which may need surgical correction, including ventricular septal defects, aortic coarctation and anomalous pulmonary venous connections. Aortic branching, pulmonary artery anatomy and patency of the ductus arteriosus may also be assessed. Shared abdominal organs and vasculature may be evaluated with a CT of the abdomen during the early aortic phase of the injected twin. Visceral organs evaluated well by CT include the spleen, pancreas, kidneys, adrenal glands and the biliary system. Early aortic phase CT scanning can help demarcate a plane of separation between the two twins in the liver. Further evaluation of delayed equilibrium can give further information on the portal and hepatic vessels, helping to assess the size and number of vessels shared between the twins. A CT angiogram of the abdomen will show visceral arteries shared between the twins that may prevent successful separation. In addition to intravenous contrast, oral contrast is used to evaluate the gastrointestinal tract. Oral contrast is typically only administered to one twin in order to discriminate shared bowel. CT scans can also provide excellent detail of bony structures to help plan for separation of axial and appendicular skeletons. CT angiography data can be translated into more and more sophisticated three-dimensional (3-D) models, which are immensely helpful for surgical guidance and planning. These models are generated from digital 3-D imaging and printed 3-D models from cross-sectional imaging. They have been used in preoperative simulation planning at multiple specialised fetal centres and can demonstrate anatomic details not immediately apparent in two-dimensional imaging.

Magnetic resonance imaging (MRI) remains superior in some respects to CT and may provide helpful information for management. The biliary system is particularly amenable to interrogation with magnetic resonance technology. Classically, hepatobiliary scintigraphy with an iminodiacetic acid (HIDA) scan including radioactive technetium-99 m has been used to visualise the gallbladders and bile ducts in conjoined twins. This evaluation of suspected shared biliary anatomy has largely been replaced with MRI through magnetic resonance cholangiopancreatography (MRCP). If two gallbladders are visualised, the twins are highly unlikely to have an extra-hepatic bile duct communication. Magnetic resonance also allows evaluation for a single common pancreas, which is most commonly identified in thoracopagus and omphalopagus conjoined twins and which, if present, adds complexity to surgical planning. MRI can also help elucidate the genitourinary system, including the number, location and extent of fusion of the kidneys, as well as identify internal genitalia and anomalous ureteral insertions.

One of the most critical organs for prognosis and patient management is the heart. A thorough cardiac examination is recommended for every set of conjoined twins, even those who typically do not present with cardiac anomalies, such as ischiopagus or craniopagus twins. A combination of postnatal electrocardiography (EKG) and echocardiography can be used to initially evaluate the extent of organ sharing, orientation and sites of fusion. If necessary, cardiac MRI can be employed. The presence of a single heartbeat on EKG indicates extensive cardiac fusion, where separation is most likely not possible.[8] Conversely, the presence of two heartbeats on EKG does not necessarily portend a better outcome or guarantee separation. Postnatal echocardiography is usually attempted in all cases, but frequently the anatomy precludes optimal pericardial views due to anatomy preventing appropriate probe placement. Therefore, if initial screening suggests cardiac fusion between the twins, a multi-detector computed tomography angiogram (CTA) and 3-D magnetic resonance angiogram (MRA) are typically obtained to track vessels, evaluate the anastomoses and assess the individual blood supply of each twin. Some centres have described different methods to determine the degree of circulatory exchange, including injection of radioactive albumin, or use of methylene blue or indigo carmine dyes.

Most commonly a combination of these radiographic modalities is used to help identify the anatomic issues associated with each type of conjoined twins. The presence of other anomalies can affect survival and should be taken into consideration, even if the anatomy of the conjoined twins suggests that separation is technically feasible. Such associated anomalies include scoliosis, congenital diaphragmatic hernia, cystic hygroma, myelomeningocele and club foot deformity. Additional gastrointestinal anomalies such as oesophageal atresia and imperforate anus have also been described. Interestingly, chromosomal abnormalities are rare in conjoined twins.

The Management Options

Women with prenatally suspected conjoined twins should be referred to a specialised fetal centre with experience in confirming and managing such patients. Prenatal counselling should be initiated in order to help with informed decision-making. Important topics that should be discussed include possible termination of pregnancy, the need for prenatal intervention, delivery considerations and postnatal work up and interventions.

If a family chooses termination of the pregnancy, it is important to take into consideration the fixed orientation of conjoined twins, which can make transvaginal termination especially difficult after 18–20 weeks of gestational age. Expertise in dilatation and curettage and fetal destructive procedures is key to avoid serious maternal injury. Second-trimester pregnancy termination via a hysterotomy may be the safest option to terminate the pregnancy.[5]

Approximately 600 sets of conjoined twins are born and undergo surgery every year.[1] These twins require close monitoring throughout their pregnancy. The presence of polyhydramnios is reported in as many as 50% of conjoined twins, and in many cases, multiple amnioreductions have been required to mitigate the attendant risks of preterm labour and rupture of membranes. The presence of hydrops may prompt early delivery for fetal indication if one or both twins are deemed viable. Because of the large placenta and fetal mass these pregnancies are at increased risk of preeclampsia and mirror syndrome, both of which may prompt delivery at any time after 20 weeks.

Postnatal management for conjoined twins can be categorised into three main categories as determined by specific anatomy. These are: (i) non-operative management, (ii) emergency separation, or (iii) planned elective separation.

Separation is typically not offered if there is significant risk to one or both twins, or if the anticipated resultant deformities following separation are regarded as too severe. Thoracopagus conjoined twins with complex cardiac fusion are typically managed with non-operative management. However, if the cardiac fusion is relatively simple, such as the presence of a single inter-atrial vessel, postnatal separation may be an option. As with major cardiac sharing, craniopagus conjoined twins with extensive cerebral fusion may not be suitable for separation. Beyond the feasibility of separating cerebral vasculature and obtaining sufficient bony and soft tissue coverage, neurologic function is always a major consideration before considering separation of inter-digitating brain matter. In these cases, there may be significant compromise of the physical abilities of one or both twin if separation is pursued, and this should be fully discussed and appropriately weighed in the development of any management plans.[9]

Emergency separation may be necessary when the anatomy of either twin is threatening the survival of the other and immediate separation presents the opportunity to save the life of one or both twins. The need for emergency separation carries significant risk with a mortality rate of 71%. This drastically contrasts with the 80% reported overall survival rate of twins undergoing planned scheduled separation. The poorer outcomes associated with immediate separation are likely a result of multiple factors, including the increased risks associated with emergency induction of general anaesthesia and the inability to fully evaluate the anatomy. Emergency separation may also preclude the use of staged separation with the added disadvantage of being unable to place tissue expanders to ensure adequate wound coverage.

Emergency separation may be inevitable and required based on prenatal findings that suggest that such separation may be lifesaving for one or both twins. Cardiac unions may result in one twin not receiving sufficient circulation with anticipated death soon after delivery. One such example might be the presence of two very different heart rates on fetal echocardiography, associated with dilated cardiac chambers in one twin, indicating a situation of significant cardiac dysfunction in one baby with the other twin supporting both itself and its twin. Following delivery, the pump baby, is likely to rapidly go into cardiac failure, and in so doing significantly increase the mortality of both. This scenario warrants consideration of the separation of the twins as soon as possible. Ex utero intra-partum treatment (EXIT) has been performed successfully in this clinical setting to facilitate separation whilst on maternal-placental circulation.[7]

Each set of twins is a unique anatomic challenge, and significant and individualised planning is needed to facilitate a safe and successful surgical separation. The best outcomes are obtained when surgical resection is staged. Another guiding principle is the combination of prenatal and postnatal diagnostic testing such that the relevant anatomy is fully understood.[10] Oftentimes, the most critical organ for the prognosis of the separation is the heart. The most commonly shared system is the gastrointestinal system, which is shared in most types of conjoined twins with the exception of craniopagus twins.

Once the affected physiologic systems are identified, the relevant subspecialists who will address these systems should be involved in early planning. Scheduled, formal, multidisciplinary meetings to discuss the separation prior to the actual operation will help to identify the critical steps of the operation and to develop contingency plans under different scenarios.

Role of Surgical Simulation

The use of surgical simulation in these high-complexity, rare cases is invaluable. It allows for care to be tailored to the specific case and helps to identify specific critical steps peculiar to that individual case. Simulation has been applied to every phase of care, including delivery, neonatal resuscitation and the various stages of separation. Simulation sessions may be facilitated with different types of aids, including 3-D-printed models or high-fidelity mannequins with custom modifications, but should be accurate in terms of anticipated gestational age, size and weight of the specific patients. This hands-on simulation helps to familiarise the team with the spatial orientation, airway management

Table 10.1 Conjoined twins anatomic classification

Type	Per cent (%)	Area of Fusion
Ventral Unions		
Cephalopagus	11	Head to umbilicus
Thoracopagus	20–40	Chest to umbilicus, always involved the heart
Omphalopagus	18–33	Lower chest to umbilicus, never involves the heart
Lateral Unions		
Ischiopagus	6–11	Umbilicus to pelvis, genitalia and anus are always involved
Parapagus	28	Umbilicus to lower abdomen/pelvis, highly variable and may extend to thorax
Dorsal Unions		
Craniopagus	2	Any portion of the skull, except face and foramen magnum
Pyopagus	18–28	Along the back with involvement of sacrococcygeal and perineal areas
Rachipagus	rare	Along the back above the sacrum

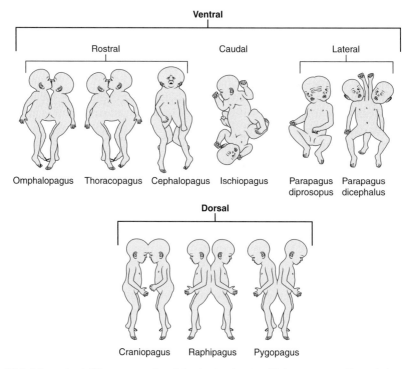

Figure 10.1 Schematic of different types of conjoined twins showing (A) thoracopagus, (B) omphalopagus, (C) pygopagus, (D) ischiopagus, (E) craniopagus, (F) parapagus, (G) cephalopagus and (H) rachipagus

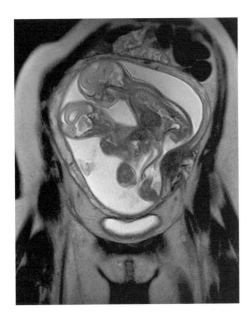

Figure 10.2 Fetal magnetic resonance imaging of omphalopagus conjoined twins at 21 weeks of gestational age showing fused liver

(a)   (b)

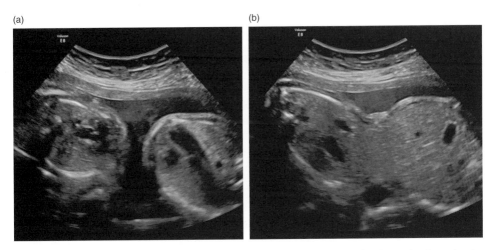

Figure 10.3 Fetal ultrasound imaging of omphalopagus conjoined twins at 21 weeks of gestational age showing separate heart and thorax (a) and fused liver parenchyma (b)

and vascular access needed in the delivery room.[11] For example, endotracheal intubation may present a significant technical challenge in the case of thoracopagus twins and warrant the availability of additional equipment, such as fibre-optic laryngoscopes in the delivery room.[12]

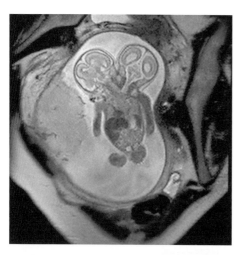

Figure 10.4 Fetal magnetic resonance imaging of dicephalic parapagus conjoined twins at 19 weeks of gestational age showing two fetal heads and a common thorax and abdomen

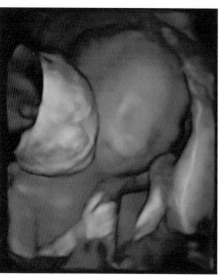

Figure 10.5 Three-dimensional ultrasound of dicephalic parapagus conjoined twins at 19 weeks of gestational age. (A black and white version of this figure will appear in some formats. For the colour version, please refer to the plate section.)

Key Points

- Conjoined twins are a rare anomaly with high in utero and perinatal mortality.
- The use of a standardised anatomic classification helps to improve consistency in diagnosis and facilitates communication between providers.
- Referral to a fetal centre with experience in the evaluation and management of conjoined twins is recommended to optimise counselling and care for these complex patients.
- Extensive prenatal and postnatal diagnostic imaging with advanced radiographic techniques help to delineate the affected anatomy.
- Postnatally, twins may be managed non-operatively, with emergency separation or with planned scheduled (staged or not) surgical separation.
- Involvement of the cardiovascular and neurovascular systems has the greatest impact on successful surgical separation and survival.

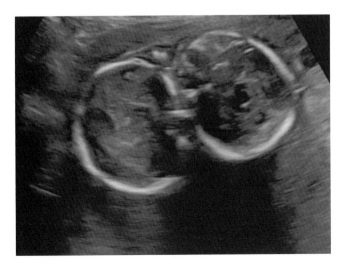

Figure 10.6 Fetal ultrasound of craniopagus conjoined twins at 18 weeks of gestational age showing shared cranium

References

1. Mian A, Gabra NI, Sharma T, Topale N, Gielecki J, Tubbs RS et al. Conjoined twins: from conception to separation, a review. Clin Anat N Y N 2017;**30**(3):385–96.

2. O'Brien P, Nugent M, Khalil A. Prenatal diagnosis and obstetric management. Semin Pediatr Surg 2015 Oct;**24**(5):203–6.

3. Pierro A, Kiely EM, Spitz L. Classification and clinical evaluation. Semin Pediatr Surg 2015 Oct;**24**(5):207–11.

4. Spencer R. Anatomic description of conjoined twins: a plea for standardized terminology. J Pediatr Surg 1996 Jul;**31**(7):941–4.

5. Pajkrt E, Jauniaux E. First-trimester diagnosis of conjoined twins. Prenat Diagn 2005 Sep;**25**(9):820–6.

6. Mehollin-Ray AR. Prenatal and postnatal radiologic evaluation of conjoined twins. Semin Perinatol 2018;**42**(6):369–80.

7. Mackenzie TC, Crombleholme TM, Johnson MP, Schnaufer L, Flake AW, Hedrick HL et al. The natural history of prenatally diagnosed conjoined twins. J Pediatr Surg 2002 Mar;**37**(3):303–9.

8. Andrews RE, Yates RWM, Sullivan ID. The management of conjoined twins: cardiology assessment. Semin Pediatr Surg 2015 Oct;**24**(5):217–20.

9. Harvey DJ, Totonchi A, Gosain AK. Separation of craniopagus twins over the past 20 years: a systematic review of the variables that lead to successful separation. Plast Reconstr Surg 2016 Jul;**138**(1):190–200.

10. Fallon SC, Olutoye OO. The surgical principles of conjoined twin separation. Semin Perinatol 2018;**42**(6):386–92.

11. Yamada NK, Fuerch JH, Halamek LP. Modification of the Neonatal Resuscitation Program Algorithm for Resuscitation of Conjoined Twins. Am J Perinatol 2016 Mar;**33**(4):420–4.

12. Parmekar S, McMullen L, Washington C, Arnold JL. Role of simulation in preparation for the care of conjoined twins: prenatal preparation to separation. Semin Perinatol 2018;**42**(6):329–39.

Chapter 11

Management of Discordant Fetal Anomaly

Rajit Narayan and Jon Hyett

Introduction

Since the advent of assisted reproductive technologies, the prevalence of twins has increased and is currently 1.7% (1 in 60 pregnancies) in our local public hospital population. Twin pregnancies may be complicated in a number of ways, including through presentation with fetal abnormality. Pregnancies that are discordant for fetal anomaly may be impacted by a range of complications that are dependent on zygosity, chorionicity and the specific anomaly concerned.

Discordance is defined as 'occurrence of a trait or disease in only one member of a matched pair of subjects, especially twins'. In this chapter, we review the prevalence of various fetal anomalies in twin pregnancies, identify means for detecting these prenatally and review a range of approaches to managing these anomalies considering the impact on the affected fetus, the co-twin and the wider family. Growth discordance does not fall within the scope of this chapter and is discussed elsewhere in this book.

Prevalence of Anomalies in Twin Pregnancies

A descriptive epidemiological review of European birth defect registries (data for 2004–7) reported that 3.6% of infants from multiple pregnancies were affected by a congenital anomaly.[1] This compared to a prevalence of 2.7% in singleton births, a relative risk (RR) of 1.31 (95%CI: 1.24–1.38). Interestingly, whilst structural anomalies were more common in multiples (RR: 1.41; 95%CI 1.34–1.48), chromosomal anomalies had a lower prevalence (RR: 0.71; 95%CI 0.60–0.78).

The observation that structural anomalies are more commonly seen in twins is well established. Structural anomalies predominantly occur within monozygotic twin pairs and have been ascribed to malformations associated with splitting of the pluripotent cell mass and with vascular disruptions resulting from monochorionicity.[1] Monozygotic twins have been estimated to have a threefold to fivefold increase in risk of anomalies compared to singleton fetuses.[2] Eighty to ninety per cent of anomalies are reported to be discordant within a twin pair, which is surprising on face value given that most events are within monochorionic twins, but it is explained by these specific mechanistic pathways.[1,2]

The most common organ systems impacted by malformation are the central nervous and cardiovascular systems (Figure 11.1).[2] Anomalies of ophthalmic and gastrointestinal systems are also more prevalent in twins than in singletons (Figure 11.2). These systems appear to be more vulnerable to errors in midline fusion/processes of laterality or to disruptive processes (such as vascular accidents). In this chapter, we limit discussion to

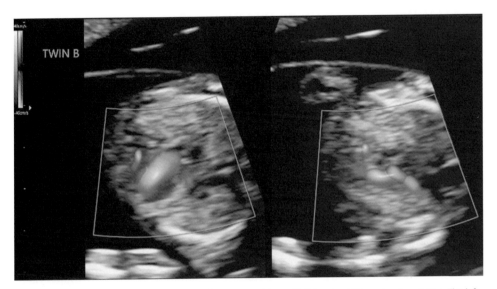

Figure 11.1 Hypoplastic left heart syndrome demonstrated in an MCDA twin at 13 weeks of gestation. The left-hand image of the four-chamber view shows univentricular filling and the right-hand image of the three-vessel view shows reversed flow in the ascending aorta. (A black and white version of this figure will appear in some formats. For the colour version, please refer to the plate section.)

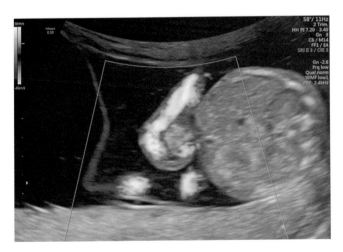

Figure 11.2 A small exomphalos seen in this MCDA twin at 14 weeks of gestation. The inter-twin membrane can be seen inserting into the monochorionic placenta. (A black and white version of this figure will appear in some formats. For the colour version, please refer to the plate section.)

'major' structural anomalies, predicted either to be lethal or to require significant postnatal intervention with risks of significant morbidity and/or mortality in the affected individual.

Whilst the genetic basis for discordant anomalies is readily recognised in dizygotic twins, a number of interesting mechanisms have been described in monozygotic twins including heterokaryotypia secondary to early post-zygotic errors, single gene defects, mitochondrial and epigenetic disorders, blood or tissue chimerism, and skewed X chromosome inactivation.[3]

Prenatal Detection of Twins Discordant for Anomaly

Ultrasound, maternal serum biochemistry and more recently cell-free DNA testing provide means for prenatal screening for both chromosomal and structural anomalies. The European registry data suggest that rates of prenatal diagnosis are similar to those seen in singleton pregnancies, but this merits further discussion.[1]

The prevalence of common chromosomal abnormalities such as trisomy 21 appears to be lower in twin than in singleton pregnancies.[4] Risk assessment is typically based on maternal age-related risks (derived in singleton populations). Parental decisions regarding continuing pregnancies may depend on whether one or both fetuses are affected. In general, monozygotic twins have the same genetic constitution and if one twin is affected, the other twin will also be affected – the a priori risk is therefore the same for both twins and is based on maternal age. In dizygotic twins, the risk that one or the other twin is affected by trisomy is essentially double the maternal age-related risk and the risk that both twins are affected is the square of the maternal age-related risk.

Ultrasound markers for trisomy 21 differ from maternal serum biochemistry and cell-free DNA as they are fetal specific rather than pregnancy specific. Risks can be adjusted accordingly, although zygosity is not determined (by ultrasound) and only monozygotic twins that are monochorionic can be adequately differentiated. All three methods of aneuploidy screening (second-trimester maternal serum biochemistry, first-trimester combined screening and cell-free DNA assessment) have lower efficacy in twin compared to singleton pregnancies. Some markers, such as fetal nuchal translucency (NT) thickness, may also be impacted by other pathologies – such as twin–twin transfusion – leading to inaccuracies in risk assessment.

A retrospective review of a series of > 1,000 twin pregnancies that had a first-trimester ultrasound assessment between 1996 and 2014 found that only 27% (95%CI: 15–43%) of structural anomalies were identified.[5] Anomalies were more prevalent and more readily recognised in twin pairs with discordant crown–rump length (CRL) and NT measures, as well as within monochorionic twins. Central nervous system abnormalities and abdominal wall defects were most readily recognised. It should be noted that this series included twins screened between 1996 and 2014 – and that the approach to a structured anatomical survey during the $11–13^{+6}$ week scan changed markedly over this time.

Current international guidelines recommend two formal structural ultrasound assessments of the fetus at $11–13^{+6}$ and 18–22 weeks of gestation. The time allocated for completion of the morphology scan should also be extended to allow for the fact that this assessment is technically more challenging. Careful assessment of the brain/neural tube, the heart, the midline structures of the face, and the anterior abdominal wall and the gastrointestinal tract should be completed given the increased prevalence of defects affecting these systems. In contrast to some other complications of twin pregnancies, chromosomal and structural anomalies can potentially be identified relatively early, providing parents with a wider range of options.

Managing Twins Discordant for an Anomaly

Defining potential outcomes and ethical implications of various management options makes decision-making difficult in complicated twin pregnancies.[6] Three parties have potentially different and competing interests: the affected fetus, whose prognosis is closely related to the severity of the anomaly; the normal co-twin, who may be impacted by complications affecting the abnormal twin or by iatrogenic preterm delivery; and the mother. Ideally, decision-making should be shared after discussion of all options and relevant risks/benefits, which typically need to be tailored to the individual situation.

Multidisciplinary input should be sought from neonatologists, paediatricians (and/or surgeons) and paediatric development physicians. Social work input should be arranged to facilitate self-exploration of moral, emotional, social, financial and/or religious values and considerations. While the mother should retain autonomy over her decision regarding management of her pregnancy, local legislative and ethical restrictions and indeed availability of clinical resources and expertise may all dictate suitability of management pathways. As a general rule, there tend to be three broad avenues of management for pregnancies affected by discordance in twins:

- Expectant: the pregnancy continues in its current form.
- Termination of the pregnancy.
- Selective reduction of the anomalous twin.

A number of fundamental concepts may impact decisions about the most appropriate way forward. One of the most central of these is the issue of chorionicity. Whilst dichorionic twins are for the most part independent, monochorionic twins almost invariably have a common placental vasculature and as a consequence any detrimental impact on an anomalous twin may be reflected in the outcome of the normal co-twin. Similarly, the extent and type of an anomaly – and the prognosis for a surviving infant – will likely have a big impact on decisions for ongoing management. The gestation at which anomalies are identified will also be important as this may impact management options. Finally, there may also be issues related to maternal health and well-being as well as the potential impact of birth of a child with significant abnormalities on the whole family.

Dichorionic Twins

The architecture of dichorionic placentas allows for some leeway in management options for discordant anomaly. This simplifies decision-making, so we address this cohort of pregnancies first. Common forms of chromosomal abnormality (such as trisomies 21, 18 or 13) and some major structural anomalies (such as anencephaly) will most likely be identified at the $11-13^{+6}$ week scan. These anomalies provide an opportunity to look at some of the principles of management outlined earlier.

The majority (likely > 75%) of fetuses identified with trisomy 21 at 11–13+6 weeks of gestation will survive pregnancy, so parents who choose expectant management should anticipate they will have a live child affected by this condition. As the pregnancy advances, other structural anomalies (such as cardiac defects and/or duodenal atresia) may be recognised, but these are unlikely to impact the course of the pregnancy, which will likely continue to a similar gestation as an unaffected twin pregnancy. As some fetuses affected by trisomy 21 have no obvious phenotype in utero, and as a proportion of dichorionic twins will be monozygous, diagnostic testing should be offered for both fetuses. An early diagnosis gives parents time to absorb information and to optimise management around and after delivery. Diagnostic testing needs to be performed with care, describing landmarks and phenotypes carefully, so that in the event selective reduction is considered this can be performed without risk to the normal co-twin.

The trajectory for a fetus identified with trisomy 18 or 13 at 11–13+6 weeks is very different. These conditions have significantly higher rates of lethality and it could therefore be argued that expectant management will in itself most likely lead to fetal demise. It should, however, be remembered that there is no certainty that this will be the case and a small proportion of live-born infants will survive weeks/months and that palliation may be very difficult whilst also managing another newborn. Another complicating factor is that in an ongoing pregnancy, the anomalous twin may develop severe polyhydramnios and this may trigger preterm delivery. This in turn might injure the normal co-twin. The dilemma here is the balance of risk: if selective termination is considered, what is the risk that this will lead to miscarriage or early preterm delivery of the normal co-twin, and how does this equate with the risk that the anomalous fetus will develop polyhydramnios leading to preterm delivery?

The third scenario involves the finding of anencephaly affecting one dichorionic diamniotic twin at 11–13+6 weeks of gestation (Figure 11.3). In this circumstance, the condition is definitely lethal and management should be focused on achieving the best outcome for the co-twin. Approximately 50% of fetuses managed expectantly with anencephaly will develop polyhydramnios, and 15–20% of dichorionic-diamniotic pregnancies that include an anencephalic fetus will deliver < 34 weeks. In contrast, selective termination is associated with an approximate 10% risk of miscarriage and 10% risk of delivery < 34 weeks.[7] Whilst it may not be immediately clear which option is least likely to cause harm, other series have suggested that risks of preterm birth with expectant management may be even higher – so intervention would be reasonable.[8]

Data describing outcomes in series of dichorionic twin pregnancies discordant for anomalies are conflicting. One study recently reported outcomes of a cohort of 56 dichorionic twin pregnancies discordant for anomaly compared to a series of 586 normal dichorionic twin pregnancies.[9] They reported similar outcomes between the two groups (preterm labour: 21.4% vs 19.1%; preterm premature rupture of the membranes (PPRoM) < 37 weeks: 17.9% vs 19.3%; intrauterine growth restriction: 7.1% vs 9.4%; fetal demise in the structurally normal twin: 0% vs 0%; composite adverse neonatal outcome (19.6% vs 15.1%)). The authors concluded that expectant management was reasonable when parents chose that option.

In contrast, another study reporting a series of 25 anomalous cases and 547 controls found a significant increase in the rate of preterm delivery < 34 weeks of gestation (76% vs

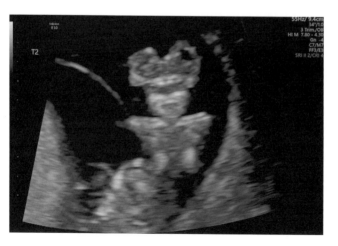

Figure 11.3 Anencephaly identified in this dichorionic twin at 11 weeks of gestation. The inter-twin membrane appears thin – which is often reported to be typical of monochorionic twins – but should not be used in isolation as a reliable sign for chorionicity.

55.4%; p = 0.042) and reported a lower mean gestation of delivery for the whole cohort (34 weeks vs 35.6 weeks; p = 0.019).[10] As described earlier, the risk appeared to be most relevant in pregnancies involving an anomaly that could affect the swallowing mechanism of the affected twin, leading to polyhydramnios such as anencephaly, a large cleft palate, tracheo-esophageal fistula, lethal skeletal dysplasia or major aneuploidies such as trisomies 13 and 18.

Several techniques for selective termination have been described. The most common approach involves ultrasound-guided percutaneous intra-cardiac injection of potassium chloride, which causes cardiac asystole. A group of eight centres with the largest known experience of selective termination worldwide published the outcome of 402 cases and found a 7% pregnancy loss rate (< 24 weeks) in twin pregnancies reduced to singletons and a further 6% preterm birth rate (< 28 weeks) with a trend towards lower pregnancy loss rates when the procedure was performed before 13 weeks of gestation.[11] Risk of maternal morbidity associated with the procedure is low.

This procedure can be performed in an office/outpatient setting. The most important issue is to complete a structured review of the pregnancy and to clearly identify both the normal and the abnormal twin prior to commencing the procedure and to confirm these findings with a second, independent, experienced sonologist. Inadvertent reduction of the normal rather than the anomalous twin has been reported on a number of occasions.

Several contemporaneous studies have reported similar or lower loss rates for twin reduction and suggest that loss rates are not as dependent on gestation as was originally thought. Indeed, some authors promote delaying the procedure to a later gestation to remove the risk of miscarriage, although this comes with its own potential legal, ethical and psychosocial complications.

Monochorionic Twins

Many of the specific risks of a fetal anomaly will be similar for dichorionic and monochorionic twins. There are some significant differences in monochorionic pregnancies, though. From an aneuploidy perspective, although monochorionic twins are monozygotic and will in most circumstances have the same karyotype, there are a number of reports of heterokaryotypia and if one fetus is anomalous and the other is apparently normal, double amniocentesis may be preferred to karyotype the pregnancy rather than chorionic villus sampling from the single placenta.[12]

A significant number of monochorionic twins will be impacted by twin–twin transfusion syndrome and/or selective intrauterine fetal growth restriction and there is a risk that the pregnancy may be impacted by two different pathologies. Similarly, almost all monochorionic pregnancies have vascular anastomoses and if a fetal anomaly is associated with an increased risk of intrauterine fetal death, this increases risk to the whole pregnancy.

Selectively reducing an anomalous twin within a monochorionic pair is technically more challenging as death of a monochorionic twin can result in secondary exsanguination of the co-twin, which has been shown to be associated with a significant risk of death (25%) or neurodevelopmental handicap (20%) in survivors.

Consequently, a procedure aiming to effect selective termination in a monochorionic twin pregnancy needs to occlude the circulation of this twin so that subsequently there can be no retrograde flow. A number of different approaches have been used for this, but three common therapies in contemporary use are bipolar cord occlusion, interstitial laser ablation and radiofrequency ablation. Each method has advantages and disadvantages.

Bipolar cord occlusion requires introduction of a single 3 mm 'vascular catheter' port into the uterus.[13] Port insertion was initially used for endoscopic laser ablation of twin–twin transfusion – in that circumstance, the port is introduced into a tense uterus with poly-hydramnios. Care has to be taken when the myometrium is typically thicker and softer; port insertion is most safely achieved using a 'Seldinger' technique and infusion of additional saline into the uterus to make room for the procedure.

Once the port is inserted, a bipolar forceps can be introduced into the uterus and, under ultrasound guidance, used to grasp the cord and apply diathermy to seal the umbilical arteries and vein. The process is normally repeated to ensure the circulation is occluded. Fetal bradycardia, cardiac asystole and death will follow over the course of several minutes.

The procedure has the advantage that it is straightforward and the equipment is cheap and readily available. Obstetricians/gynaecologists who have trained in both ultrasound and laparoscopic surgery have the skill set to complete the procedure under ultrasound guidance. The disadvantage to the procedure is that the port is relatively large (with risk of miscarriage and PPRoM) and the jaws of the instrument are limited to grasp the whole cord, making this technically challenging at more advanced gestations.

The energy for an interstitial laser is typically passed through a fine (400 um) optic fibre which can be inserted into an 18 G needle; this has the advantage of a small cross-sectional profile and can be advanced into the uterus more safely.[14] The fibre is used to heat and coagulate interstitial vessels. One disadvantage of this technique is cost – it requires access to a NdYAG/diode laser with fibres that can be used with tissue contact.

Radiofrequency ablation also requires more costly equipment, but the probes also have a smaller cross-sectional profile than bipolar forceps (Figure 11.4) and the procedure can more readily be performed under local anaesthesia.[15] We use a 17 G (1.4 mm diameter) Starburst SDE (Angiodynamics Inc., Queensbury, NY, USA) multi-tine electrode. Once the probe is inserted and the tines are advanced, a sinusoidal current is generated that agitates tissue ions, creating frictional heat and causing coagulation of the tissue. Energy levels and time of delivery are set (typically 40–60 W for 3–5 minutes to reach a target temperature of ~120°C). The probe provides temperature feedback that improves consistency of coagulation and theoretically reduces the risk of failing to occlude vessels within the 'burn radius' – which is several centimetres for most probes. Multiple cycles may be required before the desired result is achieved. As a consequence, this technique can be used for more advanced pregnancies where bipolar cord occlusion is not possible. Ultrasound assessment is used to confirm fetal cardiac asystole in the anomalous twin prior to withdrawal of the needle.

The completeness of radiofrequency or interstitial laser procedures is difficult to quantify by use of colour Doppler flow estimates, unlike post–bipolar cord occlusion, where this is quite a simple exercise. Mid-cerebral artery Doppler waveforms and cardiac filling are assessed in the surviving twin to screen for fetal anaemia consequent to ongoing haemorrhage into the dead twin.

There is also a risk heat may damage neighbouring structures using the interstitial technique – one of the proposed mechanisms for preterm rupture of membranes after these procedures. Individual circumstances may also affect choice of procedure; the length of the radiofrequency electrode limits its use in women with higher body mass index, and

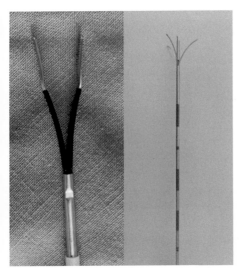

Figure 11.4 The tips of bipolar forceps (left panel) and the radiofrequency ablation (RFA) probe (right panel). The bipolar instrument is a wider diameter (3.5 mm) and the tongs open to 12 mm diameter. The RFA probe is narrower (1.5 mm) and opens to deploy multiple tines to a diameter of 2–3 cm.

bipolar cord occlusion is technically more challenging with oligohydramnios or a short cord (as is frequently seen in acardiac twin pregnancies).

Success rates vary by publication, but broadly speaking, they appear to be comparable for the two procedure types. A systematic review comparing the techniques observed that bipolar cord occlusion was preferred to radiofrequency at later gestations (21.1 vs 18.8 weeks), was associated with fewer deaths of co-twins than radiofrequency ablation (10.6% vs 14.7%), and resulted in higher live birth rates (86.7% vs 81.3%), but tended to have earlier birth in survivors (34.7 vs 35.1 weeks of gestation) and a greater PPROM risk (28.2% vs 17.7%).[16] Although there are small differences between these procedures, management of a specific pregnancy is likely best defined at the discretion of the caring clinician and will be determined by the type of anomaly, gestation, geographic features of the pregnancy and maternal body habitus.

Exceptional Circumstances

Monoamniotic Twins

The majority of monochorionic twins are diamniotic, but in the circumstance of mono-amnionicity, there is an additional post-procedural risk of cord entanglement (Figure 11.5). Post procedure, as the cord of the dead twin becomes more fibrous and the weight of the fetus pulls it taut, it is likely to be less forgiving and this can easily lead to delayed unanticipated intrauterine death of the co-twin. Transection of the cord after ablation has been proposed and several methods have been described to achieve this, including use of a contact LASER or use of endoscopic shears or a harmonic scalpel (through a second 5 mm port). Valsky et al. reported a series of 17 monoamniotic twins who underwent selective reduction plus cord transection and compared their outcomes to a cohort of 72 monochor-ionic-diamniotic twins who also underwent selective termination.[17] They observed a non-significant difference in PPROM risk (35.3% vs 20.8% before 32 weeks), preterm delivery under 32 weeks of gestation (41.2% vs 28.2%), fetal death in utero and neonatal morbidity

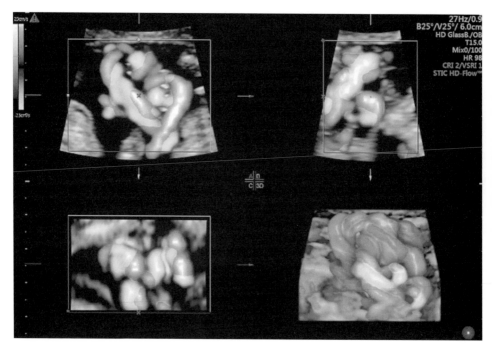

Figure 11.5 3-D multiplanar image showing cord entanglement in MCMA twins at 18 weeks of gestation (A black and white version of this figure will appear in some formats. For the colour version, please refer to the plate section.)

risk, and it is necessary to recognise that the study was likely underpowered for these outcomes. The median gestational age at delivery was 35 weeks in the monoamniotic cohort (that had cord transection) and 37^{+1} weeks in the diamniotic cohort.

Twin-Reversed Arterial Perfusion Sequence (TRAP)

Another anomaly unique to monochorionicity is twin-reversed arterial perfusion (TRAP), involving a normal 'pump' twin that also, through placental anastomoses, perfuses a parasitic tissue mass. The tissue mass represents a significantly malformed co-twin that, likely due to disrupted vascular perfusion, sustained significant errors in embryological development. Many of these masses are anencephalic as well as acardiac. Untreated, mortality in the pump twin may exceed 50% as this infant is prone to unanticipated intrauterine death during early pregnancy and later developing high-output cardiac failure and hydrops. There is also a significant risk of preterm delivery due to maternal mirror syndrome or following spontaneous onset of labour related to polyhydramnios. As first-trimester ultrasound has become more prevalent, TRAP is typically diagnosed at an early stage of pregnancy, and this provides a dilemma for management. An early intervention potentially reduces the risk of unanticipated loss of the pump twin, but intervention with substantive instrumentation (e.g. using radiofrequency ablation) has a higher risk of loss at an earlier gestation.[18] A wide range of approaches for therapeutic intervention have been reported with varying rates of success over the past 20 years. In most cases, the cord of the acardiac twin is extremely short and this fetus is held close to the placenta, making access for bipolar cord occlusion difficult. At this point in time, the two most common approaches used for treatment involve interstitial laser (particularly popular amongst those that promote an early intervention) and radiofrequency ablation.[19,20] Survival rates of the pump twin are estimated around 80%.

Higher-Order Multiples

Higher-order multiples are less common and there is little literature describing management of discordant anomalies in these pregnancies. The intervention will depend on the anomaly, gestation and pattern of chorionicity. As risks of preterm birth are inherently higher in higher-order multiples, the procedural risk and impact may be lower than that seen in twins. One systematic review, including a variety of indications for reduction, noted a reduction in preterm births from 33.3% in triplets managed conservatively to 5.5% when the pregnancy was reduced to a singleton, and 11.8–17.6% when reduced to twins.[21]

Key Points

- More than 3% of twin pregnancies will be discordant for fetal abnormality.
- Whilst anomaly rates are similar in dichorionic twins, they are three to five times more common in monochorionic twins.
- The central nervous, facial, cardiac and gastrointestinal systems are most prevalent.
- Accurate determination of chorionicity is central to management.
- Management decisions need to be made according to balance of benefits and harms and should be shared with the patient.

References

1. Boyle B, McConkey R, Garne E et al. Trends in the prevalence, risk and pregnancy outcome of multiple births with congenital anomaly: a registry-based study in 14 European countries 1984–2007. BJOG 2013;**120**:707–16.

2. Weber MA, Sebire NJ. Genetics and developmental pathology of twinning. Semin Fetal Neonatal Med 2010;**15**:313–18.

3. Silva S, Martins Y, Matias A, Blickstein I. Why are monozygotic twins different? J. Perinat Med 2011;**39**:195–202.

4. Cuckle H, Benn P. Review of epidemiological factors (other than maternal age) that determine the prevalence of common autosomal trisomies. Prenat Diagn 2020; **41**(5):536–44. Portico. https://doi.org/10.1002/pd.5822

5. D'Antonio F, Familiari A, Thilaganathan B et al. Sensitivity of first-trimester ultrasound in the detection of congenital anomalies in twin pregnancies: population study and systematic review. Acta Obstet Gynecol Scand 2016 Dec;**95**(12):1359–67.

6. Phillips T, Moore B, Posma E, Gillam L, Cuzzilla R, Cole S. Ethical considerations in multiple pregnancy: preterm delivery in the setting of discordant fetal anomaly. Twin Res Hum Genet 2019;**22**:120–3.

7. Vandecruys H, Avgidou K, Surerus E, Flack N, Nicolaides KH. Dilemmas in the management of twins discordant for anencephaly diagnosed at 11+0 to 13+6 weeks of gestation. Ultrasound Obstet Gynecol 2006;**28**:653–8.

8. Lust A, De Catte L, Lewi L, Deprest J, Loquet P, Devlieger R. Monochorionic and dichorionic twin pregnancies discordant for fetal anencephaly: a systematic review of prenatal management options. Prenat Diagn 2008;**28**:275–9.

9. Algeri P, Russo FM, Incerti M et al. Expectant management in dichorionic pregnancies complicated by discordant

anomalous twin. J. Perinat Med 2018;**46**:721–7.

10. Nassar AH, Adra AM, Gomez-Marin O, O'Sullivan MJ. Perinatal outcome of twin pregnancies with one structurally affected fetus: a case-controlled study. J Perinatol 2000;**20**:82–6.

11. Evans MI, Goldberg JD, Horenstein J et al. Selective termination for structural, chromosomal and Mendelian anomalies: international experience. AJOG 1999;**181**:893–7.

12. Egan E, Reidy K, O'Brien L, Erwin R, Umstad M. The outcome of twin pregnancies discordant for trisomy 21. Twin Res Hum Genet 2014 Feb;**17**(1):38–44.

13. Lanna MM, Rustico MA, Dell'Avanzo M et al. Bipolar cord coagulation for selective feticide in complicated monochorionic twin pregnancies: 118 consecutive cases at a single center. Ultrasound Obstet Gynecol 2012;**39**:407–13.

14. O'Donoghue K, Barigye O, Pasquini L, Chappell L, Wimalasundera RC, Fisk NM. Interstitial laser therapy for fetal reduction in monochorionic multiple pregnancy: loss rate and association with aplasia cutis congenita. Prenat Diagn 2008;**28**:535–43.

15. Paramasivam G, Wimalasundera R, Wiechec M, Zhang E, Saeed F, Kumar S. Radiofrequency ablation for selective reduction in complex monochorionic pregnancies. BJOG 2010;**117**:1294–8.

16. Gaerty K, Greer RM, Kumar S. Systematic review and meta-analysis of perinatal outcomes after radiofrequency ablation and bipolar cord occlusion in monochorionic pregnancies. Am J Obstet Gynecol 2015;**213**:637–43.

17. Valsky DV, Martinez-Serrano MJ, Sanz M et al. Cord occlusion followed by LASER cord transection in monochorionic monoamniotic discordant twins. Ultrasound Obstet Gynecol 2011;**37**:684–8.

18. Chaveeva P, Poon LC, Sotiriadis A, Kosinski P, Nicolaides KH. Optimal method and timing of intrauterine intervention in twin reversed arterial perfusion sequence: case study and meta-analysis. Eur J Obstet Gynecol Reprod Biol 2013;**166**:127–32.

19. Pagani G, D'Antonio F, Khalil A, Papageorghiou A, Bhide A, Thilaganathan B. Intrafetal laser treatment for twin reversed arterial perfusion sequence: cohort study and meta-analysis. Ultrasound Obstet Gynecol 2013;**42**:6–14.

20. Lee H, Bebbington M, Crombleholme TM. The North American Fetal Therapy Network registry data on outcomes of radiofrequency ablation for twin-reversed arterial perfusion sequence. Fetal Diagn Ther 2013;**33**:224–9.

21. Morlando M, Ferrara L, D'Antonio F et al. Dichorionic triplet pregnancies: risk of miscarriage and severe preterm delivery with fetal reduction versus expectant management. Outcome of a cohort study and systematic review. BJOG 2015;**122**:1053–60.

Single and Double Fetal Loss in Twin Pregnancy

Mark D. Kilby, Leo Gurney, Janice L. Gibson and R. Katie Morris

The Facts

First-Trimester Single Fetal Demise

Loss of a twin before 12 weeks of gestation may be referred to as 'vanishing twin syndrome'. Due to the non-viable embryo becoming incorporated into placental membranes, a proportion of such pregnancies will be unrecognised and misclassified as singleton gestations. Determining the rate of first-trimester twin loss is therefore difficult. When diagnosed, early co-twin loss does not seem to be associated with subsequent morbidity in surviving infants; however, it has an important implication for the interpretation of non-invasive prenatal chromosome anomaly screening and may contribute to an increased risk of 'false positive' results.[1]

Spontaneous Second- or Third-Trimester Fetal Loss

A single twin demise in the second or third trimester of a pregnancy (in either monochorionic (MC) twins or dichorionic twins (DC) twins) should be considered differently to earlier loss as it is associated with increased risk of late miscarriage, stillbirth, preterm birth and morbidity for the surviving twin.[2]

Rates of Second- or Third-Trimester Fetal Loss in Twin Pregnancy

Within the UK, twin stillbirth (after 24 weeks) and infant death surveillance data are presented annually within UK-MBRRACE perinatal mortality reports. The most recent publication assessed pregnancy losses in 2017 and demonstrated a stillbirth rate of twin fetuses of 6.99 per 1,000 live-born twin infants.[3] This is more than double the stillbirth rate of singleton fetuses (3 per 1,000 live-born singletons). There has, however, been a progressive reduction in UK twin stillbirth rates, with an apparent drop from 11.07 per 1,000 live twin births since 2014 documented in UK-MBRRACE reports and over the longer term from 16.7 per 1,000 live twin births in 2000 documented in preceding national perinatal surveillance programmes.[4] This provides encouragement that a number of national and international guidelines published during these time frames have had some positive effect on the outcomes of these high-risk pregnancies through the promotion of specialist and structured management.

The chorionicity of a twin pregnancy has an important influence on risk of fetal loss. National data on the rate of stillbirths in twins divided by chorionicity are difficult to obtain and are still not reported universally in multiple pregnancy research. Surveillance data of twin pregnancy outcomes collected through MBRRACE-UK now record the chorionicity of demised fetuses in more than 95% of cases. Calculations of rates of loss are hindered by the lack of linked national denominator data (live-born twins subdivided by chorionicity). However, applying an assumption that 80% of live-born twins are dichorionic to the MBRRACE-UK loss data collected between 2016 and 2018, it can be estimated that stillbirth rates fell from 27 to 19 per 1,000 live twin births in MC twins, and from 5 to 3 per 1,000 live twin births in DC twins.[4]

The reports do not calculate the rates of single compared to double in utero loss in twin pregnancies, however the majority appear to be single fetal losses.[3] The importance of more detailed data in twin pregnancies is recognised and forms the basis of a current case-based audit by UK-MBRRACE. An additional consideration when using national data to inform fetal loss rates is that although these national reports also include a separate data set on fetal losses from 22 to 24 weeks of pregnancy, complications of MC twin pregnancies, such as twin–twin transfusion syndrome (TTTS) and severe selective growth restriction (sGR), may present early in the second trimester and be associated with fetal demise at gestations earlier than 22 weeks and therefore remain hidden from national statistics.[4]

Aetiology of Fetal Loss in Twin Pregnancy

Maternal Causes of Fetal Loss

Compared to singletons, a higher incidence of pregnancy-related maternal conditions is associated with an increased risk of stillbirth, such as hypertensive disorders and gestational diabetes. Additionally, pre-existing maternal autoimmune, cardiac and renal disease can predispose to fetal loss, with such risks increased in multiple pregnancy.

Fetal Causes of Loss

Most DC twin pregnancies are dizygotic and therefore, as each embryo is associated with its own aneuploidy risk, the overall per-pregnancy aneuploidy risk is nearly twofold that of singletons. In contrast, except in rare cases of discordant chromosome anomalies (heterokaryotypic monozygotism), MC twin pregnancies have a similar per-pregnancy aneuploidy risk to singleton pregnancies (albeit with both fetuses affected). In addition to an aneuploidy causing fetal loss, a risk of loss accompanies the screening programme for such fetal chromosome anomalies. Twin pregnancies that undergo first-trimester screening for aneuploidy (by nuchal measurement, serum biochemistry or free fetal DNA) are subject to a greater false positive rate compared with singleton pregnancies, which may lead to an increased likelihood of being offered prenatal invasive testing. The risks of pregnancy loss following invasive testing are increased, with a loss rate up to 3.8% following chorionic villus sampling and 3.1% following amniocentesis, compared with rates of 0.5–1% for singletons.[5]

Monozygotic twins (all MC twins and approximately 20% of DC twins) are at increased risk of structural anomalies. The pathology reflects problems that can occur during embryonic cleavage with complex midline structures at particular risk, giving an increased risk of cardiac and neural tube abnormalities.[6] Structural anomalies may place the affected fetus and the co-twin at risk of in utero demise, with additional iatrogenic risk if selective termination of pregnancy is opted for.

Placental and Membrane Causes of Fetal Loss

Utero-placental dysfunction occurs more commonly in twin pregnancies, predisposing fetuses to intrauterine growth restriction. Although both fetuses may be affected, it is frequently selective, affecting one of the pair. Selective growth restriction is defined as a condition whereby one fetus is growth restricted, defined as < 10th centile for estimated fetal weight (EFW), alongside an inter-twin growth discordance of > 25%. At these thresholds there is a significant risk of in utero demise of the growth-restricted fetus. Management of sGR is more complex than that of growth restriction complicating a singleton pregnancy as the risks of interventions to both fetuses must be considered.

In DC twin pregnancies, if sGR is diagnosed at early viable gestations, then iatrogenic early delivery will remove the risk of in utero demise of a compromised twin, but may be associated with unacceptable risks of neonatal mortality and morbidity due to prematurity. In such a situation, a conservative approach in the interests of the appropriately grown twin may be justified. In MC twin pregnancies, the management is even more complex as in utero loss rates of individual fetuses are less independent because of the shared fetal circulations within the single placenta. Selective termination of pregnancy by vascular occlusive methods at pre-viable gestations or an earlier gestational threshold for premature delivery are options to try to reduce the risks of double fetal loss.

As well as increasing the incidence and complicating the management of severe sGR, the shared placenta of monochorionic twins places these fetuses at risk of the specific complications of TTTS, twin anaemia polycythaemia sequence (TAPS) and monoamnionicity. Twin–twin transfusion syndrome occurs in up to 15% of MCDA twin pregnancies and without interventional therapy, the risk of death for both twins is high (80–90%).

Treatments for TTTS such as fetoscopic laser ablation (FLA) (or more rarely serial amnioreduction) offer the possibility of improved survival for one or both affected twins. Fetoscopic laser ablation is associated with an improvement in survival without neurological impairment and is the recommended treatment of TTTS where available.[7] Equatorial laser 'dichorionisation' (the Solomon technique) can reduce the risk of TTTS recurrence or subsequent TAPS compared to selective ablation of anastomosis.[8] Internationally, FLA offers up to 75% overall survival rate for MC pregnancies complicated by TTTS.[9] Thus, although TTTS outcomes are greatly improved with treatment, a chance remains of single (20–25%) or double (10–15%) fetal loss from which, given the invasive nature of the procedure, there may be an iatrogenic contribution.[7]

Twin anaemia polycythaemia sequence is defined by a significant discordance in haemoglobin levels between twins without substantial differences in amniotic fluid volume. It is thought to occur from a chronic transfusion of blood from a donor to recipient fetus via miniscule (< 1 mm) artery–vein anastomoses. It affects 2% of MCDA pregnancies spontaneously, but this may increase to 13% following FLA if the Solomon technique is not utilised.[7] Twin pregnancies with this condition will be at increased risk of miscarriage and stillbirth; however, there is little evidence from prospective cohort studies regarding outcomes and optimal clinical management of this pathology.

Monochorionic-monoamniotic (MCMA) twin pregnancies are rare, constituting 5% of all monochorionic pregnancies but < 1% of all twin pregnancies.[10] They have a very high fetal and perinatal loss rate of 50% prior to 16 weeks of gestation, secondary to fetal abnormality or spontaneous miscarriage. Loss rates at later gestations have fallen from 40% to 10–15%, largely due to the management of such cases in specialist centres and delivery at an optimal preterm gestation. Monochorionic-monoamniotic twins are at increased risk of fetal loss from 34 weeks of gestation and therefore delivery via caesarean section is indicated between 32 and 33+6 weeks of pregnancy.

A reported rate of preterm, pre-labour rupture of the membranes (PPROM) in twin pregnancies of 11% versus a singleton rate of 3–4% can expose the pregnancy to ascending bacterial infection with the potential to place either twin at risk of preterm birth, stillbirth or early neonatal death. As with singletons, transplacental infections such as cytomegalovirus or parvovirus B19 are recognised causes of stillbirth for twins.

Iatrogenic Fetal Loss

The main iatrogenic cause of fetal loss in twin pregnancies is selective feticide. This may be performed in cases of discordant fetal chromosomes or structural anomaly in any twin pregnancy, or if there is evidence of severe single fetal compromise in a monochorionic twin pregnancy, such as severe early-onset sGR. The method of feticide will depend on the chorionicity of the pregnancy. Ultrasound-guided injection of an abortifactant into the fetal circulation of the affected twin is only appropriate for DC pregnancies (with discordant fetal circulations) and is associated with an incidence of overall pregnancy loss of 7% and a preterm birth risk of 14% before 32 weeks. In monochorionic twins, due to the shared feto-placental circulation, vascular occlusive procedures including ultrasound-guided intra-fetal laser (IL), usually < 16 weeks; radiofrequency ablation (RFA) up to 22 weeks; or bipolar cord occlusion (BCO) are required for selective feticide to minimise risks to the surviving co-twin. Case series have demonstrated variation in risk of further fetal loss from 12.5% to 7.7% with RFA associated with the lowest co-twin loss rate and risk of amniorrhexis.[11]

Pregnancy-Associated Risks following Spontaneous Single Intrauterine Fetal Death

The prognosis of the co-twin after spontaneous single intrauterine fetal death (sIUFD) has been analysed in systematic reviews and meta-analysis of the literature, the most recent published in 2019.[2] In this review, pregnancies were stratified to allow for separate analysis according to chorionicity of pregnancy.

As can be seen in the results summary in Table 12.1, these data indicate an approximately twofold increased risk for co-twin death in MC (41%) compared to DC pregnancy (22.4%) following a single intrauterine twin death, with rates of neonatal deaths also increased for MC pregnancies (27.8% vs 21.2%). For MC twins, when sIUFD occurred at less than 28 weeks, there was a significantly increased rate of co-twin fetal intrauterine death (OR 2.31, 95% CI 1.02–5.25) or neonatal death (OR 2.84, 95% CI 1.14–20.47) compared to twin gestations where the initial sIUFD occurred after 28 weeks of gestation.[2]

Co-twin survivors of sIUFD are also at significantly increased risk of neurodevelopmental abnormalities when compared to viable twin pregnancy controls. In cases of sIUFD, surviving co-twins are at greater risk of subsequent cerebral palsy (CP) than pregnancies where both twins survive (OR 6.3; 95% CI: 3.1–12.8)[2] and chorionicity again appears to be a key determinant of risk: epidemiological studies reviewing the rates of CP for survivors in pregnancies affected by single twin demise, using same- or different-sex twins as a surrogate means of determining chorionicity, found a rate of CP of 106 per 1,000 for same-sex twins, compared with 26 per 1,000 for different-sex twins.[12] Data from

Table 12.1 Adverse outcomes affecting surviving co-twin following single intrauterine fetal death. Adapted from Mackie et al.[2] Table includes the monochorionic and dichorionic event rates and comparative odds ratios for the following outcomes: co-twin death, preterm birth (less than 34 weeks), abnormal fetal brain MRI, other abnormal fetal brain imaging, neurodevelopmental morbidity and neonatal death.

Adverse co-twin event	Monochorionic event rate (number of studied pregnancies)	Dichorionic event rate (number of studied pregnancies)
Intrauterine fetal death	41% (379)	22% (255)
Abnormal antenatal brain fMRI	20% (116)	
Preterm birth (24+0 to 34+0 weeks of gestation)	58% (202)	54% (107)
Neonatal death	28% (206)	21% (130)
Neurodevelopmental morbidity	28% (103)	10% (62)
Abnormal postnatal brain imaging (CT, MRI or USS)	43% (140)	21% (75)

systematic reviews report event rates for neurodevelopmental abnormality of 28.5% for monochorionic twins and 10% for dichorionic twins after sIUFD.[2] However, such figures must be viewed in the context of the high risk of premature birth for twin pregnancies in general and following IUFD as prematurity can predispose towards or cause secondary neurological disability.

For both MC and DC pregnancies, there is an increased risk of preterm birth following sIUFD, with systematic reviews finding an increased risk of preterm birth between 24+0 and 34+0 weeks gestation for the remaining co-twin of 58.5% for MC and 53.7% for DC pregnancies. The limited data available suggest that iatrogenic preterm birth occurs more commonly in MC pregnancies, possibly indicating a lower threshold for clinical intervention due to the increased risks faced by these pregnancies.[6]

An increase in maternal hypertensive disorders in twin pregnancies following sIUFD has been observed when compared to viable twin pregnancy controls; however, there is no published evidence to date suggesting an increased risk of maternal coagulopathy or sepsis for a mother of a twin pregnancy complicated by a single fetal loss.

The Issues

Can Spontaneous Intrauterine Fetal Death Be Avoided?

As described earlier in this chapter, there are a broad range of predisposing factors to sIUFD, including maternal risks, fetal risks and those specifically relating to chorionicity. National guidance should be followed wherever possible and twin pregnancies should be managed within multidisciplinary teams with a specialist interest in such pregnancies. Given the potentially very high risks of stillbirth, MCMA pregnancies should be managed in fetal medicine centres with specialist expertise.

Any pre-existing maternal illness which may confer additional risk to the pregnancy (e.g. anti-phospholipid syndrome, diabetes mellitus, other autoimmune or maternal renal or cardiac disease) should be identified and management optimised prior to and during the pregnancy in specialised maternal medicine clinics. Additionally, the pregnancy-associated conditions of gestational diabetes and hypertensive disorders of pregnancy should be appropriately screened for and managed if they arise. Careful discussion and counselling regarding the dilemmas associated with twin aneuploidy and anomaly screening, including the iatrogenic risks of invasive investigations or feticide, should be fully discussed with parents prior to testing.

For all twin pregnancies, regular ultrasonographic assessment of fetal biometry, liquor volume and umbilical artery Doppler velocimetry is advised. In DC pregnancy, this can be performed every three to four weeks from 20 weeks of gestation onwards, although this may need to be more frequent and include more advanced Doppler assessments should there be concerns regarding fetal growth or well-being. Fortnightly screening for TTTS and sGR in MC pregnancies should begin at 16 weeks and continue throughout the pregnancy, to include ultrasonographic assessment of fetal biometry, liquor volume and umbilical artery Doppler velocimetry. When diagnosed using ultrasound, TTTS should be clinically staged using the Quintero system (with assessment of twin fetal cardiac function) and referred to specialist fetal medicine centres for assessment. Although routine screening for TAPS has not been recommended nationally in the UK in uncomplicated MC twins, for high-risk cases (those with TTTS or who have undergone FLA), serial middle cerebral artery peak systolic velocity (MCA-PSV) measurements should be performed on both twins.[13]

Data from systematic reviews evaluating risk of stillbirth in twins demonstrated that risk of stillbirth increases progressively with later gestations and the risk of neonatal complications diminishes to favour delivery at 36–37 weeks in uncomplicated MC pregnancies and delivery at 37–38 weeks in uncomplicated DC pregnancies.[14]

What Monitoring Should Take Place after Spontaneous Intrauterine Fetal Death?

Following sIUFD in DC pregnancy, although there is no increased risk of antenatal neurological co-twin damage, there is a twofold increased risk of co-twin death and a risk of preterm birth before 34 weeks of 53.7%.[2] There is no clear evidence base to guide clinicians on the best means of avoiding these outcomes, and therefore individuals should be managed on a case-by-case basis. Regular ultrasound surveillance of the remaining co-twin should occur to assess fetal growth, liquor volume and umbilical artery Doppler velocimetry, the timing of which can be tailored according to current fetal status and to support maternal psychological well-being. Surveillance for preterm birth should be limited to patient education regarding the risks, any signs and symptoms and an awareness of the importance of early presentation to a unit with appropriate neonatal facilities. In situations where preterm labour is suspected or preterm delivery is planned, interventions such as antenatal steroids to aid fetal lung maturity or magnesium sulphate for fetal neuroprotection should be considered based on a critical assessment of optimal benefit according to fetal gestation.

The increased risk of stillbirth and neurological morbidity for MC co-twin survivors has been explained by a 'transfusional hypothesis' whereby a single twin demise leads to a comparative fall in the vascular pressure for the chorionic unit supplying the demised twin, compared to the area supplying the surviving twin, and thus leads to an acute transfusion from the survivor to the demised twin. Evidence for this theory derives from a study examining the results of fetal blood sampling following a single twin death in a series of eight twins: samples taken from surviving twins following loss of the co-twin demonstrated significant new-onset anaemia.[15]

In MC pregnancies complicated by sIUFD, MCA-PSV Doppler studies performed on co-twin survivors before and after in utero fetal blood sampling and intrauterine transfusion (IUT) have demonstrated good correlation between MCA-PSV and pre- and post-transfusion haemoglobin concentration. Thus, surveillance of MCA PSV can be recommended from within 24 hours for surviving co-twins of monochorionic pregnancies complicated by sIUFD, and it may be suitable to continue this surveillance through the pregnancy according to an individualised plan (Figure 12.1).

Following sIUFD in MC twin pregnancies as described for DC pregnancies, regular ongoing ultrasound assessment of fetal well-being should be performed. Without evidence to guide the frequency of these ultrasound assessments, weekly assessments of liquor volume, comprehensive Doppler studies and brain structure are suggested by the authors for four weeks (with biometry performed fortnightly) following sIUFD. If reassuring, these may be spaced to fortnightly intervals with maternal anxieties taken into consideration.

Although fetal brain lesions in up to 4.9% of MC co-twin survivors may be identified by ultrasound within a week of sIUFD, in utero MRI (iuMRI) can improve this detection rate by 33%. The largest multicentre study examining antenatal iuMRI fetal brain changes in surviving MC co-twins demonstrated ventriculomegaly as the only intracranial finding in 3.4%, and other abnormalities in 9.7% of surviving twins. The pattern of neurologic acquired anomaly may range from focal ischaemic lesions (with or without reparative polymicrogyria) to global ischaemic or haemorrhagic abnormalities.[16,17] An iuMRI image demonstrating an example of reparative polymicrogyria in a surviving MC co-twin is displayed in Figure 12.2. Recent evidence supports that, where available, an assessment of brain damage can be performed with higher resolution single-shot fast-spin-echo T2-weighted MRI sequences from seven days after fetal demise.[16]

If an iuMRI for a surviving MC co-twin is performed prior to 28 weeks and is normal, then further iuMRI later in pregnancy may be considered to pick up neuronal migration disorders that may have been acquired. If a brain lesion associated with neurodevelopmental morbidity is confirmed radiologically, the option of terminating the pregnancy should be discussed with the parents in a non-judgmental fashion.

Can Co-twin Sequelae following Spontaneous Intrauterine Fetal Death Be Avoided?

Additional to the risks of preterm delivery, surviving co-twins of an MC pregnancy complicated by sIUFD are at increased risk of stillbirth and neurological insult. Due to the complex nature of decision-making involving such pregnancies, referral to a specialist centre for further management is recommended.

In a case series reporting on pregnancy outcomes following intrauterine transfusion (IUT) for MC co-twin survivors, all non-anaemic babies achieved normal outcomes. Anaemic babies receiving intrauterine transfusion demonstrated improved survival, but up to 30% of these babies had subsequent neurological abnormalities.[18] Therefore, fetal blood sampling and IUT can be offered in cases where fetal anaemia of the remaining co-twin is suspected on

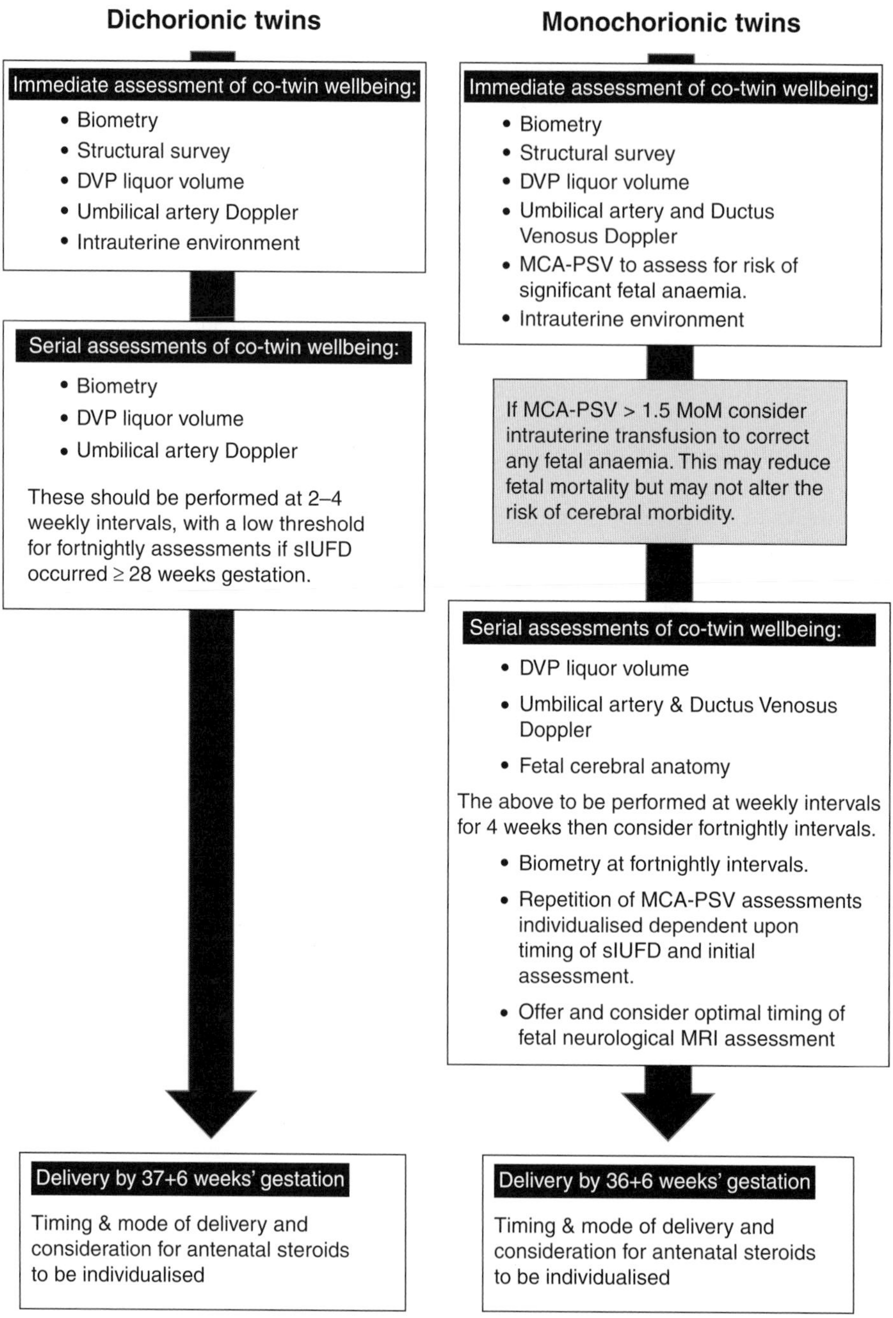

Dichorionic twins

Immediate assessment of co-twin wellbeing:

- Biometry
- Structural survey
- DVP liquor volume
- Umbilical artery Doppler
- Intrauterine environment

Serial assessments of co-twin wellbeing:

- Biometry
- DVP liquor volume
- Umbilical artery Doppler

These should be performed at 2–4 weekly intervals, with a low threshold for fortnightly assessments if sIUFD occurred ≥ 28 weeks gestation.

Delivery by 37+6 weeks' gestation

Timing & mode of delivery and consideration for antenatal steroids to be individualised

Monochorionic twins

Immediate assessment of co-twin wellbeing:

- Biometry
- Structural survey
- DVP liquor volume
- Umbilical artery and Ductus Venosus Doppler
- MCA-PSV to assess for risk of significant fetal anaemia.
- Intrauterine environment

If MCA-PSV > 1.5 MoM consider intrauterine transfusion to correct any fetal anaemia. This may reduce fetal mortality but may not alter the risk of cerebral morbidity.

Serial assessments of co-twin wellbeing:

- DVP liquor volume
- Umbilical artery & Ductus Venosus Doppler
- Fetal cerebral anatomy

The above to be performed at weekly intervals for 4 weeks then consider fortnightly intervals.

- Biometry at fortnightly intervals.
- Repetition of MCA-PSV assessments individualised dependent upon timing of sIUFD and initial assessment.
- Offer and consider optimal timing of fetal neurological MRI assessment

Delivery by 36+6 weeks' gestation

Timing & mode of delivery and consideration for antenatal steroids to be individualised

Figure 12.1 Authors' suggested management approach for co-twin survivors in cases of single in utero fetal demise for both dichorionic and monochorionic pregnancies

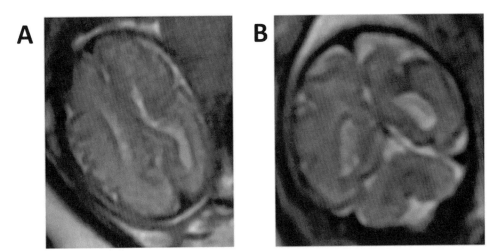

Figure 12.2 Example of reparative polymicrogyria in surviving MC co-twin. Adapted from Griffiths et al.[17] Exact time of single intrauterine demise is unknown but is after 27 weeks of gestation. The iuMRI performed here at 32 weeks shows an abnormal cleft in the left paracentral lobe lined by abnormal cortex (A axial and B coronal single-shot, fast-spin echo images). This can be interpreted as a site of previous infarct and reparative polymicrogyria.

the basis of abnormal MCA-PSV; however, parents should be aware that although the evidence supports improved survival, it may not alter the neurological prognosis.

Iatrogenic considerations can influence the subsequent prognosis of surviving co-twins following sIUFD. For dichorionic pregnancies undergoing selective feticide for fetal anomaly, it is an option to delay the procedure until advanced gestations (32–34 weeks) due to procedure-related complications (i.e. amniorrhexis) increasing risks of preterm birth. However, it should be taken into account that the anomalous twin itself may increase the risk of a preterm birth occurring and therefore the possible window for performing selective termination may be lost.

Selective feticide procedures for MC pregnancies may carry a risk to the co-twin dependent on the type of procedure with procedure-related co-twin death appearing to be higher with interstitial laser (12.5%) than with the use of bipolar cord occlusion (9.1%) or radiofrequency ablation techniques (7.5%).[11] The incidence of neurodevelopmental impairment in MC co-twin survivors following selective feticide has been reported in long-term follow-up data as 6.8%, which compares favourably with a rate of 28.5% for MC co-twin survivors of spontaneous sIUFD.[19]

Studies examining neurological outcome from MC twins following FLA for TTTS do not demonstrate differences between pregnancies where subsequent fetal loss occurs, compared to those where both twins survive. This may suggest that ablation of inter-twin placental anastomosis confers a protective effect on surviving co-twins in the event of sIUFD. Technique of ablation does not directly appear to affect risk of neurological morbidity, with data from randomised controlled trials comparing the Solomon technique with standard anastomotic ablation reporting similar subsequent rates of severe cerebral injury (5% and 6% respectively).[8] Despite this, the Solomon technique is shown to reduce rates of recurrent TTTS and post-laser TAPS and theoretically this should have a neuroprotective benefit for surviving co-twins.

How and When Should Delivery Take Place after Spontaneous Intrauterine Fetal Death?

Dichorionic twins do not share a circulation and there is not an increased risk of antenatal neurological damage to the surviving co-twin following sIUFD, and therefore preterm birth is the most prominent risk faced by such pregnancies. Although limited outcome data are available for preterm twin pregnancies, it is recognised that for singleton pregnancies, moderate to late preterm deliveries (32–36 weeks) can exhibit mild developmental delay at two years of age when compared to full-term controls. Therefore, in the absence of evidence of maternal or fetal compromise, aiming to prolong the pregnancy towards 37 weeks of gestation is advisable.

For MC pregnancies complicated by sIUFD, the initial management dilemma is whether to choose conservative surveillance of the pregnancy in order to advance fetal gestation or opt for immediate delivery. There is little evidence to guide the obstetrician as to whether immediate delivery is of benefit or harm. Several considerations must be balanced: co-twin demise appears more likely within seven days of sIUFD, large placental vascular anastomoses predispose to adverse outcome and detailed ultrasound assessment of the surviving co-twin is the primary indicator as to whether the fetus is at imminent risk of loss. The exact timing of neurological insult in MC surviving co-twins following sIUFD is unknown and it is possible that such damage may occur immediately. Therefore, immediate delivery may not be of value in reducing the risk of neurodevelopmental delay in surviving co-twins, even at advanced gestations.

For MC twins, therefore, any decision regarding immediate delivery upon diagnosis of sIUFD will depend upon the current gestational age, available information concerning the surviving fetal condition or maternal well-being, and a weighing up of the ongoing risk of in utero demise compared to the iatrogenic preterm delivery risks of neonatal mortality and morbidity. Where conservative management is implemented, then delivery is likely to be justified earlier than 36–37 weeks with precise timing individualised by the complex interplay of obstetric and maternal concerns.

Vaginal delivery may be considered in twin pregnancies where sIUFD has occurred and decisions regarding mode of delivery can be individualised in discussion with the woman. If the demised twin is presenting, then there is the potential for intra-partum dystocia or obstruction and delivery by caesarean section is typically preferred. For MC pregnancies, there is an increased risk of planned delivery between 34 and 36 weeks of gestation and therefore such pregnancies are more likely to be delivered by caesarean section.

Pregnancy Management following Spontaneous Intrauterine Fetal Death

As with prognosis, the management of sIUFD is highly dependent on chorionicity and gestation. There remains a lack of a strong evidence base for management in cases of sIUFD in multiple pregnancy, with recommendations largely based on case reports, case studies and expert opinion. A suggested approach to the management of such pregnancies is outlined in Figure 12.1. For multiple pregnancies complicated by sIUFD in the first trimester, there is minimal ongoing risk to the remaining co-twin in MC or DC pregnancies other than an increased risk of miscarriage to the whole pregnancy; therefore, a conservative approach throughout the remaining pregnancy is warranted.

Once sIUFD has been confirmed, rhesus-negative mothers should have a Keilhauer test and an appropriate volume of anti-D should be administered to minimise risk of allo-immunisation. The mother should have close surveillance for hypertensive disorders of pregnancy and should be educated about signs and symptoms of preterm labour with advice to present early for assessment if she has any concerns. Ideally, the ongoing monitoring of her pregnancy should be provided though a named multidisciplinary team to whom she can promptly self-refer.

Following delivery, parents should be encouraged to consider the benefits of post-mortem and placental histology to investigate or help confirm the cause of single or double in utero death. Surviving neonates should be assessed for the need of neonatal and paediatric follow-up. Infants delivered preterm and those with known abnormal antenatal neurological findings should have specialised neurodevelopmental follow-up.

Parents should be offered postnatal follow-up with a senior obstetrician, ideally the clinician managing their case prenatally. This discussion should cover what occurred during the pregnancy, review the results of any investigations, talk about any implications for future pregnancies and ensure that parents are managing emotionally and have multidisciplinary support. Loss of a twin is a devastating emotional experience for parents. Educating parents about support and counselling services is important, and referral to perinatal mental health services should be considered if there are risk factors for or evidence of postnatal depression.

Key Points

- Defining rates of single and double twin stillbirth in national surveillance reports is challenging; however, there appears to be an overall trend towards twin stillbirth reduction from UK reported data.
- The causes of twin single or double fetal loss can be considered as maternal causes, fetal causes, causes related to the chorionic and amniotic status of the pregnancy and iatrogenic causes.
- The key determinants of risk posed to the surviving co-twin are chorionicity and gestation.
- Risk of preterm birth is increased following sIUFD for both DC and MC co-twin survivors.
- Monochorionic co-twin survivors are at additional risk of stillbirth, neonatal death and neurological morbidity.
- Management should be tailored to individual pregnancies with chorionicity and gestation at sIUFD key factors in determining approach.
- Post-delivery investigations including full post-mortem should be offered.
- Postnatal follow-up is essential with emotional and bereavement support for parents a vital component of this.

References

1. Van der Meij KRM, Sistermans EA, Macville MVE et al. TRIDENT-2: national implementation of genome-wide non-invasive prenatal testing as a first-tier screening test in the Netherlands. *Am J Hum Genet* 2019 Dec 5;**105**(6):1091–1101.

2. Mackie FL, Rigby A, Morris RK, Kilby MD. Prognosis of the co-twin following

spontaneous single intrauterine fetal death in twin pregnancies: a systematic review and meta-analysis. BJOG 2019 Apr;**126**(5):569–78.

3. MBBRACE-UK. Perinatal Mortality Surveillance Report. 2019. www.npeu.ox.ac.uk/mbrrace-uk/reports

4. Kilby MD, Gibson JL, Ville Y. Falling perinatal mortality in twins in the UK: organisational success or chance? BJOG 2019 Feb;**126**(3):341–7.

5. Agarwal K, Alfirevic Z. Pregnancy loss after chorionic villus sampling and genetic amniocentesis in twin pregnancies: a systematic review. Ultrasound Obstet Gynecol 2012 Aug;**40**(2):128–34.

6. Glinianaia SV, Rankin J, Wright C. Congenital anomalies in twins: a register-based study. Hum Reprod 2008 Jun;**23**(6):1306–11.

7. Roberts D, Neilson JP, Kilby MD, Gates S. Interventions for the treatment of twin-twin transfusion syndrome. *Cochrane Database Syst Rev.* 2014 Jan 30;(1): CD002073. https//:doi.org/10.1002/146518 58.CD002073.pub3. PMID: 24482008.

8. Slaghekke F, Lopriore E, Lewi L et al. Fetoscopic laser coagulation of the vascular equator versus selective coagulation for twin-to-twin transfusion syndrome: an open-label randomised controlled trial. Lancet 2014;**383**(9935):214–51.

9. Müllers SM, McAuliffe FM, Kent E et al. Outcome following selective fetoscopic laser ablation for twin to twin transfusion syndrome: an 8 year national collaborative experience. *Eur J Obstet Gynecol Reprod Biol* 2015;**191**:125–9.

10. Litwinska E, Syngelaki A, Cimpoca B, Frei L, Nicolaides KH. Outcome of twin pregnancy with two live fetuses at 11–13 weeks' gestation. *Ultrasound Obstet Gynecol* 2020;**55**(1):32–8.

11. Nobili E, Paramasivam G, Kumar S. Outcome following selective fetal reduction in monochorionic and dichorionic twin pregnancies discordant for structural, chromosomal and genetic disorders. *Aust NZ J Obstet Gynaecol* 2013;**53**(2):114–18.

12. Pharoah PO, Adi Y. Consequences of in-utero death in a twin pregnancy. Lancet 2000 May 6;**355**(9215):1597–1602.

13. RCOG. Management of monochorionic twin pregnancy: Green-Top Guideline No. 51. BJOG 2017 Jan;**124**(1):e1–e45.

14. Cheong-See F, Schuit E, Arroyo-Manzano D et al. Prospective risk of stillbirth and neonatal complications in twin pregnancies: systematic review and meta-analysis. *BMJ* 2016;**354**:i4353.

15. Nicolini U, Pisoni MP, Cela E, Roberts A. Fetal blood sampling immediately before and within 24 hours of death in monochorionic twin pregnancies complicated by single intrauterine death. Am J Obstet Gynecol 1998 Sep; **179**(3 Pt 1):800–3.

16. Conte G, Righini A, Griffiths PD et al. Brain-injured survivors of monochorionic twin pregnancies complicated by single intrauterine death: MR findings in a multicenter study. Radiology 2018 Aug;**288**(2):582–90.

17. Griffiths PD, Sharrack S, Chan KL, Bamfo J, Williams F, Kilby MD. Fetal brain injury in survivors of twin pregnancies complicated by demise of one twin as assessed by in utero MR imaging. Prenat Diagn 2015 Jun;**35**(6):583–91.

18. Tanawattanacharoen S, Taylor MJ, Letsky EA, Cox PM, Cowan FM, Fisk NM. Intrauterine rescue transfusion in monochorionic multiple pregnancies with recent single intrauterine death. Prenat Diagn 2001 Apr;**21**(4):274–8.

19. Van Klink J, Koopman H, Middeldorp J et al. Long-term neurodevelopmental outcome after selective feticide in monochorionic pregnancies. BJOG 2015;**122**(11):1517–24.

Chapter 13

Management of Twin–Twin Transfusion Syndrome

Christian Bamberg and Kurt Hecher

Introduction

Twin–twin transfusion syndrome (TTTS) is a serious complication of monochorionic (MC) multiple gestations. Monochorionicity is the fundamental underlying prerequisite for TTTS because the fetuses share a single placenta, and almost all cases exhibit placental vascular communications between the umbilical circulations. Three different types of anastomoses have been described (arterio-venous, arterio-arterial and veno-venous), and the type, number and calibre of these anastomoses determine the risk profile for TTTS development.[1] Twin–twin transfusion syndrome usually occurs between 16 and 26 weeks of gestation. Arterio-arterial anastomoses with bidirectional blood flow between the two cord insertions seem to be partially protective against TTTS development and are significantly less common in TTTS cases compared to uncomplicated MC pregnancies. Additionally, compared to uncomplicated MC pregnancies, the artery-to-artery connections in TTTS placentas exhibit a significantly thinner median diameter and a more central location.[2]

The process of placental angiogenesis in MC placentas remains elusive. In the first trimester, multiple anastomoses are present in a random and balanced pattern. It has been hypothesised that in cases of TTTS, during the second trimester, vascular connections are progressively and asymmetrically reduced, leading to dominance of arterio-venous vessels from donor to recipient, allowing a shift of blood.[3] Twin–twin transfusion syndrome results from the imbalanced chronic blood flow through placental anastomoses. The donor commonly exhibits hypovolemia, oliguria and oligohydramnios, while the recipient exhibits hypervolemia, polyuria and polyhydramnios as an expression of fluid overload. These observations emphasise the unique role of the angio-architecture of MC placentation in TTTS development, and may explain why TTTS complicates only 10–15% of MC twin pregnancies during mid-gestation. In the present chapter, we discuss TTTS pathophysiology, diagnosis and optimal treatment,[4] as well as long-term outcomes after laser intervention.

Twin–Twin Transfusion Syndrome Diagnosis

Twin–twin transfusion syndrome is diagnosed by ultrasound, and all MC pregnancies should be screened biweekly by sonography starting at a gestational age of 16 weeks until 26 weeks for this specific complication.[5] Delayed TTTS detection results in deterioration of prognosis in terms of worse perinatal outcome. The main sonographic finding in cases of TTTS is a huge discrepancy in the amount of fluid between the twins' amniotic sacs. The donor twin presents with a small or invisible urinary bladder and oligo- or anhydramnios (deepest vertical pocket of < 2 cm), and often becomes stuck to the uterine wall or placenta. The recipient twin displays an oversized urinary bladder and polyuric polyhydramnios, defined by a deepest vertical pocket of > 8 cm before 20 weeks and > 10 cm after 20 weeks. These amniotic fluid cut-off values are recommended by the Eurofoetus group, but in the United States, most fetal medicine specialists use a cut-off of 8 cm regardless of gestational age. Several pitfalls are faced in amniotic fluid evaluation. Sometimes the donor twin may be wrapped within its membranes and floating freely in an amniotic sling in the polyhydramnios of the recipient twin (cocoon sign). Additionally, the single largest vertical pocket must be measured free from fetal parts or umbilical cord and is dependent on uterine tension. The probe should be gently positioned on the maternal abdomen, perpendicular to the longitudinal axis of the uterus and without tilting.

Monochorionic-monoamniotic (MCMA) twin pregnancies rarely develop TTTS (2–6% prevalence) because there are usually plenty of anastomoses between the umbilical cord insertions, which are often placentally inserted close to each other. In cases of MCMA TTTS, the common amniotic sac exhibits polyhydramnios. The donor twin presents with absent or minimal bladder filling while the recipient twin has a large bladder.

To encourage early detection, healthcare providers should inform mothers about the clinical symptoms of TTTS, which include sudden maternal abdominal swelling disproportionate to gestational age, abdominal discomfort, back pain, a tense and oversized uterus and early contractions. If a woman reports these signs, an ultrasound should be performed immediately and she should be referred to a fetal surgery unit if TTTS is diagnosed.

Twin–Twin Transfusion Syndrome Prediction in the First Trimester

All women carrying a multiple pregnancy should be offered a prenatal ultrasound examination at 11–13 gestational weeks to assess viability, chorionicity, crown–rump length, ductus venosus Doppler velocity waveforms and nuchal translucency. First-trimester identification of MC twins with a high risk for the development of TTTS enables improved surveillance. A recent small prospective study demonstrated that the best predictive marker for TTTS was nuchal translucency discordance of $\geq$ 20% (AUC, 0.79; 95% CI, 0.59–0.99).[6] However, the positive predictive value was only 36%, meaning ultrasound screening is still mandatory. In a large retrospective study including 1,274 MC diamniotic twin pregnancies, the authors analysed data from routine ultrasound examinations at 11–13 gestational weeks.[7] The rate of fetal loss or need for endoscopic laser surgery at < 20 gestational weeks was 24.1% in the subgroup of fetuses with NT $\geq$ 95th percentile and 40.5% in those with NT $\geq$ 99th percentile. Moreover, a systematic review and meta-analysis found that TTTS development was significantly predicted by discrepancy in NT and crown–rump length of > 10%, NT > 95th percentile or abnormal ductus venosus flow on first-trimester ultrasound examination.[8] We performed a prospective study, using three-dimensional ultrasound with colour Doppler imaging to investigate the umbilical coiling index in untreated TTTS cases[9]. On the day of laser surgery, the coiling index was quantified in 65 recipients and 56 donors, revealing that the median coiling index was two-fold higher in recipient twins compared to donor twins (0.55 vs. 0.26; p < 0.0001). This discordance of umbilical cord coiling in TTTS may reflect the recipient's hypervolemia and the donor's hypovolemia. Further investigation is required to evaluate whether evaluation of the inter-twin first trimester coiling index may be useful as an early TTTS predictor.

Twin–Twin Transfusion Syndrome Staging

Prenatal ultrasound staging systems have been developed to provide a standardised method of describing TTTS severity and predicting perinatal outcome. These categorical staging systems were designed to describe a heterogeneous and dynamic clinical entity. The Quintero classification was introduced more than 20 years ago and remains the most frequently used system owing to its simplicity.[10]

At all Quintero stages, polyhydramnios is present in the recipient twin and oligo/anhydramnios is present in the donor twin. The donor twin's bladder is visible during stage I and cannot been seen at stage II. Stage III is characterised by critically abnormal Doppler findings, including absent or reversed end-diastolic flow in the umbilical artery, and/or absent or reversed flow during a-wave in the ductus venosus. Stage IV includes

Table 13.1 The Quintero Staging Classification

Quintero stage	Ultrasound findings	Total (n = 1,020)
I	Oligo- and polyhydramnios sequence, visible donor bladder filling, normal Doppler findings in both twins	184 (18)
II	No visualisation of fetal bladder in donor twin	360 (35.3)
III	Absent or reversed umbilical artery diastolic flow, reversed ductus venosus a-wave, and/or pulsatile umbilical vein	427 (41.9)
IV	Hydrops in one or both fetuses	49 (4.8)

Data are shown as n (%).

hydrops. Table 13.1 summarises the Quintero staging criteria and the prevalence of each stage in our own TTTS laser surgery population.[11]

The Quintero system has several important limitations. For instance, a donor twin may have a visible bladder but abnormal Doppler findings. Two research groups from the United States have incorporated additional cardiovascular parameters for neonatal outcome prediction, based on findings that recipient twins may show signs of heart failure even at early TTTS stages.[12,13] In contrast, donor twins generally show normal echocardiograms. Importantly, the stage may remain stable, regress or rapidly progress, and TTTS often does not progress in a predictable or chronological manner. Intrauterine fetal death can occur at stage I without deterioration to more advanced stages.

Twin–Twin Transfusion Syndrome Treatment

Cases of mild-to-moderate TTTS show amniotic fluid discordance but do not fulfil the criteria of severe TTTS. Membrane folding is frequently observed, but the donor twin is not stuck to the uterine wall. In such cases, weekly ultrasound follow-up is required until the presence or absence of severe TTTS is clear. Most moderate cases remain stable and do not necessitate intervention.

Fetoscopic Laser Surgery

Without treatment, severe TTTS carries an 80–90% risk of perinatal mortality due to intrauterine fetal death, miscarriage or extremely preterm delivery.[14] For severe TTTS, fetoscopic laser surgery is the first-line therapy because it is the only causal therapy by a single intervention. On the other hand, serial amnioreduction of the recipient's polyhydramnios is a symptomatic treatment that reduces the intrauterine pressure and may prolong the pregnancy. However, amniodrainage does not solve the causative problem of the disease. Notably, amnioreduction should be avoided prior to fetoscopy as it may reduce the feasibility and success of laser surgery due to bleeding, chorioamniotic separation or membrane rupture.

Evidence clearly indicates that fetoscopic laser coagulation of placental vascular anastomoses is superior to serial amniodrainages in severe TTTS cases. Senat and co-workers conducted a multicentre randomised controlled trial (RCT) comparing fetoscopic laser therapy with serial amnioreductions in cases of TTTS at between 15 and 26 gestational weeks.[15] The trial was stopped early because interim analysis revealed that compared to serial amnioreductions (n = 70), fetoscopic laser therapy (n = 72) resulted in higher survival of at least one twin, higher gestational age at delivery and better neurological outcomes at all stages.

Technique

Fetoscopy should only performed by highly experienced fetal medicine experts. In preparation for the intervention, careful ultrasound scanning provides the surgeon with essential information such as the extent of the placenta with both cord insertions, localisation of the stuck twin and the expected vascular equator on the placental surface. Twin–twin transfusion syndrome is not associated with an increased risk of chromosomal abnormalities, but fetuses with MC placentation exhibit an increased incidence of congenital abnormalities. Therefore, a detailed fetal anomaly scan including fetal echocardiogram and brain evaluation should always be performed before laser intervention.

Before surgery, a single shot of prophylactic antibiotics is administered and magnesium is administered intravenously to inhibit contractions. After 24 gestational weeks, we administer tractocile as a tocolytic agent, combined with a course of antenatal steroids. Following local anaesthesia of the skin and myometrium, an operating sheath with obturator is inserted percutaneously into the recipient's sac under ultrasound guidance. An optimal insertion site is essential for visualising the entire vascular equator, and should be selected opposite the assumed vascular anastomoses. In cases with an anterior placenta, the entry site should be chosen lateral to the placental margin. Special endoscopes have been developed with a 30° optical system and integrated steering levers for bending of the laser fibre tip upwards to the placenta, as well as curved operating sheaths After insertion of the scope through the sheath, the fetal surgeon will identify several important landmarks such as the cord insertion site of the recipient twin and the inter-twin membrane on the chorionic plate. This is followed by placental mapping, in which the different types of anastomoses are characterised. Diode or Nd:YAG lasers have optimal energy absorbance in the spectrum of haemoglobin and are commonly used to coagulate the anastomoses selectively.

During fetoscopy, the surgeon should also visualise the limbs of the recipient twin because this fetus will sometimes also have polycythaemia and may show signs of thrombosis, primarily in the lower extremities. The laser procedure is completed by draining excess amniotic fluid through the cannula to achieve a deepest vertical pocket of 5–6 cm. The patient is usually discharged between 24 and 48 hours after the procedure and then undergoes weekly ultrasound follow-up examinations. These should always include Doppler blood flow studies of the umbilical artery, middle cerebral artery peak systolic velocity and ductus venosus.

Complications of Fetoscopic Twin–Twin Transfusion Syndrome Treatment

Maternal Complications

Fetoscopy is considered safe for the mother when performed by an experienced specialist. Sacco et al. recently summarised the outcomes of 9,403 fetoscopic surgery patients and reported a severe maternal complication rate of ~2% and a minor complication rate of ~4%.[16] However, due to the lack of standardised evaluation of maternal complications, the incidence of complications may by underreported.

Fetal Complications

Laser surgery may lead to single (21.7%) or double (3.0%) intrauterine fetal demise.[11] In up to 60% of cases, TTTS is accompanied by selective intrauterine growth restriction due to unequal placental sharing.[17] The main risk factors for intrauterine donor death are growth discordance > 30%, reverse end-diastolic flow in the umbilical artery after laser surgery and a marginal or velamentous cord insertion.[18] Risk factors for death of the recipient twin include a reversed a-wave in the ductus venosus and hydrops.[19]

The most common complication of fetoscopic laser surgery is iatrogenic preterm premature rupture of the membranes (PPROM), which mainly occurs due to a persistent membrane defect at the trocar insertion site. Many experts in this field share the opinion that the amniotic access is the Achilles' heel of operative fetoscopy. Stirnemann and colleagues reported the follow-up of 1,017 cases after TTTS treatment with percutaneous fetoscopic laser.[20] Gestational age at surgery before 17 weeks was a significant risk factor for PPROM. However, reducing the diameter of the inserted instruments has decreased the PPROM risk. Observational management is recommended, but preterm delivery occurs on average two weeks earlier than in cases without PPROM. Membrane separation may occur at the entry site of the trocar, and this is associated with increased risk of PPROM and consecutively with a higher risk of preterm delivery before 32 weeks. As mentioned earlier, prematurity is a major challenge in TTTS and the most important risk factor for neonatal mortality and morbidity.

After fetoscopic laser surgery in TTTS, residual placental anastomoses may lead to post-laser twin anaemia-polycythemia sequence (TAPS) and recurrent TTTS. Twin anaemia-polycythemia sequence is defined as a chronic feto-fetal net transfusion of erythrocytes owing to a few missed minuscule arterio-venous anastomoses, which may occur in 3–16% of cases depending on the laser technique.[21,22] It is characterised by large inter-twin haemoglobin differences without discrepancy in amniotic fluid volume. Prenatal diagnosis is made by Doppler ultrasound revealing a significant discordance of peak systolic velocities in the middle cerebral arteries of both twins. There is recurrence of TTTS with a prevalence of 5%, which is characterised by either ongoing or inversed discrepancies in amniotic fluid volumes and bladder fillings, owing to missed larger arterio-venous anastomoses.

Outcomes after Laser Treatment for Twin–Twin Transfusion Syndrome

Perinatal Survival

A recent systematic review summarised 25 years of fetoscopic laser coagulation for TTTS.[23] The authors reported the outcomes of 3,868 women from 34 studies and highlighted the large variations in caseloads and outcomes among different fetal medicine centres. Over the review time period, the mean survival of both twins significantly increased from 35% to 65% and the mean survival of at least one twin significantly increased from 70% to 88%. The average gestational age at birth was 32.4 ± 1.3 weeks.

In 2017, we published a single-centre study of laser therapy in 1,020 pregnancies with severe TTTS.[11] The rate of survival of both twins significantly increased from 50% in the first group of 200 cases to 69.5% in the last group of 220 cases (p = 0.018) and reached a plateau after 600 procedures. The rate of at least one survivor showed a non-significant trend of increase from 80.5% to 91.8% (p = 0.072). The mean gestational age at delivery with at least one live-born twin was 33.7 ± 3.2 weeks. The introduction of 30° scopes with a special mechanism to deflect the laser fibre for anterior placentas led to an improvement of the double survival rate, which was no longer different from posterior placentas.

Neurodevelopment and the Cardiovascular System

We recently published a detailed review of long-term outcomes for MC twins after laser therapy for TTTS, which includes neurodevelopmental and cardiovascular outcomes, growth, renal function and ischemic events.[24] Approximately 2% of survivors after fetoscopic laser surgery exhibit fetal brain lesions (equally distributed between donors and recipients), which may be ischemic or haemorrhagic.[25] Significant risk factors include recurrent TTTS and post-laser TAPS following incomplete laser surgery. Importantly, follow-up studies of TTTS cases treated with laser surgery have reported varying rates of cerebral palsy and neurodevelopment impairment, possibly due to differences in methodology, heterogeneity within small case series and lack of uniform criteria regarding outcome. A review of 13 studies reported a 6.1% prevalence of cerebral palsy and a 9.8% prevalence of neurodevelopmental impairment.[26] Preterm delivery was an independent risk factor for neurodevelopmental impairment after laser treatment. Other important risk factors included increased gestational age at intervention, higher Quintero stage, perinatal severe cerebral injury and low birthweight. In a recent investigation of 434 children who underwent laser surgery for TTTS, follow-up at two years of age revealed a 3% incidence of severe neurodevelopment impairment and a 2% incidence of cerebral palsy.[27] Increased survival rates after TTTS laser surgery have not been associated with a rising risk of neurological damage, suggesting that an improvement of the technique with growing experience is shown at some specialised high volume centres.

Congenital heart defects are more frequent among twins with TTTS compared to uncomplicated MC twins and singletons. Cohort studies have examined the prevalence of heart disease in children after laser therapy for TTTS. Herberg and co-workers analysed 62 survivors at the age of 10 years and found that 6 (9.7%) exhibited structural heart defects.[28] The main finding was pulmonary stenosis, which may affect both former recipient and donor twins.

Management of Stage I Twin–Twin Transfusion Syndrome

Stage I TTTS is defined as discordance of amniotic fluid between the two fetuses, combined with a still visible bladder in the donor twin and normal fetal Doppler blood flow findings in both twins. We currently lack important data regarding the natural history of stage I TTTS cases. Between 10% and 50% of cases (pooled average, 27%) show disease progression to more advanced stages but, unfortunately, there are no clear indicators for predicting progression.[29]

Management of stage I TTTS remains controversial. A systematic review and meta-analysis suggested that the pooled overall survival was 79% with expectant treatment, 77% with amnioreduction, 68% with laser treatment performed after progression and 84% with laser surgery as the first-line choice.[29] In the absence of maternal complications, conservative management with weekly surveillance may be offered at stage I.

A multicentre RCT has been conducted to compare conservative management to immediate laser surgery in stage I TTTS cases between 16+0 and 26+6 gestational weeks. The women were randomly assigned to undergo primary laser surgery within 72 hours or conservative management with weekly ultrasound follow-up. Within the conservative management group, laser treatment was performed in cases that exhibited progression to stage II or higher, severe maternal discomfort due to polyhydramnios and/or cervical shortening < 15 mm. Recently, this study was prematurely completed after 117 inclusions. Intact survival at 6 months was seen in 84 of 109 (77%) expectant cases and in 89 of 114 (78%) immediate surgery cases (p=0.88). In patients followed expectantly, 41% remained stable with a dual intact survival of 86%, whereas it was 78% and 71% followed immediate or rescue surgery, respectively., although these differences were not statistically significant. The authors could not identify any meaningful predictors of progression. (Stirnemann J et al., Am J Obstet Gynecol 2021).

From a practical point of view and based on our experience, visualisation of the donor twin's bladder filling at stage I is often dependent on the duration of the examination. Slight bladder filling without dynamic changes indicates absent voiding due to impaired urine production. Therefore, in our unit, we usually offer laser treatment in all cases with stage I TTTS, particularly in the presence of maternal symptoms and a short cervix.[30]

Premature Cervical Shortening

Cervical shortening in TTTS may presumably be caused by excessive uterine distension due to polyhydramnios. However, the definition of a short cervix is inconsistent (< 10, 20 or 25 mm), and the optimal management (vaginal progesterone, cervical pessary or cerclage) is unclear due to the lack of randomised trials. A multicentre retrospective cohort study (n = 163) evaluated the benefit of cervical cerclage in cases with a cervical length of < 25 mm at the time of fetoscopic laser coagulation. Approximately half of the women received a cerclage, but cerclage placement did not significantly prolong pregnancy (28.8 weeks vs 29.1 weeks at delivery with and without cerclage, respectively) or improve survival rates.[31] Two smaller single-centre studies investigated cerclage performance after laser surgery in TTTS patients with an extremely short cervix (< 10 mm or < 15 mm).[32,33] Both research groups demonstrated that emergency cerclage placement was feasible and improved perinatal outcome. Overall, the benefit of cerclage for TTTS patients with a short cervix remains controversial. Notably, it is clear that premature cervical shortening should not be an exclusion criteria for laser treatment.

Optimal Laser Technique

Although it is a consensus that all vascular anastomoses should be ablated during the fetoscopic laser procedure, it is questionable whether all connecting vessels can be identified and coagulated. Patent anastomoses have been detected in up to one-third of placentas after treatment using standard fetoscopic laser technique.[34] This prompted the development of a modified laser method called the Solomon technique. After identification and selective sequential coagulation of the anastomoses, the laser is used to draw a thin line from one placental edge to the other, connecting the laser dots. The rationale underlying this method is that coagulating the entire vascular equator (dichorionisation) minimises the risk of residual anastomoses that are not visible to the eye.

In the RCT Solomon trial, 274 women were randomly assigned to treatment with the Solomon technique (n = 139) or the standard selective laser method (n = 135).[34] The Solomon technique was associated with significant reductions of recurrent TTTS (1% vs 7%) and post-laser TAPS (3% vs 16%), and the treatment groups did not differ in perinatal mortality or severe neonatal morbidity. The procedure time was identical in both groups; however, the total amount of laser energy was approximately twofold higher with the Solomon technique (9,275 Joule vs 4,933 Joule; p < 0.0001).

Concerns have been raised about whether it is justified to laser healthy placental tissue between the anastomoses, resulting in a greater extent of placental injury.[36] Additionally, a recent report described an increased risk of placental abruption after Solomon laser treatment.[37] The authors concluded that the greater risk of placental abruption with the Solomon technique might be due to more extensive tissue damage of the thinner areas at the placenta edges. The results of these studies must be interpreted cautiously and further long-term investigations are required to determine the correct use of the Solomon technique. In our clinical experience, we favour a partial Solomon technique in which we coagulate an area of neighbouring anastomoses by drawing a line along the vascular equator without unnecessarily sacrificing placental tissue where no vessels at all are detectable on the chorionic plate.

Twin–Twin Transfusion Syndrome in Triplets, before Gestational Week 17 and after Gestational Week 26

Monochorionic triplets may also develop TTTS and such cases should be treated with laser intervention. Among triplet pregnancies, 75% are dichorionic-triamniotic. In MC triplets, the number of donors and recipients varies depending on the placental architecture. If there are two recipients, both amniotic cavities have to be entered to gain access to all anastomoses. D'Antonio and co-workers summarised the perinatal outcomes of triplets after laser treatment for TTTS. Their analysis included eight studies and a total of 126 triplet pregnancies (104 dichorionic triamniotic and 22 monochorionic-triamniotic).[38] Perinatal survival rates of at least one triplet, at least two triplets and all three triplets were 94.1%, 80.2% and 51%, respectively. In general, these pregnancies carried higher risks for extremely preterm birth and for fetal and perinatal loss than twins.

Some evidence suggests that laser treatment for TTTS at a gestational age of < 17 weeks or > 26 weeks is feasible and safe and may improve perinatal outcome.[39] However, only 2.5% of all TTTS patients are affected before 17 gestational weeks. In such cases, the perinatal outcome after conventional laser therapy is comparable to that between 17 and 26 weeks; there is an increased risk of PPROM within one week after laser treatment and a hypothetical chance of spontaneous regression. The prevalence of TTTS after a gestational age of 26 weeks is 4–8%. In such cases, laser therapy may lead to delayed delivery, recovery of both twins in utero and improved neonatal outcome. The presence of turbid amniotic fluid and the increased difficulty of coagulating larger placental vessels may occur at higher gestational weeks.

Timing and Mode of Delivery after Laser Treatment

From our perspective, in the absence of post-laser complications, delivery can be scheduled at between 36/0 and 37/0 gestational weeks. Some experts suggest delivery at 34 gestational weeks, but evidence is lacking for such management. In terms of delivery mode, we offer a vaginal delivery for cases meeting the following criteria: > 32 gestational weeks, vertex presentation of the first twin, appropriate fetal weight and absence of severe weight discordance, normal Doppler and fetal heart tracing results, presence of a trained maternal fetal medicine specialist who is familiar with internal manoeuvres and signed informed consent.

Conclusion

In conclusion, TTTS occurs due to chronic unbalanced blood shunting between MC multiples across placental vascular connections. The treatment of choice is fetoscopic laser coagulation of the anastomoses. For stage I TTTS, some fetal medical centres offer conservative management with close surveillance, but laser treatment is recommended for cases involving a short cervix, maternal discomfort and increasing polyhydramnios. Perinatal survival has significantly improved over the past 30 years since the introduction of fetoscopic laser surgery for TTTS. High-volume centres achieve 70% double twin survival and > 90% survival of at least one twin. Laser therapy should be offered in specialised fetal medicine centres that perform at least 20 procedures per surgeon annually. We have demonstrated that centralisation of TTTS laser treatment improves the survival rates for both twins and the individual learning curve. The ultimate goal of TTTS laser surgery should be double survival with normal long-term neurodevelopment by avoidance of very preterm delivery. There remains a need for prospective studies with standardised evaluation of long-term outcomes.

Key Points

- Severe TTTS affects 10–15% of MC multiples and usually occurs between 16 and 26 gestational weeks.
- All MC pregnancies should be screened and monitored by ultrasound every two weeks until delivery.
- Large discordance of amniotic fluid volume is the main ultrasound finding in TTTS.
- Evidence suggests that fetoscopic laser coagulation of placental anastomoses is the gold standard for TTTS treatment, which is the most frequently performed intrauterine surgery nowadays.
- Specialised laser centres achieve double and at least one survival rates of 70% and > 90%, respectively.
- Centralisation of specialised care for TTTS results in reduced complications and increased intact double survival.
- Long-term studies show incidences of severe neurodevelopmental impairment of 3–13%, which is independently associated with low gestational age at delivery.

References

1. Benirschke K, Masliah E. The placenta in multiple pregnancy: outstanding issues. Reprod Fertil Dev 2001;**13**:615–22.

2. Zhao DP, de Villiers SF, Slaghekke F et al. Prevalence, size, number and localization of vascular anastomoses in monochorionic placentas. Placenta 2013;**34**:589–93.

3. Sebire NJ, Talbert D, Fisk NM. Twin-to-twin transfusion syndrome results from dynamic asymmetrical reduction in placental anastomoses: a hypothesis. Placenta 2001;**22**:383–91.

4. Bamberg C, Hecher K. Twin-to-twin transfusion syndrome: Controversies in the diagnosis and management. Best Pract Res Clin Obstet Gynaecol 2022; doi: 10.1016/j.bpobgyn.2022.03.013. Online ahead of print.

5. Khalil A, Rodgers M, Baschat A et al. ISUOG practice guidelines: role of ultrasound in twin pregnancy. Ultrasound Obstet Gynecol 2016;**47**:247–63.

6. Mogra R, Saaid R, Tooher J, Pedersen L, Kesby G, Hyett J. Prospective validation of first-trimester ultrasound characteristics as predictive tools for twin–twin transfusion syndrome and selective intrauterine growth restriction in monochorionic diamniotic twin pregnancies. Fetal Diagn Ther 2020;**47**(4):321–7.

7. Cimpoca B, Syngelaki A, Litwinska E, Muzaferovic A, Nicolaides KH. Increased nuchal translucency at 11–13 weeks' gestation and outcome in twin pregnancy. Ultrasound Obstet Gynecol 2020;**55**:318–25.

8. Stagnati V, Zanardini C, Fichera A et al. Early prediction of twin-to-twin transfusion syndrome: systematic review and meta-analysis. Ultrasound Obstet Gynecol 2017;**49**:573–82.

9. Bamberg C, Diemert A, Glosemeyer P, Tavares de Sousa M, Hecher K. Discordance of umbilical coiling index between recipients and donors in twin-twin transfusion syndrome. Placenta 2019;**76**:19–22.

10. Quintero RA, Morales WJ, Allen MH, Bornick PW, Johnson PK, Kruger M. Staging of twin–twin transfusion syndrome. J Perinatol 1999;**19**:550–5.

11. Diehl W, Diemert A, Grasso D, Sehner S, Wegscheider K, Hecher K. Fetoscopic laser coagulation in 1020 pregnancies with twin–twin transfusion syndrome demonstrates improvement in double-twin survival rate. Ultrasound Obstet Gynecol 2017;**50**:728–35.

12. Michelfelder E, Gottliebson W, Border W et al. Early manifestations and spectrum of recipient twin cardiomyopathy in twin-twin transfusion syndrome: relation to Quintero stage. Ultrasound Obstet Gynecol 2007;**30**:965–71.

13. Rychik J, Tian Z, Bebbington M et al. The twin–twin transfusion syndrome: spectrum of cardiovascular abnormality and development of a cardiovascular score to assess severity of disease. Am J Obstet Gynecol 2007;**197**(392):e1–e8.

14. Berghella V, Kaufmann M. Natural history of twin–twin transfusion syndrome. J Reprod Med 2001;**46**:480–4.

15. Senat MV, Deprest J, Boulvain M, Paupe A, Winer N, Ville Y. Endoscopic laser surgery versus serial amnioreduction for severe twin-to-twin transfusion syndrome. N Engl J Med 2004;**351**:136–44.

16. Sacco A, Van der Veeken L, Bagshaw E et al. Maternal complications following open and fetoscopic fetal surgery: a systematic review and meta-analysis. Prenat Diagn 2019;**39**:251–68.

17. Groene SG, Tollenaar LSA, Van Klink JMM et al. Twin–twin transfusion syndrome with and without selective fetal growth restriction prior to fetoscopic laser surgery: short- and long-term outcome. J Clin Med 2019 Jul 3;**8**(7):969.

18. Snowise S, Moise KJ, Johnson A, Bebbington MW, Papanna R. Donor death after selective fetoscopic laser surgery for twin–twin transfusion syndrome. Obstet Gynecol 2015;**126**:74–80.

19. Skupski DW, Luks FI, Walker M et al. Preoperative predictors of death in twin-to-twin transfusion syndrome treated

with laser ablation of placental anastomoses. Am J Obstet Gynecol 2010;203(388):e1–e11.

20. Stirnemann J, Djaafri F, Kim A et al. Preterm premature rupture of membranes is a collateral effect of improvement in perinatal outcomes following fetoscopic coagulation of chorionic vessels for twin–twin transfusion syndrome: a retrospective observational study of 1092 cases. BJOG 2018;125:1154–62.

21. Habli M, Bombrys A, Lewis D et al. Incidence of complications in twin–twin transfusion syndrome after selective fetoscopic laser photocoagulation: a single-center experience. Am J Obstet Gynecol 2009;201(417):e1–e7.

22. Robyr R, Lewi L, Salomon LJ et al. Prevalence and management of late fetal complications following successful selective laser coagulation of chorionic plate anastomoses in twin-to-twin transfusion syndrome. Am J Obstet Gynecol 2006;194:796–803.

23. Akkermans J, Peeters SH, Klumper FJ, Lopriore E, Middeldorp JM, Oepkes D. Twenty-five years of fetoscopic laser coagulation in twin–twin transfusion syndrome: a systematic review. Fetal Diagn Ther 2015;38:241–53.

24. Hecher K, Gardiner HM, Diemert A, Bartmann P. Long-term outcomes for monochorionic twins after laser therapy in twin-to-twin transfusion syndrome. Lancet Child Adolesc Health 2018;2:525–35.

25. Stirnemann J, Chalouhi G, Essaoui M et al. Fetal brain imaging following laser surgery in twin-to-twin surgery. BJOG 2018;125:1186–91.

26. Van Klink JM, Koopman HM, Rijken M, Middeldorp JM, Oepkes D, Lopriore E. Long-term neurodevelopmental outcome in survivors of twin-to-twin transfusion syndrome. Twin Res Hum Genet 2016;19:255–61.

27. Spruijt MS, Lopriore E, Tan R et al. Long-term neurodevelopmental outcome in twin-to-twin transfusion syndrome: is there still room for improvement? J Clin

Med 2019 Aug 15;8(8):1226. https://doi.org /10.3390/jcm8081226

28. Herberg U, Bolay J, Graeve P, Hecher K, Bartmann P, Breuer J. Intertwin cardiac status at 10-year follow-up after intrauterine laser coagulation therapy of severe twin–twin transfusion syndrome: comparison of donor, recipient and normal values. Arch Dis Child Fetal Neonatal Ed 2014;99:F380–F385.

29. Khalil A, Cooper E, Townsend R, Thilaganathan B. Evolution of stage 1 twin-to-twin transfusion syndrome (TTTS): systematic review and meta-analysis. Twin Res Hum Genet 2016;19:207–16.

30. Bamberg et al. Neither the differentiation between twin-twin transfusion syndrome Stages I and II nor III and IV makes a difference regarding the probability of double survival after laser therapy. Ultrasound Obstet Gynecol 2020.

31. Papanna R, Habli M, Baschat AA et al. Cerclage for cervical shortening at fetoscopic laser photocoagulation in twin–twin transfusion syndrome. Am J Obstet Gynecol 2012;206(425):e1–e7.

32. Salomon LJ, Nasr B, Nizard J et al. Emergency cerclage in cases of twin-to-twin transfusion syndrome with a short cervix at the time of surgery and relationship to perinatal outcome. Prenat Diagn 2008;28:1256–61.

33. Aboudiab MS, Chon AH, Korst LM, Llanes A, Ouzounian JG, Chmait RH. Management of twin–twin transfusion syndrome with an extremely short cervix. J Obstet Gynaecol 2018;38:359–62.

34. Lopriore E, Middeldorp JM, Oepkes D, Klumper FJ, Walther FJ, Vandenbussche FP. Residual anastomoses after fetoscopic laser surgery in twin-to-twin transfusion syndrome: frequency, associated risks and outcome. Placenta 2007;28:204–8.

35. Slaghekke F, Lopriore E, Lewi L et al. Fetoscopic laser coagulation of the vascular equator versus selective coagulation for twin-to-twin transfusion syndrome: an

open-label randomised controlled trial. Lancet 2014;**383**:2144–51.

36. Quintero RA, Kontopoulos E, Chmait RH. Laser treatment of twin-to-twin transfusion syndrome. Twin Res Hum Genet 2016;**19**:197–206.

37. Lanna MM, Faiola S, Consonni D, Rustico MA. Increased risk of placental abruption after Solomon laser treatment of twin–twin transfusion syndrome. Placenta 2017;**53**:54–6.

38. D'Antonio F, Thilaganathan B, Toms J et al. Perinatal outcome after fetoscopic laser surgery for twin-to-twin transfusion syndrome in triplet pregnancies. BJOG 2016;**123**:328–36.

39. Baud D, Windrim R, Keunen J et al. Fetoscopic laser therapy for twin–twin transfusion syndrome before 17 and after 26 weeks' gestation. Am J Obstet Gynecol 2013;**208**(197):e1–e7.

Management of Twin Anaemia-Polycythaemia Sequence

Liesbeth Lewi and Enrico Lopriore

The Facts

Twin anaemia polycythaemia sequence (TAPS) is a unique complication of monochorionic multiple pregnancies characterised by a severe difference in haemoglobin levels with an anaemic donor and a polycythaemic recipient. It is caused by a chronic transfusion of red blood cells across minuscule (1 mm or less) placental vascular anastomoses.[1,2]

Before birth, we can detect TAPS by an elevated middle cerebral artery peak systolic velocity (MCA-PSV) at or above 1.5 multiples of the median (MoM) in the donor in combination with a decreased MCA-PSV at or below 0.8 MoM in the receptor. Also, an inter-twin discordance between MCA-PSV values of 1 MoM or more indicates the presence of TAPS. After birth, we make the diagnosis of TAPS if the haemoglobin difference is at least 8 g/dL. To indicate a chronic transfusion imbalance, the donor must show signs of increased erythropoiesis with an elevated reticulocyte count. In contrast, the recipient must demonstrate a suppressed erythropoiesis with a decreased reticulocyte count, resulting in a donor: recipient reticulocyte count ratio of 1.7 or more.[3] Alternatively, the presence of only minuscule anastomoses proves the transfusion imbalance must have occurred over a long time.[1,2]

On ultrasound scan, additional signs commonly point towards the presence of TAPS. Typically, there is a striking discrepancy in the echogenicity and thickness between the two placental parts. As such, the donor share is usually white and thick whereas the recipient's part is dark and thin (Figure 14.1A). The anaemic donor often has cardiomegaly whereas the polycythaemic recipient typically has a 'starry sky' aspect of the liver (Figure 14.1B).[4]

Twin anaemia polycythaemia sequence can occur in a previously uncomplicated pregnancy or after fetoscopic laser surgery for twin–twin transfusion syndrome (TTTS) if small anastomoses remain open.[1,2] Spontaneous TAPS is rare and its incidence is probably only around 3% in monochorionic-diamniotic twin pregnancies.[5] Similarly, the incidence of post-laser TAPS is also 3% if the Solomon technique is used.[6] In monoamniotic pairs, TAPS is extremely rare as usually these twins have proximate cord insertions with large anastomoses. If a transfusion imbalance occurs in a monoamniotic pregnancy, it is usually an acute and substantial transfusion leading to unexpected and usually double demise before any amniotic fluid or haemoglobin discordances appear.

In contrast to TTTS, which is typically diagnosed between 16 and 26 weeks of gestation, spontaneous TAPS can occur at any time during pregnancy from as early as the first trimester to late into the third trimester.[2,7] Post-laser TAPS usually occurs one to four weeks after the surgery. Twin anaemia polycythaemia sequence is classified according to severity into five stages (Table 14.1).[8] Although TAPS has a more benign course than TTTS,

Table 14.1 Antenatal twin anaemia polycythaemia sequence staging[8]

Staging	Findings on prenatal ultrasound examination
Stage 1	MCA-PSV donor > 1.5 MoM and MCA-PSV receptor < 1.0 MoM with no other signs of compromise
Stage 2	MCA-PSV donor > 1.7 MoM and MCA-PSV receptor < 0.8 MoM with no other signs of compromise
Stage 3	Cardiac compromise of the donor with critically abnormal Doppler
Stage 4	Hydrops of donor
Stage 5	Fetal demise of donor or receptor with TAPS

TAPS = twin anaemia-polycythaemia sequence; MCA-PSV = middle cerebral artery – peak systolic velocity; MoM = multiple of the median

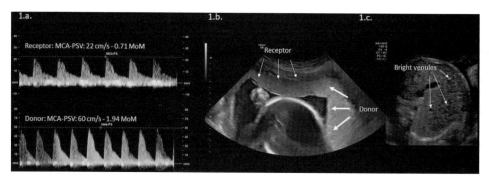

Figure 14.1 Ultrasound images of a spontaneous TAPS at 24 weeks of gestation. (a) The receptor has decreased MCA-PSV. The donor twin's MCA-PSV is increased. (b) The receptors' placental part is dark and thin (thin arrows) whereas the donor's part is white and thickened (thick arrows). (c) The receptor also has a 'starry sky' aspect of the liver due to bright venules (arrows). Both have normal amniotic fluid. This patient underwent a fetoscopic laser coagulation of five tiny anastomoses followed by a Solomon line combined with an intrauterine transfusion of the donor for a haemoglobin of 4 g/dL. She delivered two healthy boys at 34 weeks of gestational age.

TAPS may lead to fetal and neonatal demise. As such, fetal loss occurs in about 10–15% whereas the neonatal mortality rate is around 5–10%.[9,10]

Severe anaemia may also lead to growth restriction, hydrops and cerebral haemorrhage. Likewise, hyperviscosity in the receptor may cause cerebral insults or vascular occlusion with limb necrosis and amputations. Babies with TAPS are born early, around 32 weeks, and hematologic complications are common in the neonatal period with the need for transfusion and exchange transfusion in the donor and receptor, respectively.[9,10] Because of these increased risks and because antenatal treatment is available, we should screen all monochorionic twin pregnancies with a fortnightly (biweekly) scan not only for TTTS, but also for TAPS by measuring the MCA-PSV in both twins from 20 weeks onwards, in pregnancies with selective growth restriction, after fetoscopic laser surgery for TTTS or whenever there is a sonographic suspicion of TAPS.[11,12]

Twin anaemia polycythaemia sequence is characterised by a haemoglobin difference. In TAPS, the amniotic fluid may differ between the twins, but the deepest vertical pocket is more than 2 cm in the donor and less than 8 cm in the recipient. If the amniotic fluid discordance complies with the TTTS criteria, we classify and treat the pregnancy as TTTS. The hallmark of TTTS is a discrepancy in amniotic fluid and generally, both twins have similar haemoglobin levels. Nevertheless, a minority of TTTS pregnancies (about 10–15%), are accompanied by TAPS with a polycythaemic recipient and an anaemic donor.[13] In TAPS, as in TTTS, the donor is commonly smaller than the recipient because the transfusion imbalance affects the growth in monochorionic pregnancies. If growth is concordant, then the recipient usually has the smaller placental share and the more marginal cord insertion. Twin anaemia polycythaemia sequence must be excluded in growth-discordant monochorionic pairs as management will differ.

Twin anaemia polycythaemia sequence is a chronic inter-twin transfusion imbalance and must be differentiated from an acute inter-twin transfusion. An acute transfusion may happen during pregnancy, generally leading to the demise of both twins, or during labour. Acute inter-twin transfusion requires a low-resistance artery-to-artery anastomosis that permits rapid exsanguination of one twin into the other twin. Before birth, a large artery-to-artery anastomosis, proximate cord insertions, a similar echogenicity of the placental territories or a type 3 selective growth restriction decrease the likelihood of TAPS. After birth, colour injection of the placenta with the demonstration of a large artery-to-artery anastomosis confirms an acute inter-twin transfusion. Also, if the maternal side of the placenta has a similar colour, this indicates an acute rather than a chronic transfusion imbalance because TAPS placentas characteristically have a clear colour difference between the two placental territories (Figure 14.2).[14] Other reasons for an elevated MCA-PSV or an inter-twin MCA-PSV discordance of 1 MoM or more must be excluded too. As such, in selective growth restriction, the smaller twin commonly has a higher MCA-PSV than the appropriately growing twin in the context of brain sparing.

The Issues

Twin anaemia polycythaemia sequence was described for the first time only ten years ago, first as a complication after fetoscopic laser surgery for TTTS[1] and second as a transfusion imbalance in previously uncomplicated twin pregnancies.[2] Because of its recent discovery and rarity, many uncertainties remain about its pathophysiology, natural history, diagnostic criteria and management.

We do not know why a transfusion imbalance sometimes presents as a discrepancy in amniotic fluid, like in TTTS, and at other times as a haemoglobin difference, like in TAPS. It seems the number and type of anastomoses are similar in TTTS and TAPS placentas, but their size differs. Compared to uncomplicated monochorionic placentas, TTTS and TAPS placentas have fewer anastomoses, and typically the artery-to-artery anastomosis is missing. An artery-to-artery anastomosis allows flow in both directions and compensates for any imbalances in inter-twin transfusion. In contrast, in TTTS and TAPS, usually, only artery-to-vein connections are present, which allow flow in one direction only and may cause an inter-twin transfusion imbalance. In contrast to TTTS, the anastomoses in TAPS are significantly smaller (less than 1 mm) and require colour injection to make them visible to the naked eye. This also explains why TAPS may occur after laser surgery for TTTS if we only coagulate the visible anastomoses. By coagulating the large anastomoses, TTTS will disappear, but TAPS may become apparent several weeks later if tiny anastomoses are missed.[15]

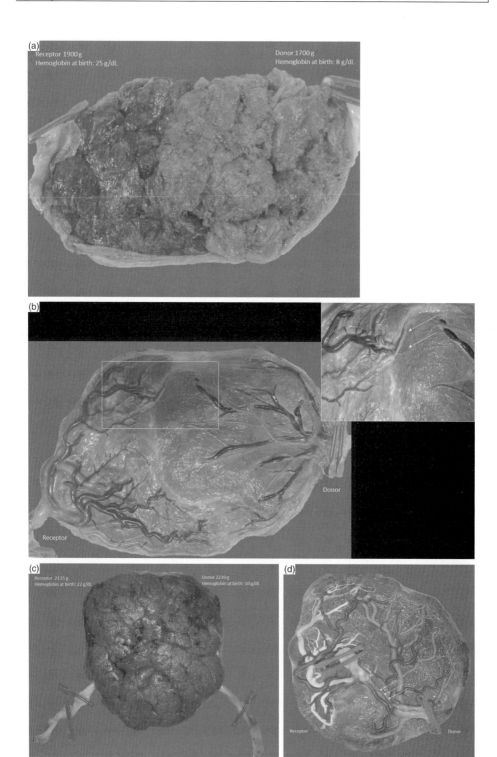

Figure 14.2 (a) Image of the maternal side from a monochorionic placenta of a spontaneous TAPS diagnosed at 30 weeks of gestation. This patient received one intrauterine transfusion at 31 weeks and was delivered electively at 32

The larger the anastomoses, the larger the placental part shared by the twins. In TTTS, the twins have a larger shared part than in TAPS, where the twins are connected by minuscule vessels. The size of this shared placental part probably determines if an imbalance results in TTTS rather than TAPS. Although both TTTS and TAPS are due to imbalanced blood flow, the large shared territory in TTTS allows the recipient to recruit fluid into its vascular compartment, which masks its polycythaemia but leads to polyuria and polyhydramnios. On the other hand, the large shared territory allows the donor to contract its vascular compartment and mask the anaemia, which leads to oliguria and oligohydramnios. When we coagulate all visible anastomoses, we eliminate the shared part, but when tiny communications are left, a chronic net transfer of blood will occur for which the twins can no longer compensate (Figure 14.3).[15]

The natural history of TAPS is also not well documented. The data currently available are from tertiary referral centres and the outcomes may be biased as it is likely that more severe TAPS cases are included.[9,10] As such, it is uncertain what proportion of mild TAPS cases, diagnosed in the first or early second trimester, resolve spontaneously without any intervention.[7] Also, data on long-term neurodevelopment are limited and based on small cohorts from tertiary referral centres only. These studies suggest a similar risk of severe neurological impairment of 9% after spontaneous and post-laser TAPS. However, in spontaneous TAPS, the donor had a four times higher risk of impairment than the recipient. Also, one in eight donors had bilateral hearing loss.[10] Although these numbers underscore the need to organise neurodevelopmental follow-up for these infants, because of possible selection bias of tertiary referral cases, the real impairment rate is likely somewhat lower.

The antenatal criteria to define TAPS have changed repeatedly. As such, for the recipient, a cut-off of 1.0 rather than 0.8 MoM has been proposed. The discordance between the MCA-PSV values may be more accurate than the individual MCA-PSV values of donor and recipient, but it is uncertain whether we best use a discordance of 1 MoM, as is currently recommended, or 0.5 MoM. Another limitation with the current antenatal definition is that it does not distinguish between an acute or chronic inter-twin transfusion imbalance and that an elevated MCA-PSV in the context of brain sparing may lead to a wrong TAPS diagnosis. Additional criteria, such as a difference in placental echogenicity, cardiomegaly in the donor or starry sky liver in the recipient, may improve diagnostic accuracy.

Also, we do not have data from controlled studies on the best management of TAPS. The results from a small observational study comparing fetoscopic laser surgery with intrauterine transfusion did not show a difference in survival and severe neonatal morbidity. However, laser surgery prolonged the interval between diagnosis and birth and decreased the risk of respiratory distress syndrome.[9] At present, we decide management for each case individually based on the gestational age, the severity of the disease, the feasibility to perform an intervention and the preference of the patient. We discuss the four different management options next.

Caption for Figure 14.2 (cont.)

weeks. There is a striking colour difference between the two parts. Also, the larger receptor had the smaller part of the placenta, indicating that TAPS influences fetal growth. (b) Image of the fetal side after colour injection. There were tiny artery-to-vein anastomoses (arrows). (c) Image of the maternal side from a monochorionic placenta of an acute peri-partum inter-twin transfusion. The babies were born vaginally at 34 weeks. There is no colour difference between the placental shares. (d) Placental injection showed a large artery-to-artery anastomoses (arrow), confirming an acute intra-partum transfusion as the cause of the haemoglobin difference. (A black and white version of this figure will appear in some formats. For the colour version, please refer to the plate section.)

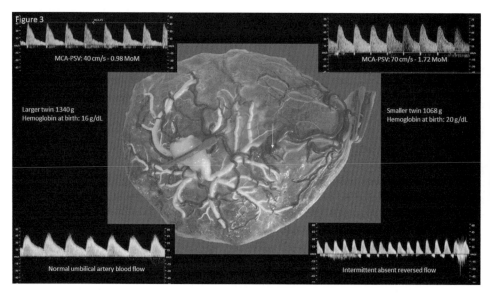

Figure 14.3 Monochorionic twin pair with type 3 selective growth restriction at 30 weeks of gestational age. Because of brain sparing, the MCA-PSV was increased in the smaller twin and normal in the larger twin. The typical intermittent absent or reversed end-diastolic flow pattern in the umbilical artery of the smaller twin indicates the presence of a large artery-to-artery anastomosis, which precludes the diagnosis of TAPS. The placenta showed the typical features of a type 3 growth restriction with a large artery-to-artery anastomosis (arrows) and little individual territory for the smaller twin with the marginal insertion. (A black and white version of this figure will appear in some formats. For the colour version, please refer to the plate section.)

The Management Options

As mentioned previously, the proposed management (Figure 14.4) is not validated by controlled studies. For each case, a dedicated plan must be developed that weighs the risks and benefits, taking into account the characteristics of each case.[8]

Expectant Management

Expectant management is currently preferred for stage 1 TAPS.[8] Usually, we review the patient within one week to confirm the diagnosis and assess the evolution. Also, we manage stage 2 before 18 weeks and after 28 weeks expectantly. In the early second trimester, the natural history is not well documented, and TAPS may disappear spontaneously when the minuscule TAPS vessels close spontaneously with rapid placental growth.[7] Moreover, fetoscopic laser surgery or intrauterine transfusion carries higher loss rates when performed at these early gestational ages. After 28 weeks, the aim is to gain a week or two to attain the 30- to 32-week limit when the risks of severe neonatal morbidity decrease. Fetoscopic laser surgery is usually no longer performed for TAPS after 28 weeks, and intrauterine transfusions should be well timed and limited in number, as each transfusion of the anaemic donor will increase the polycythaemia of the receptor. Therefore, after 28 weeks, we first administer a course of steroids for lung maturation and follow these pregnancies twice a week to timely detect any signs of cardiac decompensation in the donor twin.

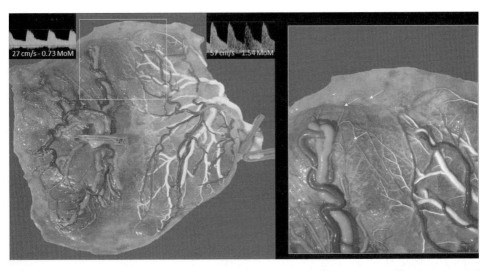

Figure 14.4 Images of a monochorionic pair with TTTS and coexistent TAPS at 28 weeks. The deepest vertical pocket was 11 cm in the receptor and 1.3 cm in the donor. At 28 weeks, we coagulated a visible artery-to-vein anastomosis and three tiny, unspecified anastomoses. We could not draw a Solomon line on the placenta because of intra-amniotic bleeding. After the surgery, TTTS disappeared but TAPS persisted. At 29 weeks, we gave an intrauterine transfusion to the donor for a haemoglobin of 6 g/dL and a partial exchange transfusion of the recipient for a haemoglobin of 21 g/dL. She was delivered electively at 32 weeks. The placenta showed minuscule, residual artery-to-vein anastomoses from the donor (2 clamps) to the receptor (1 clamp). (A black and white version of this figure will appear in some formats. For the colour version, please refer to the plate section.)

Fetoscopic Laser Coagulation of the Vascular Anastomoses

Fetoscopic laser coagulation of the anastomoses cures TTTS and is currently the preferred treatment modality for mid-trimester TTTS. The shared circulation is also the underlying cause of TAPS, and therefore fetoscopic laser surgery may be the best treatment for TAPS in the second trimester. However, controlled studies are not yet available and the intervention is more challenging in TAPS for several reasons. First, there is no poly-oligohydramnios in TAPS. In the absence of a stuck donor, the septum floats freely between the twins and the anastomoses may be behind the inter-twin septum, which then necessitates a septostomy to occlude all anastomoses. Additionally, in the absence of polyhydramnios, the amniotic fluid is more turbid, which hampers visibility, and if the placenta is anterior, there may be no placenta-free access to insert a trocar. Second, the placental territory of the donor is thickened and folded, which does not help to visualise the tiny anastomoses (Figure 14.5). Finally, a second surgery for post-laser TAPS is especially challenging as anastomoses were missed under the best surgical conditions. The first intervention may have caused membrane separation or blood-stained amniotic fluid, hampering a re-intervention.

Amnioinfusion of 1 to 2 litres warmed saline almost certainly improve the operative conditions. Most experts would draw a Solomon line between the vascular territories of both twins from one edge of the placenta to the other, which is usually sufficient to occlude all anastomoses, except when velamentous vessels skip the coagulation line to communicate across the membranes to the other placental territory. At present, laser coagulation is usually offered for stage 2 or above between 18 and 28 weeks, when we anticipate that complete separation is technically feasible.[8]

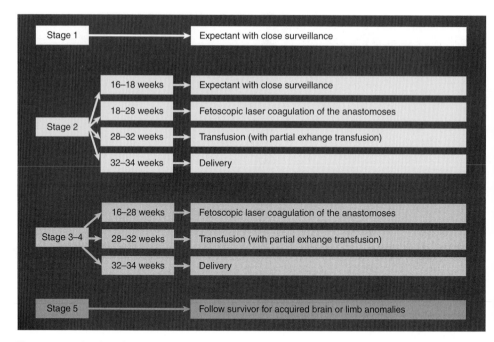

Figure 14.5 Flowchart for the proposed management according to stage and GA at presentation. These recommendations are only indicative, and obviously technical limitations, clinical characteristics and patient preference need to be taken into account too. As such, before 28 weeks, an intrauterine transfusion with partial exchange transfusion may be the best option if fetoscopic laser surgery is not feasible.

Intrauterine Transfusion, Exchange Transfusion

Intrauterine transfusion of the donor with/without a partial exchange transfusion of the receptor does not cure the disease and is only a temporary solution to gain time to deliver the babies or to perform a fetal intervention. As such, intrauterine transfusion–exchange transfusion is the preferred treatment between 28 and 32 weeks for stage 3. A cordocentesis also confirms the TAPS diagnosis, and in experienced hands, it is a safe procedure. For severe TAPS in the early second trimester, an intra-peritoneal transfusion may be a safer alternative because an intravascular transfusion is technically challenging and associated with greater risks. Although each transfusion of the donor worsens the polycythaemia of the receptor, it is uncertain if a simultaneous partial exchange transfusion is of benefit. Here, the blood of the receptor is progressively replaced by saline to reduce the hyperviscosity.[4] Usually, we start with partial exchange transfusions to the recipient, when we give a second or third intrauterine transfusion to the donor.

Selective Reduction

In the absence of an anomaly, the place of a selective reduction for TAPS is not well established. Like fetoscopic laser coagulation of the anastomoses, a selective reduction will undoubtedly arrest the inter-twin transfusion imbalance. However, especially the anaemic donor is at risk of dying, and theoretically, because of the minuscule anastomoses, the risk of acute exsanguination with subsequent demise or brain damage in the recipient should be

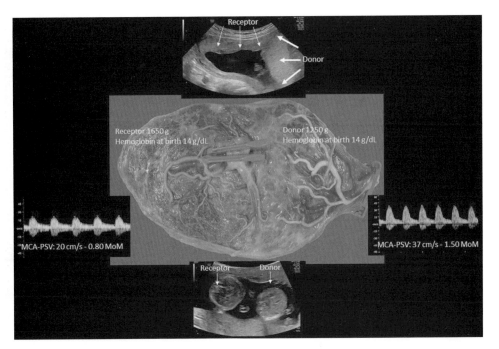

Figure 14.6 Ultrasound image of twin anemia-polycythemia at 15 weeks. The donor had the thick white part of the placenta, whereas the receptor had the thin, dark part. The receptor had a starry sky aspect of the liver. The pregnancy was managed expectantly. The MCA-PSV discordance improved spontaneously, and by 20 weeks, the MCA-PSV was concordant. She delivered at 31 weeks after spontaneous rupture of the membranes. The placenta did not show any anastomoses, as if we had performed a laser coagulation of all the anastomoses. (A black and white version of this figure will appear in some formats. For the colour version, please refer to the plate section.)

small. Therefore, if the donor is hydropic in the early second trimester, expectant management may avoid the iatrogenic risks of a probably unnecessary selective reduction.

Elective Birth

At 32 weeks, we usually deliver for stage 3 TAPS or above.[14] For the milder TAPS cases, the time of birth depends on the rate of progression and clinical characteristics, but after 34 to 35 weeks, there seems no benefit of delaying birth. Since the risk of an acute intra-partum transfusion is low, we allow a vaginal birth for cases with stage 1 or 2, especially if patients already had a vaginal birth and fetal well-being is acceptable.

Key Points

- Twin anaemia-polycythaemia sequence is characterised by a severe inter-twin haemoglobin discordance.
- Twin anaemia-polycythaemia sequence is caused by a chronic transfer of blood through minuscule anastomoses.
- Twin anaemia-polycythaemia sequence is diagnosed before birth by a discrepancy in MCA-PSV.
- Usually, additional ultrasound features are present, such as a discordance in placental echogenicity.
- Spontaneous TAPS is rare and occurs in about 3% of previously uncomplicated monochorionic twin pairs.

- Post-laser TAPS may occur after fetoscopic laser surgery for TTTS if small anastomoses are missed.
- Twin anaemia-polycythaemia sequence may lead to fetal and neonatal demise and long-term impairment.
- Fetoscopic laser coagulation of the minuscule anastomoses or intrauterine transfusion with partial exchange transfusion may improve the outcome and prolong the pregnancy.
- We should screen monochorionic twin pregnancies for the occurrence of TAPS by measuring the MCA-PSV in both twins.

References

1. Lewi L, Jani J, Cannie M et al. Intertwin anastomoses in monochorionic placentas after fetoscopic laser coagulation for twin-to-twin transfusion syndrome: is there more than meets the eye? Am J Obstet Gynecol 2006;**194**(3):790–5.
2. Lopriore E, Middeldorp JM, Oepkes D, Kanhai HH, Walther FJ, Vandenbussche FP. Twin anemia-polycythemia sequence in two monochorionic twin pairs without oligo-polyhydramnios sequence. Placenta 2007;**28**(1):47–51.
3. Khalil A, Gordijn S, Ganzevoort W et al. Consensus diagnostic criteria and monitoring of twin anemia polycythemia sequence: a Delphi procedure. Ultrasound Obstet Gynecol 2019.
4. Tollenaar LSA, Lopriore E, Middeldorp JM et al. Prevalence of placental dichotomy, fetal cardiomegaly and starry-sky liver in twin anemia polycythemia sequence. Ultrasound Obstet Gynecol 2019.
5. Couck I, Ponnet S, Deprest J, Devlieger R, De Catte L, Lewi L. Outcome of selective intrauterine growth restriction in monochorionic twin pregnancies at 16, 20 or 30 weeks according to the new consensus definition. Ultrasound Obstet Gynecol 2020.
6. Slaghekke F, Lopriore E, Lewi L et al. Fetoscopic laser coagulation of the vascular equator versus selective coagulation for twin-to-twin transfusion syndrome: an open-label randomised controlled trial. Lancet 2014;**383**(9935):2144–51.
7. Couck I, Valenzuela I, Russo F, Lewi L. Spontaneous regression of twin anemia-polycythemia sequence presenting in the first trimester. Ultrasound Obstet Gynecol 2019.
8. Tollenaar LS, Slaghekke F, Middeldorp JM et al. Twin anemia polycythemia sequence:

current views on pathogenesis, diagnostic criteria, perinatal management, and outcome. Twin Res Hum Genet 2016;**19**(3):222–33.
9. Slaghekke F, Favre R, Peeters SH et al. Laser surgery as a management option for twin anemia-polycythemia sequence. Ultrasound Obstet Gynecol 2014;**44**(3):304–10.
10. Tollenaar LSA, Lopriore E, Slaghekke F et al. High risk of long-term neurodevelopmental impairment in donor twins with spontaneous twin anemia-polycythemia sequence. Ultrasound Obstet Gynecol 2020;**55**(1):39–46.
11. Khalil A, Rodgers M, Baschat A et al. ISUOG practice guidelines: role of ultrasound in twin pregnancy. Ultrasound Obstet Gynecol 2016;**47**(2):247–63.
12. NICE guideline [NG137]: twin and triplet pregnancy 2019. Available from www.nice.org.uk/guidance/ng137
13. Donepudi R, Papanna R, Snowise S, Johnson A, Bebbington M, Moise KJ, Jr. Does anemia-polycythemia complicating twin–twin transfusion syndrome affect outcome after fetoscopic laser surgery? Ultrasound Obstet Gynecol 2016;**47**(3):340–4.
14. Tollenaar LSA, Zhao DP, Middeldorp JM, Oepkes D, Slaghekke F, Lopriore E. Can color difference on the maternal side of the placenta distinguish between acute peripartum twin–twin transfusion syndrome and twin anemia-polycythemia sequence? Placenta 2017;**57**:189–93.
15. Couck I, Lewi L. The placenta in twin-to-twin transfusion syndrome and twin anemia polycythemia sequence. Twin Res Hum Genet 2016;**19**(3):184–90.

Chapter 15

Management of Twin-Reversed Arterial Perfusion (TRAP) Sequence

Werner Diehl

The Facts (What We Know)

Twin-reversed arterial perfusion (TRAP) sequence is a rare complication of monochorionic twinning characterised by reverse (retrograde) perfusion of one of the twins via abnormal placental arterio-arterial anastomoses, with the consequence of completely disrupted and malformed fetal development. Typically, the affected fetus has an absent or rudimentary heart and is therefore referred to as the 'acardiac twin' and the unaffected twin is known as the 'pump twin' since it haemodynamically supplies the acardiac twin completely. As a consequence of this burden, there is a high risk of heart failure and intrauterine death of the pump twin, as well as development of polyhydramnios, preterm birth and neonatal death. As a result, the survival rate of the pump twin is approximately only 50–60%. Twin-reversed arterial perfusion can also occur in monochorionic triplets or higher-order monochorionic pregnancies.

Historically, the incidence of TRAP sequence has been reported as a very rare abnormality affecting 1 in 35,000 pregnancies or 1% of monochorionic twins. However, a recent study concluded that the incidence is higher at around 1 in 10,000 pregnancies or 2.6% of monochorionic twins.[1] The study found that when taking into account recent more robust statistics and the effect of assisted reproductive therapy on the increased rate of multiple pregnancies seen in recent decades in general, and the increased proportion of monochorionic twins in particular, this diagnosis can be expected more frequently than previously assumed.

Furthermore, among the fundamental conditions believed to be required for an acardiac twin pregnancy to occur, one is the existence of at least a set of one arterio-arterial (AA) and one veno-venous (VV) placental anastomoses, as further discussed later in this chapter. When seen from the embryological perspective of placental vascular development, one in eight monochorionic twins with a placenta with this particular configuration of anastomoses could be affected by TRAP sequence. However, early spontaneous cessation of retrograde perfusion to the acardiac twin or demise of the pump twin and pregnancy loss may contribute to the reported lower incidence of 2.6%.

The precise mechanisms involved in the development of acardiac twin malformation are not well known, as only snapshot observations of early embryonic and fetal pathology specimens are available. However, as mentioned earlier, some fundamental prerequisites appear to be required for the occurrence of an acardiac twin. Before going into these prerequisites, it is important to look at the timeline of post-zygotic twinning and the point in time at which a splitting occurs, since in monozygotic twins this is of key importance in the understanding of different types of chorionicity and amnionicity.

It is generally accepted that splitting of the fertilised oocyte leads to monozygotic (MZ) 'identical' twins and that if cleavage occurs as early as within the first three days post conception (i.e. before differentiation of cells that will contribute to the placenta), two separate placentae with two separate amniotic sacs will develop, leading to monozygotic dichorionic (DC) diamniotic (DA) twins. Around 20–30% of MZ twins are believed to have this origin. In contrast, if splitting occurs between day 3 and day 9 (after differentiation of chorionic precursor cells, but before development of amnion precursor cells), one common placenta with two separate amniotic cavities will be the result. This gives rise to mono-chorionic (MC) diamniotic (DA) twins, and 70–80% of MZ twins have this origin. If splitting occurs between days 9 and 12 (after differentiation of amnion cells), separation into two amniotic sacs then is no longer possible and the result will be monoamniotic (MA) twins.[2] Around 5% of MZ twins will have this origin. Although the exact point in time and mechanism of origin in conjoined twins is controversial, it is hypothesised that an even later splitting after 12 days may be involved in their origins, if following the fission theory (incomplete separation of embryonic structures). However, due to the different anatomical sites of non-separation observed in conjoined twins, fusion processes in monoamniotic embryos seem plausible as well (fusion theory). Conjoined twinning and other forms of aberrant twinning (e.g. extra-parasitic twins, endo-parasitic twins) are beyond the scope of this chapter but are in general most likely related to intrinsic embryonic developmental disorders. Although the majority of acardiac twins are diamniotic, a number of them prove to be monoamniotic and therefore other factors different than the timing of their splitting process are most likely involved in their genesis.

It is increasingly accepted that the process of MZ twinning rather rarely results in an equal splitting of the inner cell mass in the stage of the blastocyst. Presumably due to intrinsic genetic, epigenetic and intercellular processes not all yet elucidated, it is more likely that if a splitting is to occur, the majority of events will result in unequal number of cells that will thereafter be available to develop the corresponding future embryos.[3] This fact, apart from contributing to the general observation that MZ twins rarely are 'truly' identical, may have the consequence that one of the future embryos, although initially having the potential to develop normally, would display a slightly more 'retarded' evolution. This may result in significant differences in vascularisation, cardiac development and perfusion that may underlie the spectrum of complications typical to MC twins, ranging from twin–twin transfusion syndrome (TTTS) to selective fetal growth restriction (sIUGR). But in the case of acardiac twinning, an unequal number of cells as embryonic precursors may lead to either intrinsic cardiac abnormalities in the affected embryo or the development of aberrant placental vascular anastomoses, or even both. Furthermore, it is possible that an unequal inner cell mass segregation may also affect development of the corresponding chorionic vascular territories, later resulting in unequal placental sharing (as underlying cause of selective growth restriction and as contributing cause in TTTS).

Another prerequisite is the coexistence of a haemodynamically dominant set of one AA and one VV anastomoses (see earlier in this chapter) on the placenta, and it is then the combination of all these factors that may lead to a progressive retrograde perfusion of the smaller embryo. Favoured by a lower resistance, transfusion of deoxygenated blood via the AA anastomosis from the dominant pump twin to the smaller embryo in a reversed fashion is the most likely cause for major structural abnormalities in the affected twin. As a consequence, typically the acardiac twin shows some normal development of lower extremities but severe and bizarre malformations of the upper body (missing/abnormal upper limbs and acrania). After arterial retrograde perfusion of the acardiac mass, further desaturated blood returns to the pump twin via the VV anastomosis, bypassing the placenta and increasing its cardiac preload. This hemodynamic burden results in chronic hyperdynamic heart failure in the pump twin, causing hydrops and intrauterine death, polyhydramnios and preterm birth.

In some cases, perhaps due to increasing oedema and increasing vascular resistance within the acardiac mass, spontaneous cessation of retrograde flow can occur. In a series of 24 cases of TRAP, it was found that after diagnosis during first trimester and subsequent re-evaluation at 16 to 18 weeks, in 21%, there was spontaneous arrest of flow to the acardiac twin.[4] However, during this period of time, there was demise of the pump twin in 33% of cases and persistent flow to the acardiac twin in 46% of cases. This important observation has strengthened the rationale for intervention in the first trimester.

Advances in ultrasound technology and high-resolution imaging have allowed a shift in the diagnosis of TRAP sequence from the second to the first trimester. But irrespective of gestational age, the ultrasound diagnosis of TRAP sequence can be established when in a monochorionic twin pregnancy besides a structurally normal co-twin, a hydropic mass of tissue with some skeletal structures (in particular vertebral structures, pelvis and lower limbs) and colour Doppler evidence of retrograde blood flow is visualised. Although in some cases, an inter-twin membrane may be absent due to monoamnionicity, amniotic fluid can be reduced in the sac of the acardiac twin in a diamniotic setting and the inter-twin membrane may be difficult to identify. However, careful identification of the inter-twin membrane is important, as this does have major implications for therapeutic options. Additional typical findings include that the umbilical cord of the acardiac twin is frequently thinner and shorter than that of the pump twin and contains only two vessels in the majority of cases. However, if gestational age is more advanced, the cord can be thickened by hydropic changes and this too may have implications for therapeutic options. A more detailed examination of the placental topography will reveal in most of the cases one AA and one VV anastomosis between both cord insertions. Cord insertions frequently are close to each other, although in more rare cases, the cord of the acardiac inserts laterally onto the cord of the pump twin.

Although the use of colour Doppler in the first trimester should be limited to the minimum necessary, in the presence of an intra-amniotic hydropic tissue mass aside of a normal co-twin, its use is key for the diagnosis of TRAP sequence since it will demonstrate retrograde perfusion of the acardiac twin. Key ultrasound diagnostic features, signs of poor prognosis and their descriptions are summarised in Tables 15.1 and 15.2 respectively.

The Issues (What We Do Not Know)

Our current understanding of the origin of the acardiac twinning process is still incomplete. As discussed earlier in this chapter and inherent to the limited possibilities of accurate observation of early human development, the process of monochorionic splitting and distribution of inner cell masses of the future embryos and their placental sharing escapes our capabilities. However, multiple factors certainly are involved when the outcome of the splitting process is adverse as in acardiac twinning. Not only the point in time of splitting, but also an unequal number of cells splitting off in the inner mass and destined to develop into future embryos, as well as development and coexistence of AA and VV anastomoses in

Table 15.1 Key ultrasound signs for diagnosis of twin-reversed arterial perfusion sequence

Diagnostic signs of TRAP sequence	Description
MC placenta (MC twin pregnancy)	Presence of a single placenta
Presence of hydropic tissue mass AND (normal) co-twin	Besides a structurally normal co-twin, a hydropic mass of tissue with some skeletal structures can be seen (vertebrae, pelvic bones, lower limbs) with absence of a heartbeat (caveat: rudimentary cardiac structures are possible) and absence of a cranial vault (hence the term 'acardius acranius').
Retrograde perfusion of acardiac twin (colour Doppler)	Colour Doppler demonstrates retrograde perfusion of acardiac twin: Typically blood flow is seen entering the acardiac tissue mass at the abdominal region and ascending along the abdominal aorta to reach the thoracic area. In some cases, intrinsic pulsations of rudimentary heart structures can be seen. Blood flow then is seen to return via a former intra-fetal umbilical vein to the cord of this acardiac twin. Some cases may present already without any demonstrable blood flow in the acardiac twin (spontaneous cessation of retrograde perfusion).
Close cord insertions	Cord insertions of the pump twin and the acardiac twin are topographically close together in most cases. In rare cases, cord insertion of the acardiac twin may even arise directly from cord insertion of pump twin in a lateral fashion.
Placental AA and VV anastomoses	Detailed assessment of the chorionic plate between both cord insertions using colour Doppler may reveal the presence of at least one AA and one VV anastomoses.
Thin umbilical cord with two vessels	The umbilical cord of the acardiac twin can be thinner as compared to the pump twin. However, if the acardiac twin is hydropic, its umbilical cord may be thick and hydropic as well.

Table 15.2 Signs of poor prognosis in twin-reversed arterial perfusion sequence

Signs of poor prognosis	Description
Large acardiac twin	The acardiac twin's largest diameters can be used to compare its estimate weight with the pump twin's weight. If it is more than 50% of the weight of the pump twin, its haemodynamic effect is most likely to negatively impact the pump twin.
Signs of cardiac decompensation of pump twin (abnormal ductus venosus flow, tricuspid regurgitation, hydrops)	The presence of reverse flow (reversed a-wave) in the ductus venosus (DV) in the pump twin may be interpreted as a sign of cardiac distress in the context of TRAP sequence. Cardiac decompensation is even more likely if the pump twin shows signs of hydrops (ascites, pericardial or pleural effusions, skin oedema) or abnormal umbilical Doppler flow.
Monoamniotic pregnancy	Cord entanglement is known to be present in almost all monoamniotic twins as early as the first trimester. As in all monoamniotic twins, cord complications most likely accounts for the majority of fetal losses in acardiac twins.
Low resistance in umbilical artery of acardiac twin	Low-resistance umbilical blood flow in the acardiac twin or within its tissue mass (i.e. increased end-diastolic flow) makes spontaneous cessation of flow less likely and confirms haemodynamic burden of the pump twin's circulation.

the future chorionic plate, most likely need to coincide with and contribute to this abnormal phenomenon.

Although the study mentioned before points to the rationale for early intervention, we don't exactly know when and how this should be undertaken.[4] Heterogeneity of existing studies and paucity of robust statistics with limited number of cases do not allow a conclusive management strategy.

A case series and meta-analysis on optimal method and timing of interventions for TRAP found that when the diagnosis is established in the first trimester and intervention delayed until the second trimester, there is 60% spontaneous cessation of blood flow to the acardiac twin. However, in these cases, there is death of the pump twin or brain damage thereafter in up to 61%. Along with the lack of predictive ultrasound signs for subsequent fetal demise if expectantly managed, and the lack of benefit of delaying an intervention in terms of improved survival rates, elective intervention at 12–14 weeks appears to be indicated in TRAP.[5] Addressing the method of choice, the study concludes that intra-fetal laser appears to be the technique most likely to prevail.

In an attempt to definitively shed light on the best time for intervention, an international multicentre randomised trial is underway and will recruit women with a first-trimester diagnosis of TRAP and compare early intervention between 12 and 14 weeks (intra-fetal coagulation) versus late intervention between 16 and 19 weeks (intra-fetal or fetoscopic coagulation) (TRAPIST = TRAP Intervention Study).[6] To optimise outcomes and reproducibility, the procedures will be undertaken by experienced operators and the techniques standardised.

Long-term neurodevelopmental outcomes after TRAP sequence also need further investigation, taking into account if managed with early or late intervention, and as compared to expectant management. Again here, standardisation not only of procedure type and timing is of key importance, but also of neurodevelopmental tests to allow definitive conclusions.

Management Options

A variety of intrauterine interventions have been used in the treatment of TRAP. Historically, second-trimester ultrasound guided interventions and posteriorly fetoscopic approaches have been implemented with the aim of coagulation of the umbilical cord of the acardiac twin. Intra-fetal techniques targeting vessels within the body of the acardiac have successfully been used as well. However, in recent years, the tendency to earlier and less invasive techniques has become stronger, mostly involving ultrasound guided intra-fetal laser or radiofrequency coagulation of vessels within the acardiac twin. However, it is the gestational age at which the diagnosis of TRAP is established in a particular case that will define the treatment options available.

Expectant Management

Gestational age at diagnosis plays a key role in the management of TRAP sequence. When diagnosed during the first trimester (11–13 +6 weeks), in around one-third of cases, demise of the pump twin will occur if managed expectantly.[4] This observation has led to the implementation of earlier and less invasive therapeutic options than fetoscopy, and a number of recent studies have shown that early intervention may result in improved survival rates and perinatal outcomes.

However, in selected cases, expectant management may achieve satisfactory outcomes. In particular, a small size of the acardiac twin at diagnosis has been used as criteria for this option.[7] For instance, a survival rate of 88% was reported if the calculated weight of the acardiac twin was less than 50% the weight of the pump twin. However, the numbers in these series were very small and no definitive conclusion can be drawn from these findings. Spontaneous flow arrest may be likely in these cases and invasive interventions with their inherent risks could be avoided, but spontaneous demise of pump twins with small acardiac twins has also been reported. However, if a small-sized acardiac twin presents in combination with high-resistance umbilical flow or intra-fetal blood flow shows low peak velocities, expectant management may be justified since spontaneous cessation of retrograde perfusion is likely. Close surveillance to detect deterioration of the pump twin or increasing retrograde perfusion to the acardiac twin may, however, indicate the need for intervention, as does rapid growth of the acardiac mass. Regardless of gestational age at diagnosis, and especially in the presence of signs of poor prognosis (Table 15.2), most parents may opt for intervention, more so if the diagnosis is established during the first trimester.

If no retrograde flow to the acardiac twin is detected by colour Doppler (at diagnosis or after spontaneous cessation in a follow-up review), expectant management is indicated as the goal of any invasive treatment – that is, the interruption of flow to the acardiac twin – has spontaneously occurred. Perinatal outcomes are very good with survival rates reaching 100% and gestational age at delivery beyond 36 weeks.[7] However, the patient needs to be aware that sudden demise of the pump twin may still occur, especially in monoamniotic TRAP. Invasive cord transection in monoamniotic acardiac twins, even with arrested flow to the acardiac at presentation or during follow-up should be discussed with the parents, since there is persistent risk of tightening of cord entanglement due to retraction of necrotising cord tissues.[8] In monoamniotic TRAP, with active retrograde perfusion of the acardiac at diagnosis during the first trimester, expectant management is not recommended, but the intervention should be delayed until beyond 16 weeks, when fetoscopy with cord coagulation and cord transection becomes feasible. When compared to cord occlusion in monoamniotic discordant twins, additional cord transection appears not to have a significant impact on outcomes apart from a longer operative time.[9]

Early Intervention (12–14 Weeks)

The aim of this minimally invasive procedure is to coagulate and stop blood flow in the acardiac twin by means of laser or radiofrequency energy, with the use of a needle which is much thinner than a fetoscope. In order to achieve this, usually a 17G or 18G needle is percutaneously inserted under ultrasound guidance, using maternal local anaesthesia, into the body of the acardiac twin (intra-fetal) at the level of its abdominal cord insertion and pelvic area. This is undertaken in tertiary centres with appropriate equipment and expertise. Although a transamniotic approach is preferred, leaving the sac of the pump twin intact, sometimes an extensive anterior placenta cannot be avoided, resulting in transplacental access to the acardiac fetus. Since it is unclear whether the latter has an impact on outcomes in this procedure, maternal safety and a clear needle path and target entry justify this approach. Once the needle tip is in close proximity of the target vessels, a 400 nm laser fibre or radiofrequency (RF) device is passed through and activated. Colour Doppler is used to determine and confirm retrograde blood flow arrest before retrieving the laser fibre or RF device. After needle extraction, fetal heart rate in the pump twin should be documented and again cessation of retrograde flow to the acardiac twin should be confirmed. Although incomplete coagulation with persistence of flow may require a repeated procedure, this is unlikely in expert hands.

Most centres using early intra-fetal laser coagulation (between 12 and 14 weeks) have reported an overall survival rate of 80–90%. A recent small retrospective series reported survival rates of up to 91.7% with the majority of pregnancies reaching 39 weeks at delivery.[10] When compared with late intervention, another study found a reduced rate of premature rupture of membranes, a lower incidence of delivery before 34 weeks and significantly higher birthweight, at comparable survival rates and rate of demise of the pump twin.[11] Although with statistically limited power, these outcomes are adding evidence in favour of early intervention as compared to second-trimester intervention. A recent review on current treatment options also comes to the conclusion in favour of early intervention.[12]

Late Intervention (after 16 Weeks)

If after early diagnosis expectant management until a second-trimester intervention is chosen, or if first establishment of the diagnosis of TRAP is during the second trimester, most commonly an intra-fetal radiofrequency ablation or fetoscopic laser coagulation is offered. Although a number of different techniques have been used, these two approaches have become the most frequently used. Although intra-fetal laser coagulation may also be used in second-trimester intervention, it rather is preferred for first-trimester treatment. However, the use of intra-fetal radiofrequency ablation at this gestational age has reported survival rates of 80% and gestational ages at delivery beyond 36 weeks.[13] Ultrasound-guided or fetoscopic bipolar coagulation also represents a common alternative, especially for cases where advanced hydrops of the acardiac and its cord anticipate limitations of laser coagulation.

Inherent to the procedure, fetoscopy is more invasive than intra-fetal coagulation as it involves insertion of fetoscopes of 2–2.8 mm in diameter with a working channel for a laser fibre, similarly as used for the management of severe mid-trimester TTTS. Preoperative evaluation of amnionicity and placental topography are key to a successful procedure. Once vascular anastomoses (AA and VV) on the chorionic plate have been visualised at fetoscopy, laser coagulation is undertaken to stop retrograde perfusion to the acardiac fetus. This is confirmed intraoperatively with the use of colour Doppler. However, if fetoscopic access to the anastomosis is impaired or the cord to the acardiac directly arises from the cord of the pumping twin, cord coagulation is undertaken. This may be more difficult to achieve as the cord to the acardiac may be thick or hydropic or the flow is high due to advanced gestational age. In this situation, bipolar coagulation may be used primarily (if technical complications are anticipated at the time of diagnosis), or secondarily (during fetoscopy). If so, a second entry trocar may be inserted to pass the bipolar forceps. It is used either to electro-coagulate the cord or just to compress it to reduce flow and then use laser energy to coagulate cord vessels. A second entry may not significantly increase the rate of premature rupture of membranes or miscarriage, as shown in a series and the likelihood of its necessity was reported to be 15% if the procedure was undertaken after 18 weeks.[14]

As previously discussed, in monoamniotic acardiac twins the aim of intervention is not only to stop retrograde perfusion, but additionally to address the risk of cord complications. Therefore, after coagulation of two segments of the cord of the acardiac twin (usually close to its abdominal insertion to ensure identification), cord transection between these segments is undertaken using laser energy. Thereafter, cord disentanglement should be undertaken to minimise the risk of tightening of true knots or twists by retraction of necrotic cord tissues.[8]

When looking at data from the largest series and meta-analysis, in general, survival rates of fetoscopy range from 76% to 83% with the majority of pregnancies delivering after 36 weeks. The rate of procedure-related premature rupture of membranes can be estimated at around 7% and the rate of severe preterm birth (before 32 weeks) at around 7–20%.[5,14,15]

Management Options Conclusion

Although there is large heterogeneity in the available data and therefore only ranges of survival rates can be used for counselling patients, what we can say is that intervention has changed the natural course of these pregnancies, which otherwise would have a high risk of poor outcome. Current thinking is in favour of early intervention, but this has not been proven definitively. See Figure 15.1, which illustrates a common management approach.

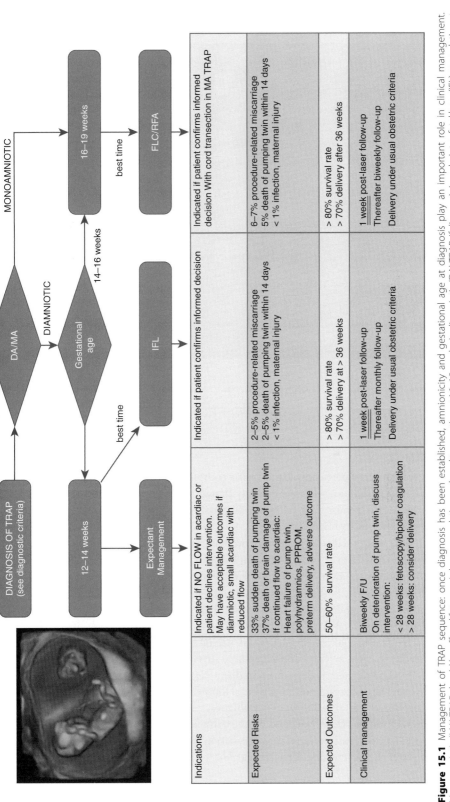

	12–14 weeks	14–16 weeks	16–19 weeks
	Expectant Management	IFL	FLC/RFA
Indications	Indicated if NO FLOW in acardiac or patient declines intervention. May have acceptable outcomes if diamniotic, small acardiac with reduced flow	Indicated if patient confirms informed decision	Indicated if patient confirms informed decision With cord transection in MA TRAP
Expected Risks	33% sudden death of pumping twin 37% death or brain damage of pump twin If continued flow to acardiac: Heart failure of pump twin, polyhydramnios, PPROM, preterm delivery, adverse outcome	2–5% procedure-related miscarriage 2–5% death of pumping twin within 14 days < 1% infection, maternal injury	6–7% procedure-related miscarriage 5% death of pumping twin within 14 days < 1% infection, maternal injury
Expected Outcomes	50–60% survival rate	> 80% survival rate > 70% delivery at > 36 weeks	> 80% survival rate > 70% delivery after 36 weeks
Clinical management	Biweekly F/U On deterioration of pump twin, discuss intervention: < 28 weeks: fetoscopy/bipolar coagulation > 28 weeks: consider delivery	1 week post-laser follow-up Thereafter monthly follow-up Delivery under usual obstetric criteria	1 week post-laser follow-up Thereafter biweekly follow-up Delivery under usual obstetric criteria

Figure 15.1 Management of TRAP sequence: once diagnosis has been established, amnionicity and gestational age at diagnosis play an important role in clinical management. Monoamniotic (MA) TRAP should be offered fetoscopic laser coagulation and cord transection at 16–19 weeks. In diamniotic (DA) TRAP, if diagnosis is early, intra-fetal laser (IFL) coagulation at 12–14 weeks most likely represents the best treatment option. If diagnosis is made later, fetoscopic laser coagulation (FLC) of placental anastomoses or cord coagulation can be offered. Intra-fetal radiofrequency ablation (RFA) represents an alternative with comparable outcomes as well. If diagnosis is established between 14 and 16 weeks, expectant management until safer FLC or RFA can be undertaken is indicated, as higher rates of procedure-related rupture of membranes and miscarriage are observed.

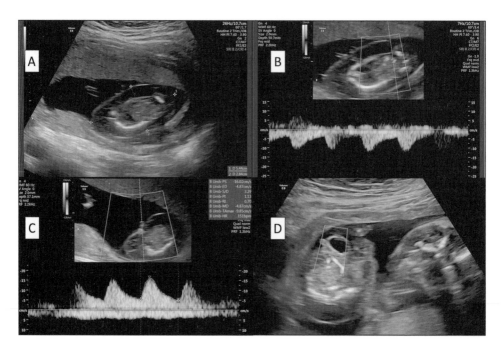

Figure 15.2 Ultrasound images of TRAP sequence: an acardiac twin with marked hydrops is seen (A). Low-resistance retrograde perfusion within the body of the acardiac is clearly seen in (B) in colour Doppler. Retrograde perfusion at the abdominal cord insertion can be detected in (C). Optimal target for interstitial laser coagulation is the abdominal area of the acardiac due to confluence of vessels (D).

Key Points

- Twin-reversed arterial perfusion sequence is a complication of monochorionic twinning that occurs more frequently than previously thought.
- With increasing awareness, first-trimester diagnosis should be aimed for, as the latter is of key importance in its management.
- Intervention is associated with better outcomes compared with expectant management.
- Even if the acardiac twin is small, there is a lack of reassuring predictive factors and intervention is advocated in view of the risk of death or brain damage of the pump twin.
- Although still unclear whether early intervention (i.e. in the first trimester) leads to better perinatal outcomes, recent data support this management.
- First-trimester intra-fetal laser coagulation is likely to become treatment of choice supported by its minimal invasiveness (18G needle technique, short operative time, outpatient/day-surgery setting) and acceptable survival rates.
- If diagnosis is late or there is deterioration during expectant management, intervention with fetoscopic laser coagulation of placental anastomoses or acardiac fetus cord coagulation or intra-fetal radiofrequency ablation can be offered with comparable outcomes, and the choice will depend on the clinician's preference and expertise.
- The TRAPIST trial of early versus late intervention is expected to definitively answer the question about the best timing for intervention.

- In monoamnionicity, intervention can only be late as in addition to cord coagulation, cord transection is required.

References

1. Van Gemert MJ, Van den Wijngaard JP, Vandenbussche FP. Twin reversed arterial perfusion sequence is more frequent than generally accepted. Birth Defects Res A Clin Mol Teratol 2015;**103**(7):641–3.

2. Benirschke K. The monozygotic twinning process, the twin–twin transfusion syndrome and acardiac twins. Placenta 2009;**30**(11):923–8.

3. Machin G. Non-identical monozygotic twins, intermediate twin types, zygosity testing, and the non-random nature of monozygotic twinning: s review. Am J Med Genet Part C Semin Med Genet 2009;**151**C:110–27.

4. Lewi L, Valencia C, Gonzalez E, et al. The outcome of twin reversed arterial perfusion sequence diagnosed in the first trimester. Am J Obstet Gynecol 2010;**203**:213.e1–e4.

5. Chaveeva P, Poon LC, Sotiriadis A, Kosinski P, Nicolaides KH. Optimal method and timing of intrauterine intervention in twin reversed arterial perfusion sequence: case study and meta-analysis. Fetal Diagn Ther 2014;**35**:267–79.

6. TRAP Intervention STudy (TRAPIST). ClinincalTrials.gov: NCT02621645.

7. Jelin E, Hirose S, Rand L et al. Perinatal outcome of conservative management versus fetal intervention for twin reversed arterial perfusion sequence with a small acardiac twin. Fetal Diagn Ther 2010;**27**:138–41.

8. Berg C, Koenninger A, Gembruch U, Geipel A. Twin arterial reversed arterial perfusion (TRAP) sequence: does monoamnionicity preclude early intervention? Ultrasound Obstet Gynecol 2014;**44**:241–2.

9. Valsky DV, Martinez-Serrano MJ, Sanz M et al. Cord occlusion followed by laser cord transection in monochorionic monoamniotic discordant twins. Ultrasound Obstet Gynecol 2011;**37**:684–8.

10. Tavares de Sousa M, Glosemeyer P, Diemert A, Bamberg C, Hecher K. First-trimester intervention in twin reversed arterial perfusion sequence. Ultrasound Obstet Gynecol 2020;**55**:47–9.

11. Berg C, Holst D, Mallmann MR, Gottschalk I, Gembruch U, Geipel A. Early vs late intervention in twin reversed arterial perfusion sequence. Ultrasound Obstet Gynecol 2014;**43**:60–4.

12. Vitucci A, Fichera A, Fratelli N, Sartori E, Prefumo F. Twin reversed arterial perfusion sequence: current treatment options. Int J Womens Health 2020;**12**:435–43.

13. Lee H, Bebbington M, Crombelholme TM, North American Fetal Therapy Network. The North American Fetal Therapy Network Registry data on outcomes of radiofrequency ablation for twin-reversed arterial perfusion sequence. Fetal Diagn Ther 2013;**33**(4):224–9.

14. Diehl W, Hecher K. Selective cord coagulation in acardiac twins. Semin Fetal Neonatal Med 2007;**12**(6):458–63.

15. Pagani G, D'Antonio F, Khalil A, Papageorghiou A, Bhide A, Thilaganathan B. Intrafetal laser treatment for twin reversed arterial perfusion sequence: cohort study and meta-analysis. Ultrasound Obstet Gynecol 2013 Jul;**42**(1):6–14. https://doi.org/10.1002/uog .12495

Chapter 16

Management of Fetal Growth Pathology in Multiple Pregnancy

Nikolaos Antonakopoulos and Asma Khalil

Introduction

The advances in assisted reproductive techniques combined with the advanced age of women trying to conceive has led to increased implementation of these techniques in order to overcome fertility barriers. An inevitable consequence of assisted reproduction is the raised incidence of multiple pregnancies, mainly twin pregnancies.[1]

Twin pregnancies are known to have significantly higher rates of perinatal morbidity and mortality than singleton pregnancies. This is related not only to the high rate of preterm delivery of these pregnancies, but also to the high risk of fetal growth disturbances. It is well established that twin pregnancies with evident growth discordance have poorer perinatal outcomes, independently of gestational age at delivery.[2]

Prevalence

The prevalence of fetal growth restriction (FGR) in twins depends on the definition used. The incidence is 48%, 27% or 16% if the definition denotes at least one twin with birthweight < 10th centile, < 5th centile or a birthweight discrepancy ≥ 20%, respectively. In recent years, the diagnostic convention for selective fetal growth restriction (sFGR) has become an estimated fetal weight < 10th centile in one twin with an inter-twin discordance of ≥ 25%.

Monochorionic (MC) twin pregnancies are more likely to be complicated by growth restriction than dichorionic (DC) twin pregnancies, with nearly twice the rate of FGR at 19.7% compared to 10.5% and a higher incidence of associated perinatal mortality with a rate of 7.5% compared to 3.3%.[3] Selective growth restriction may have similar prevalence between MC and DC twins, but neurological complications and morbidity in the co-twin are more common in affected MC pregnancies than in DC pregnancies.[3] In an attempt to standardise the management of sFGR in MC pregnancies, a consensus was recently published on the diagnostic criteria of sFGR in DC and MC twin pregnancies. The diagnosis of sFGR is made if the estimated fetal weight (EFW) of the small twin is less than the 3rd centile or if two of the following criteria are met: EFW of one twin < 10th centile, AC of one twin < 10th centile, EFW discordance ≥ 25% or umbilical artery pulsatility index (PI) of the smaller twin > 95th centile (Table 16.1).[4,5]

Aetiology

Although FGR is usually thought to be placental in origin, it is important to rule out intrauterine infection (cytomegalovirus, toxoplasmosis and rubella) and discordance due to chromosomal or congenital anomalies. The incidence of discordant anomalies is around 4% in DC twin pregnancies compared to 6.7% in MC twin pregnancies.[3]

Table 16.1 Diagnostic criteria for selective fetal growth restriction in twin pregnancy as determined by experts[4]

	Monochorionic twin pregnancy	Dichorionic twin pregnancy
Solitary	EFW of one twin < 3rd centile	EFW of one twin < 3rd centile
Contributory	Two out of four of the following contributory parameters are required (irrespective of which parameter) EFW of one twin < 10th centile	Two out of three of the following contributory parameters are required (irrespective of which parameter) EFW of one twin < 10th centile
	AC of one twin < 10th centile	EFW discordance ≥ 25%
	EFW discordance ≥ 25%	UA-PI of smaller twin > 95th Centile
	UA-PI of smaller twin > 95th centile	

AC, abdominal circumferences; EFW, estimated fetal weight; PI, pulsatility index; UA, umbilical artery

Chorionicity and amnionicity also determine the aetiology of fetal growth discordance in twins to a large extent. In MC twins, differences are largely attributed to twin-to-twin transfusion syndrome (TTTS) or to unequal share of placental mass between the fetuses. There is also evidence from the ESPRiT study cohort relating to the cord insertion site and its relation to both birthweight discordance and small-for-gestational age (SGA) status in MC twins.[2]

On the other hand, in DC twins, differences may be attributed to different genetic growth potential, but underlying pathology may also be present, leading to adverse neonatal outcomes, similar to singleton cases. In DC twins, in contrast to MC twins, both discordant birthweight and SGA status are associated with underlying placental histological abnormalities. For DC twins, growth discordance can be related to underlying placental insufficiency selectively affecting one twin.[2]

Fetal Biometry in Twin Pregnancies

The inter-twin biometry discordance, as well as the difference in size between twin and singleton pregnancies, is more pronounced in the third trimester and is seen earlier in MC pregnancies. A problematic common practice is to plot the growth of twin fetuses on growth charts created from data of uncomplicated singleton pregnancies. The issue is whether the observed differences in growth between twins and singletons represent physiological adaptation to the intrauterine environment or growth restriction to less than optimal growth. Thus, if twins are physiologically adapted, then comparing them to singletons may increase unnecessary interventions and prematurity for suspected fetal compromise without actual benefit.[3]

Management Dilemma

The management of FGR in multiple pregnancy, particularly where only one fetus is affected, is complicated by the need to consider the interests of both twins. A policy which relies on the fetal size alone to identify fetuses at risk is unlikely to be very effective in preventing stillbirth at term. There is a need for better markers to identify fetuses at risk of adverse perinatal outcome among those which are SGA, as the majority of small fetuses have normal outcome.

Equally important, a more challenging task is to identify the fetuses at risk of adverse perinatal outcome among those which are presumed to be at low risk, simply due to the fact that their size is within normal range. It may be the case that in both singleton and twin pregnancies, the addition of Doppler parameters is of benefit in distinguishing the growth-restricted fetus from the 'normally' small baby.[3]

Selective FGR represents a management dilemma which is unique to twin pregnancies, where one twin appears to be compromised while the other is growing normally. The best interests of the twins may diverge, but the management chosen, whether intervention or conservative, will affect both.

Management Options

Regular ultrasound monitoring of fetal growth is an essential part of antenatal care in multiple pregnancies and the frequency of monitoring depends on chorionicity (Figures 16.1 and 16.2).[6]

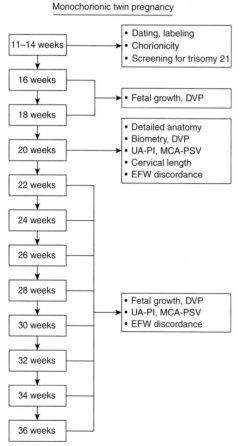

Figure 16.1 Sonographic monitoring of fetal growth and well-being in monochorionic twin pregnancies[6]

Dichorionic twin pregnancy

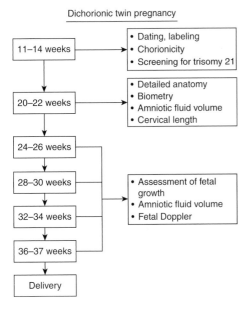

Figure 16.2 Sonographic monitoring of fetal growth and well-being in dichorionic twin pregnancies[6]

The management of the growth-restricted dichorionic twin is similar to that of a growth-restricted singleton, with the added factor of aiming to continue the pregnancy as long as possible in the interests of the appropriately grown co-twin. In same-sex twins, greater discordance is associated with increased risk of intrauterine death for both the smaller and the larger twin, while intrauterine death and the prognosis of the larger twin are unrelated to discordance when the twins are of different sexes.[7]

In certain highly selected cases, selective reduction can be the most appropriate management in a DC twin pregnancy. For example, early-onset severe pre-eclampsia may be associated with severe growth restriction in one of the twins. Selective reduction of the affected twin may be associated with resolution of the pre-eclampsia and can allow continuation of the pregnancy to achieve improved outcomes in the appropriately grown twin. In DC pregnancies, the death of the affected twin introduces a low risk of harm to the co-twin, mainly the risk of preterm delivery; therefore, expectant management is usually preferred.[3]

The management of sFGR in MC twins is based on the MC placental structure and interdependent fetal circulations. There is only scant evidence on how best to manage this condition, based on observational studies, and current practice varies among centres and clinicians. In MC pregnancies, the connected placental circulations put the healthy co-twin at risk of death and serious neurological impairment in addition to the risk of preterm delivery. Demise of one twin is associated with a 15% risk of death and 25% risk of neurodevelopmental impairment in the co-twin due to the acute feto–fetal transfusion that can result from the sudden fall in vascular resistance in the circulation of the demised twin. Any intervention should precede the fetal demise in order to prevent these consequences. Selective reduction is technically challenging as the vascular communications preclude the use of potassium chloride. Intrauterine fetal therapy has introduced a range of potential interventions for the antenatal management of these cases, including cord occlusion of the affected twin, intra-fetal laser ablation or radiofrequency ablation (RFA) of communicating vessels. With either of the latter techniques, the outcome for the co-twin looks similar, so the choice depends on operator preference and expertise.[3]

Doppler assessment seems to offer reliable information to determine the management type and timing. In DC pregnancies, similar to singletons, Dopplers are expected to follow a pattern of deterioration that can be used to guide the timing of intervention, but in MC pregnancies, the typical pattern of deterioration may not be observed. The compensatory effect of the co-twin's circulation may delay or even fully obscure the deterioration of the affected twin.[3]

In MC pregnancies, the presence or absence of umbilical artery Doppler end-diastolic flow in the affected twin at the time of diagnosis forms the basis of the classification system by Gratacos et al. (Figure 16.3).[8] Positive end-diastolic flow is reassuring (type I) whereas absent or reversed end-diastolic flow is a poor prognostic indicator (type II). The third category of intermittent absent or reversed end-diastolic flow (type III) is unique to MC pregnancies. In this group, the presence of large-diameter arterio-arterial anastomoses permits a compensatory flow from the normal twin, promoting longer survival of the growth-restricted twin. Unfortunately this is also the cause of acute transfusion events that is unpredictable and can lead to unexpected intrauterine death or neurological damage in both the growth-restricted and normally grown twin. It must be noted that this Doppler pattern is most likely to be close to the placental cord insertion site of the umbilical cord and can be missed unless low-sweep-speed pulsed Doppler is used.

The outcome of sFGR in MC twin pregnancies is dependant on the type. Type I sFGR has a good prognosis and elective delivery at around 34 weeks, and sometimes even up to 36 weeks is possible. A proportion of these cases can progress, underlining the importance of regular ultrasound surveillance. Types II and III have a poorer prognosis and are more likely to require intervention. Type II tends to progress in about 60% of cases, necessitating earlier delivery at 30–32 weeks, and has a worse prognosis compared with types I and III, particularly for the smaller fetus. In type III, deterioration of fetal status occurs in about 10% of cases, necessitating delivery at 31–33 weeks, and the larger fetus can have abnormal brain imaging and periventricular leukomalacia in up to 20% of cases due to the unpredictable acute transfusion events mentioned earlier. See Tables 16.2 and 16.3 for more detailed outcome data for each type derived from a systematic review and meta-analysis of 13 studies.[9]

Timing of Delivery in Dichorionic Twins with Selective Fetal Growth Restriction

There is little consensus about the optimal time of delivery. Early delivery carries the risks associated with prematurity, but delay may increase hypoxic damage.[10] In very early-onset severe FGR (< 28 weeks), particularly where the estimated weight of the growth-restricted fetus is not viable or is borderline viable (< 500–600 g), one option is no intervention, accepting that the growth-restricted fetus may die in utero but optimising gestation and hence outcome for the normal fetus. Where the growth-restricted fetus is viable and live birth is desirable, management decisions follow the same principle as for singleton FGR, but given that it is generally advised that uncomplicated dichorionic twins are delivered at 37–38 weeks of gestation and this is considered 'term', for late-onset growth pathology, an earlier gestational threshold is advised – that is, 35–36 weeks.

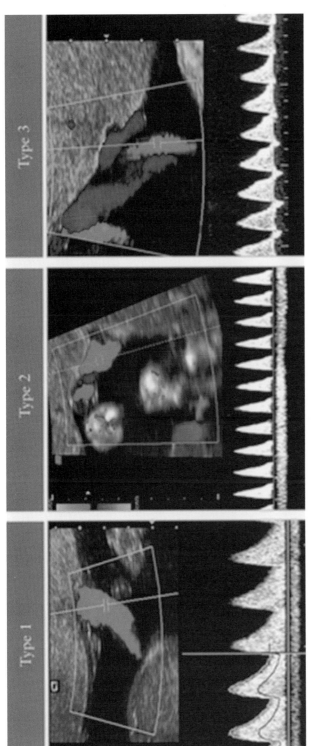

Figure 16.3 Gratacos et al. classification system for sFGR in twin pregnancies. In type I, the umbilical artery Doppler waveform has positive end-diastolic flow, while in type II, there is absent or reversed end-diastolic flow (AREDF). In type III, there is a cyclical/intermittent pattern of AREDF.[7] (A black and white version of this figure will appear in some formats. For the colour version, please refer to the plate section.)

Table 16.2 Outcomes in monochorionic twin pregnancies with selective fetal growth restriction (sFGR) according to type of sFGR) (adapted from systematic review and meta-analysis Buca et al. 2017)[9]

	Type I sFGR	Type II sFGR	Type III sFGR
Deterioration of fetal status	16.2%	58.9%	10.1%
Mean gestational age at delivery in weeks (95% CI)	33.7 (33.0–34.3)	30.9 (30.0–31.8)	32.0 (31.3–32.8)
% Birthweight discordance (95% CI)	23% (14.7–31.4)	44.3% (36.8–51.8)	32.5% (28.5–36.6)
Fetal outcomes (%)			
Perinatal mortality	6.3	21	11
Intrauterine death	2.5	13.2	8.9
Neonatal death	3.1	9.2	2.7
Double fetal loss	1	7.8	3.4
Abnormal brain imaging	2.5	13.8	12
IVH	0	8.2	4.9
PVL	2.1	13.9	11.7
Admission to NICU	38	93.4	58.3
RDS	30.1	45.7	91.7
Composite adverse outcome*	4.8	26.3	18.6

* Composite adverse outcome defined as presence of any mortality or abnormal brain findings
IVH = intraventricular haemorrhage; PVL = periventricular leukomalacia; RDS = respiratory distress syndrome; NICU = neonatal intensive care unit

For early-onset FGR, a few prospective multicentre studies have addressed the timing of delivery issue based on Doppler flow parameters. The Growth Restriction Intervention Trial (GRIT) investigated the timing of delivery for FGR in singleton pregnancy.[11] Pregnant women between 24 and 36 weeks of gestation with FGR were randomly assigned to immediate or delayed delivery if the obstetrician was uncertain about when the FGR fetus should be delivered based on umbilical artery Doppler parameters. There was no difference in overall mortality between the two groups. Although the GRIT study could not provide standard criteria for determining the timing of delivery, the lack of a difference in overall mortality between immediate and delayed delivery suggests that it may be important for parents or obstetricians to consider prolonging the time in utero for the normal twin of DC twins with sFGR, even for a short period. This is further supported by the fact that in a subgroup analysis of those delivered before 31 weeks, delayed delivery was associated with less neurodevelopmental morbidity and disability at age two.[12] Since publication of the GRIT study, the Trial of Umbilical and Fetal Flow in Europe (TRUFFLE) investigated in singleton pregnancy which method of fetal assessment should be used to trigger delivery in preterm fetal growth restriction – early or late changes in the fetal ductus venosus Doppler

Table 16.3 Outcomes in monochorionic twin pregnancies with selective intrauterine growth restriction (sFGR) according to type of sFGR, for smaller and larger fetus (adapted from systematic review and meta-analysis Buca et al. 2017)[9]

%	Type I sFGR		Type II sFGR		Type III sFGR	
	Smaller fetus	Larger fetus	Smaller fetus	Larger fetus	Smaller fetus	Larger fetus
Perinatal mortality	7.7	4.8	28	14.3	15.6	6.4
Intrauterine death	3	2	16.3	10.1	14.4	3.4
Neonatal death	4.1	2	12.6	4.4	2.3	3.8
Abnormal brain imaging	2	2.9	19.4	8.8	5.6	17.8
IVH	0	0	11.4	5.7	7.1	2.9
PVL	2.1	2.1	28.6	2.3	2	19.7
Composite adverse outcome*	7	4.8	35	17.5	18.2	16.7

* Composite adverse outcome is defined as the presence of any mortality or abnormal brain findings.
IVH = intraventricular haemorrhage; PVL = periventricular leukomalacia

waveform or cardiotocograph (CTG) short-term variation.[13] There was no difference in the primary outcome of the trial or the proportion of children free from neurological impairment at two years old, but the findings suggested that waiting for late ductus venosus changes (or severe CTG changes, which were used as safety net indication for delivery) was associated with more favourable developmental outcomes at two years of age. Current guidance is that a combination of sonographically evaluating growth velocity and Doppler flow parameters in umbilical artery, middle cerebral artery and the ductus venosus, using biophysical profile and/or computerised CTG should trigger gestational cut-offs to consider delivery.[14] See Tables 16.4 and 16.5.

Timing of Delivery in Monochorionic Twins with Selective Fetal Growth Restriction

The most recent guidelines on twin pregnancy have highlighted the lack of evidence. The ISUOG guidance states that 'there is limited evidence to guide the management of MC twins affected by sFGR',[6] while the Royal College of Obstetricians and Gynaecologists (RCOG) guidance on twin pregnancy states that 'due to a lack of available high quality evidence, there is no clear guidance on how to manage sFGR in twin pregnancies'.[15]

Based on expert opinion, these pregnancies should have follow-up ultrasound examinations at least weekly. In cases in which ductus venosus Doppler shows absent or reversed a-wave before 26 weeks of gestation, indicating a substantial risk of fetal demise of the

Table 16.4 Thresholds for timing of delivery in fetal growth restriction in dichorionic twins

Threshold for delivery	Parameters
< 30 weeks	Expectant management
30 weeks	DV absent or reversed 'a' wave
30–32 weeks	UA REDF
32–34 weeks	UA AEDF
> 34 weeks	MCA low PI
34–36 weeks	UA high PI
Triggers for considering earlier delivery at any gestation when EFW of FGR fetus > 500–600g	Static growth in a 2 week period, repeated persistent unprovoked decelerations on CTG or abnormal STV on cCTG, maternal indication eg. severe fulminating pre-eclampsia

DV = ductus venosus, UA = umbilical artery, REDF = reversed end diastolic flow, AEDF = absent end diastolic flow, MCA = middle cerebral artery, PI = pulsitility index, STV = short term variation, CTG = cardiotocograph, cCTG = computerized CTG

Table 16.5 Computerised cardiotocograph short-term variation (STV) thresholds (adapted from ISUOG Practice Guidelines)[12]

Gestation	STV (ms)
26–28+6 weeks	< 2.6
29–31+6 weeks	< 3.0
32–33+6 weeks	< 3.5
>/= 34 weeks	< 4.5

smaller twin, selective termination should be considered in order to protect the normally grown fetus from serious harm should the smaller twin die in utero.

When sFGR presents with an umbilical artery positive end-diastolic flow – that is, type I sFGR – the prognosis is usually good, and therefore it is a consensus that the expectant management based on a weekly Doppler evaluation (umbilical artery, middle cerebral artery and ductus venosus) and biweekly growth evaluation should be undertaken to look for progression to more severe stages, which can occur in up to 16% of cases.[8] Delivery should be timed for around 34 weeks if there is satisfactory growth velocity and no Doppler abnormality deterioration.

In types II and III sFGR, evaluation of ductus venosus Doppler and/or use of computerised CTG drives management. If ductus venosus Doppler (absent or reversed a-wave) or computerised CTG STV are abnormal (see Table 16.5), delivery will be indicated if the gestation is above 26 weeks. In cases in which the ductus venosus Doppler is normal and the growth velocity is acceptable, early delivery at or beyond 32 weeks, after a course of steroids, is indicated.[15]

Role of Intrauterine Fetal Intervention in Monochorionic Twins with Selective Fetal Growth Restriction

In general, after 26–28 weeks, the risks of preterm delivery are less than the risks of fetal intervention, depending on the locally available neonatal services. Only those sFGR pregnancies identified prior to the third trimester and with a high risk of intrauterine complications may be considered for fetal intervention. The available choices are laser coagulation of the anastomotic connections between the fetal circulations, selective reduction or termination of the whole pregnancy.[3]

Selective Reduction of the Smaller Twin

One management option, where expectant management is felt to carry an unacceptable risk of intrauterine demise of the smaller twin and the associated risks of mortality and neurological morbidity in the larger twin, is selective reduction of the smaller twin. This procedure is relatively straightforward to perform, the clinical outcomes are well described and most fetal intervention centres have a high degree of familiarity with both RFA (radiofrequency ablation) and bipolar cord occlusion. The survival of the larger twin after selective reduction in cases of type II sFGR is 87–90.9%, giving an overall survival rate of 43.8–45.4%. The most recent prospective cohort of severe types II and III sFGR reported an overall survival rate of 46.6% with survival of the larger twin at 93.3%.[16,17]

Fetoscopic Laser Photocoagulation of Connecting Vessels

Laser photocoagulation of connecting placental vessels is an established treatment for TTTS and there is growing interest in the benefit of using this technique in the management of sFGR in MC pregnancies. There are a number of theoretical advantages, including achieving separation of the fetal circulations and protecting the larger twin without necessarily sacrificing the smaller twin. Unlike in TTTS, however, the anastomotic connections are not the root cause of the growth restriction and in fact may be of net benefit to the smaller twin. Removing from the smaller twin the compensation afforded by the larger twin's circulation may only hasten the intrauterine demise of the smaller twin while protecting the larger twin from the effects of that event.

The procedure is technically difficult to perform because the normally grown twin does not have polyhydramnios and the growth-restricted twin is not stuck – that is, may have oligohydramnios but not anhydramnios, which makes it more difficult to visualise the placental vascular equator. In one study of laser photocoagulation of connecting placental vessels for type III sFGR, only 88.9% of procedures were completed because of technical difficulties and 12.5% of them required a second procedure.[18] The procedure carries a risk of preterm premature rupture of the membranes (PPROM), preterm labour and chorioamnionitis. Furthermore, perforation of the inter-twin membrane may occur either deliberately to facilitate access to the vascular equator or incidentally during the procedure, and cases of iatrogenic monoamniotic pregnancies have been reported.[18] Chorioamniotic separation may occur in up to 20% of cases treated fetoscopically and is associated with worse pregnancy outcomes.

Type II sFGR has the worst clinical prognosis and pregnancies with it comprised the first target group for trials of laser therapy. The survival of the larger twin seems to be less than after laser therapy (67.6–73.9%), but 30.4–38.7% of the smaller twins survive, contributing to a slight increase in overall survival compared to cord occlusion. The sFGR pregnancies most at risk of acute feto–fetal transfusion events are type III cases where large AA anastomoses render each twin vulnerable to ischaemic brain damage during even short periods of bradycardia and hypotension in their co-twin. Although the overall survival rate is higher than in type II, the difficulty in predicting deterioration in this group means they might be expected to benefit most from the 'dichorionisation' effect of laser treatment.[3]

Prediction of Growth Restriction

In terms of prediction, discordance in the crown–rump length is associated with the development of growth discordance and sFGR later in pregnancy. Crown–rump length discordance in the first trimester is also associated with a number of adverse pregnancy outcomes, including preterm delivery and pregnancy loss, thus pregnancies affected by a CRL discordance of > 20% should be discussed with a fetal medicine expert for consideration of additional monitoring. Recent studies have reported that the predictive accuracy is poor, however. In the second trimester, if the EFWs are concordant, it is highly unlikely that sFGR will develop, and this finding can be used to guide frequency of monitoring in later pregnancy. The presence of discordance at 21–24 weeks has been shown to be a poor predictor of the development of growth discordance and sFGR later in pregnancy.[3]

Conclusion

As twin pregnancies increase in frequency, general obstetricians need to develop a detailed appreciation of the physiological differences and subsequent challenges of managing FGR in twin pregnancies. Increased antenatal surveillance in twins is necessary to identify growth impairment early and to facilitate timely intervention. Concerning MC twins, despite the widespread use of fetoscopic intervention for TTTS, the therapeutic value of fetal intervention for sFGR is yet to be established. No randomised controlled trials have yet been reported, and there is therefore a lack of clarity on where the balance of risk and benefit lies when considering intervention in this group. Current best evidence suggests that selective reduction and fetoscopic laser therapy offer similar overall survival chances but laser therapy carries a higher risk of mortality and lower risk of morbidity.

Key Points

- At every ultrasound assessment of a twin pregnancy beyond 20 weeks of gestation, the EFW discordance should be calculated.
- Regular monitoring of fetal growth is fundamental.
- Chorionicity determines the aetiology of fetal growth discordance in multiple pregnancy.
- Selective fetal growth restriction in MC twins is related to placental share or TTTS.
- Selective FGR in DC twins is attributed to different genetic growth potential or underlying placental pathology, similar to singleton cases.

- Management of growth restriction in twin pregnancy needs to balance the competing interests of the larger and smaller fetuses.
- The Gratacos classification of sFGR in MC twin pregnancies is strongly correlated to the adverse perinatal outcomes.
- The management of the growth-restricted DC twin is similar to that of a growth-restricted singleton, with the added factor of aiming to continue the pregnancy as long as possible in the interests of the appropriately grown co-twin.
- The management of sFGR in MC pregnancies is complex and depends on type and severity of sFGR.
- In MC pregnancies, the typical pattern of Doppler deterioration may not be observed.
- Fetoscopic laser coagulation for sFGR is technically challenging and its therapeutic value is yet to be established.
- Twin pregnancies presenting with a CRL discordance of > 20% in the first trimester should be discussed with a fetal medicine specialist.

References

1. Kulkarni AD, Jamieson DJ, Jones HW Jr et al. Fertility treatments and multiple births in the United States. N Engl J Med 2013;369(23):2218–25.

2. Kent EM, Breathnach FM, Gillan JE et al. Placental pathology, birthweight discordance, and growth restriction in twin pregnancy: results of the ESPRiT Study. Am J Obstet Gynecol 2012;207(220):e1–e5.

3. Townsend R, Khalil A. Fetal growth restriction in twins. Best Pract Res Clin Obstet Gynaecol 2018;49:79–88.

4. Khalil A, Beune I, Hecher K et al. Consensus definition and essential reporting parameters of selective fetal growth restriction in twin pregnancy: a Delphi procedure. Ultrasound Obstet Gynecol 2019;53:47–54.

5. Khalil A, Thilaganathan B. Selective fetal growth restriction in monochorionic twin pregnancy: a dilemma for clinicians and a challenge for researchers. Ultrasound Obstet Gynecol 2019;53:23–5.

6. Khalil A, Rodgers M, Baschat A et al. ISUOG practice guidelines: the role of ultrasound in twin pregnancy. Ultrasound Obstet Gynecol 2016;48:669–70.

7. Demissie K, Ananth CV, Martin J et al. Fetal and neonatal mortality among twin gestations in the United States: the role of intrapair birth weight discordance. Obstet Gynecol 2002;100(3):474–80.

8. Gratacós E, Lewi L, Muñoz B et al. A classification system for selective intrauterine growth restriction in monochorionic pregnancies according to umbilical artery Doppler flow in the smaller twin. Ultrasound Obstet Gynecol 2007;30:28–34.

9. Buca D, Pagani G, Rizzo G, et al. Outcome in monochorionic twin pregnancies with selective intrauterine growth restriction according to the umbilical artery Doppler pattern of the smaller twin: a systematic review and meta-analysis. Ultrasound Obstet Gynecol 2017;50:559–68.

10. Kaku S, Kimura F, Murakami T. Management of fetal growth arrest in one of dichorionic twins: three cases and a literature review. Obstet Gynecol Int 2015;2015:289875.

11. GRIT Study Group. A randomised trial of timed delivery for the compromised preterm fetus: short term outcomes and Bayesian interpretation. BJOG 2003;110(1):27–32.

12 Thornton JG, Hornbuckle J, Vail A, Spiegelhalter DJ, Levene M. GRIT Study Group. Infant wellbeing at 2 years of age in the Growth Restriction Intervention Trial (GRIT): multicentred randomised controlled trial. Lancet 2004 7–13 Aug;364

(9433):513–20. https://doi.org/10.1016/S01
40-6736(04)16809-8. PMID: 15302194.

13. Lees CC, Marlow N, Van Wassenaer-
Leemhuis A et al. 2 year
neurodevelopmental and intermediate
perinatal outcomes in infants with very
preterm fetal growth restriction
(TRUFFLE): a randomised trial. Lancet
2015;385(9983):2162–72. https://doi.org/
10.1016/S0140-6736(14)62049-3

14. Khalil A, Rodgers M, Baschat A et al.
ISUOG practice guidelines: diagnosis and
management of small-for-gestational-age
fetus and fetal growth restriction.
Ultrasound Obstet Gynecol
2020;56:298–312. Published online in
Wiley Online Library (wileyonlinelibrary.
com). https://doi.org/10.1002/uog.22134

15. Royal College of Obstetricians and
Gynaecologists (RCOG). Management of
monochorionic twin pregnancy. Green-top
Guideline No. 51. RCOG: London, 2016.
www.rcog.org.uk/en/guidelines-research-
services/guidelines/gtg51

16. Bebbington MW, Danzer E,
Moldenhauer J, Khalek N, Johnson MP.
Radiofrequency ablation vs bipolar
umbilical cord coagulation in the
management of complicated
monochorionic pregnancies. Ultrasound
Obstet Gynecol 2012;40(3):319–24.

17. Parra-Cordero M, Bennasar M,
Martínez JM, Eixarch E, Torres X,
Gratacós E. Cord occlusion in
monochorionic twins with early
selective intrauterine growth
restriction and abnormal umbilical
artery Doppler: a consecutive series of
90 cases. Fetal Diagn Ther 2016 Jan;39
(3):186–91.

18. Gratacós E, Antolin E, Lewi L, et al.
Monochorionic twins with selective
intrauterine growth restriction and
intermittent absent or reversed
end-diastolic flow (Type III): feasibility and
perinatal outcome of fetoscopic placental
laser coagulation. Ultrasound Obstet
Gynecol 2008;31(6):669–75.

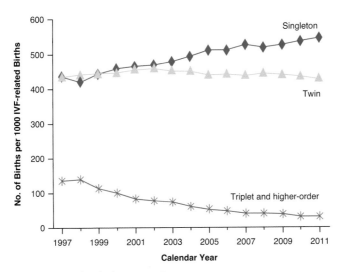

Figure 1.1 Changing incidence of multiple pregnancies
(Kulkarni AD, Jamieson DJ, Jones HW Jr, Kissin DM, Gallo MF, Macaluso M, Adashi EY. Fertility treatments and multiple births in the United States. *N Engl J Med* 2013; 369(23):2218–25. doi: 10.1056/NEJMoa1301467)

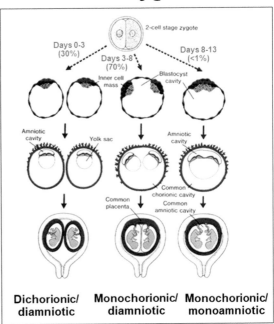

Figure 1.2 Zygosity and chorionicity of twin pregnancies

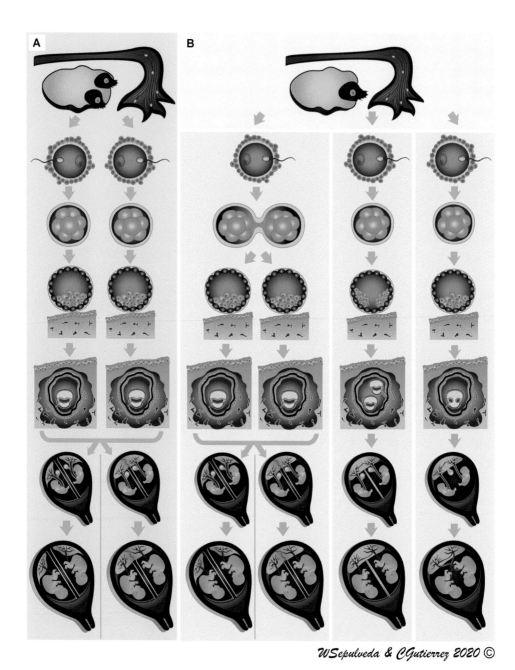

WSepulveda & CGutierrez 2020 ©

Figure 3.1 Classical representation of the three types of placentation in twin pregnancies according to zygosity. (A) Dizygotic twins develop from two separate eggs that are fertilised by two sperm; all have dichorionic-diamniotic placentation. (B) Monozygotic twins develop from a single zygote that subsequently splits and forms two embryos. Depending on the timing of splitting, they can be dichorionic-diamniotic, monochorionic-diamniotic or monochorionic-monoamniotic.

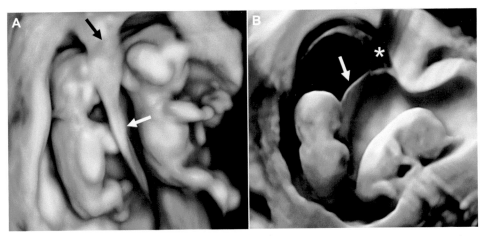

Figure 3.8 Surface-rendering three-dimensional ultrasound views of first-trimester twin pregnancies show the differences between dichorionic-diamniotic and monochorionic-diamniotic twins at the level of the dividing membrane (white arrows). **(A)** In dichorionic twins, the dividing membrane is thicker than in monochorionic-diamniotic twins and the 'lambda' sign is clearly seen at the inter-twin membrane–placental junction (black arrow). **(B)** In monochorionic-diamniotic twins, the dividing membrane is thin and is devoid of interposing chorion, which is also reflected at the level of the chorionic cavity (asterisk).

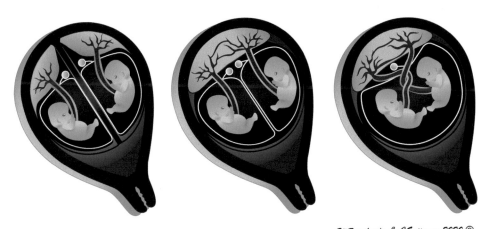

WSepulveda & CGutierrez 2020 ©

Figure 3.12 Schematic representation of the relation between yolk sac number and amnionicity in early pregnancy. In all dichorionic-diamniotic twin pregnancies, the yolk sacs are separated by chorionic tissue (left panel). In monochorionic-diamniotic twin pregnancies, two yolk sacs are present in the single chorionic cavity (middle panel). In monochorionic-monoamniotic twin pregnancies, only one yolk sac is usually identified (right panel).

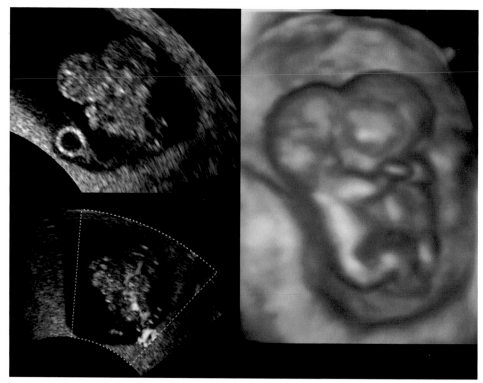

Figure 3.14 Amnionicity in early first-trimester monochorionic-monoamniotic twins. In this set of monochorionic-monoamniotic conjoined twins (thoracopagus type), there is only one yolk sac in the common chorionic cavity.

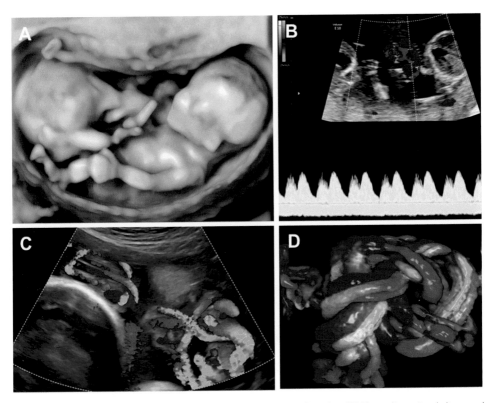

Figure 3.15 Monochorionic-monoamniotic twin pregnancy at 12 weeks 6 days. **(A)** Three-dimensional ultrasound shows two fetuses lying close together. The amniotic membrane was not identified. (B) Entanglement of the umbilical cords confirmed monoamnionicity. Spectral Doppler ultrasound demonstrates the two cardiac beats in the area of entanglement of the umbilical cords. (C) At 30 weeks, entanglement of the umbilical cords is evident as visualised with colour flow mapping. D, Three-dimensional HD live flow mapping demonstrates entanglement of the umbilical cords.

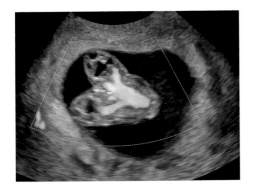

Figure 7.8 These images represent conjoined monochorionic-monoamniotic at 9 weeks. Colour Doppler is used to clarify the anatomy and identification of the conjoined twins which are thoracopagus (fusion from thorax to umbilicus).

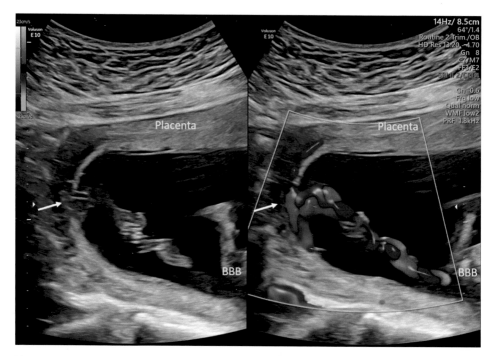

Figure 8.2 Split-screen ultrasound demonstrating a velamentous PCI (arrows) by two-dimensional (left) and colour flow (right) imaging with the anterior placenta several centimetres from the cord insertion.

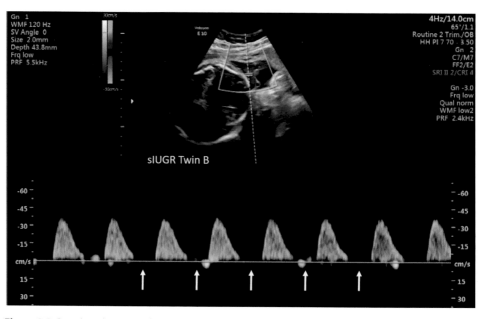

Figure 8.3 Doppler velocimetry of an MCDA twin with sIUGR demonstrating persistent absent end-diastolic flow (arrows)

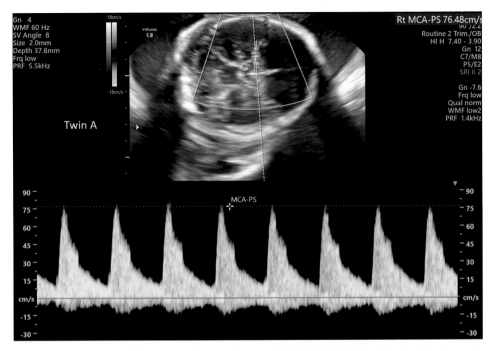

Figure 8.4 Elevated MCA-PSV in an MCDA twin pregnancy complicated by TAPS at 29 weeks after laser therapy for stage III TTTS at 21 weeks of gestation.

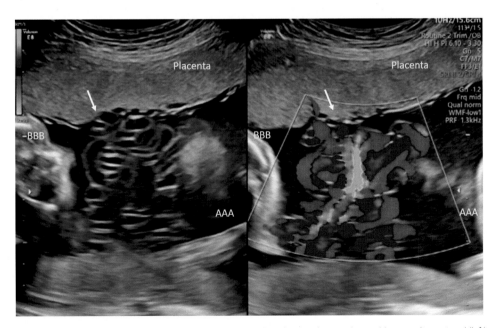

Figure 8.6 Split-screen ultrasound demonstrating umbilical cord entanglement (arrows) by two-dimensional (left) and colour flow (right) imaging in monoamniotic twins.

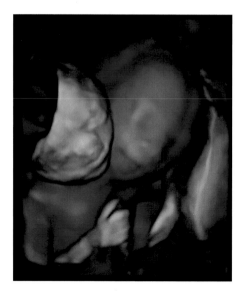

Figure 10.5 Three-dimensional ultrasound of dicephalic parapagus conjoined twins at 19 weeks of gestational age.

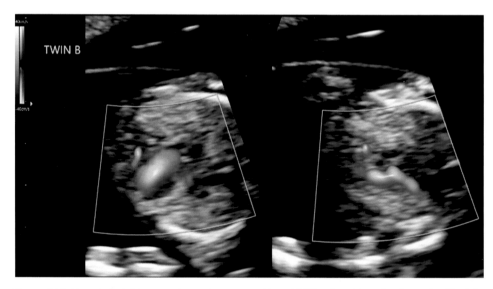

TWIN B

Figure 11.1 Hypoplastic left heart syndrome demonstrated in an MCDA twin at 13 weeks of gestation. The left-hand image of the four-chamber view shows univentricular filling and the right-hand image of the three-vessel view shows reversed flow in the ascending aorta.

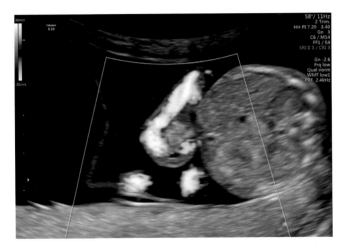

Figure 11.2 A small exomphalos seen in this MCDA twin at 14 weeks of gestation. The inter-twin membrane can be seen inserting into the monochorionic placenta.

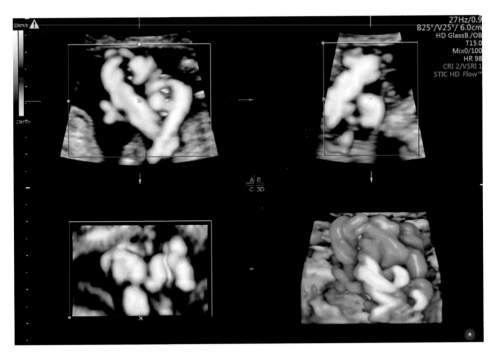

Figure 11.5 3-D multiplanar image showing cord entanglement in MCMA twins at 18 weeks of gestation

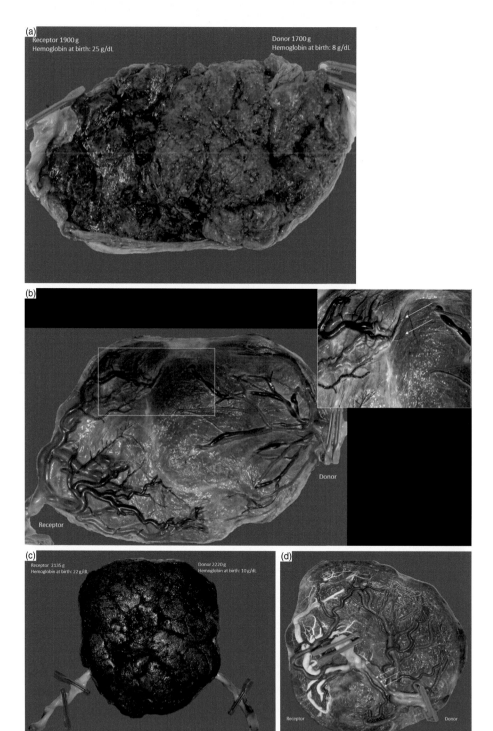

Figure 14.2 (a) Image of the maternal side from a monochorionic placenta of a spontaneous TAPS diagnosed at 30 weeks of gestation. This patient received one intrauterine transfusion at 31 weeks and was delivered electively at 32 weeks. There is a striking colour difference between the two parts. Also, the larger receptor had the smaller part of the placenta, indicating that TAPS influences fetal growth. (b) Image of the fetal side after colour injection. There were tiny artery-to-vein anastomoses (arrows). (c) Image of the maternal side from a monochorionic placenta of an acute peri-partum inter-twin transfusion. The babies were born vaginally at 34 weeks. There is no colour difference between the placental shares. (d) Placental injection showed a large artery-to-artery anastomoses (arrow), confirming an acute intra-partum transfusion as the cause of the haemoglobin difference.

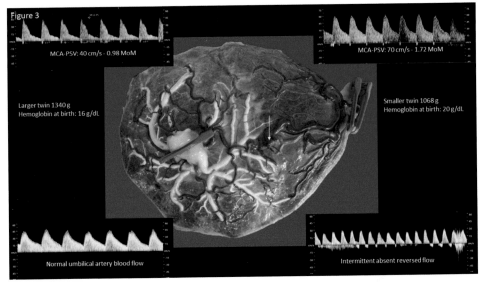

Figure 14.3 Monochorionic twin pair with type 3 selective growth restriction at 30 weeks of gestational age. Because of brain sparing, the MCA-PSV was increased in the smaller twin and normal in the larger twin. The typical intermittent absent or reversed end-diastolic flow pattern in the umbilical artery of the smaller twin indicates the presence of a large artery-to-artery anastomosis, which precludes the diagnosis of TAPS. The placenta showed the typical features of a type 3 growth restriction with a large artery-to-artery anastomosis (arrows) and little individual territory for the smaller twin with the marginal insertion.

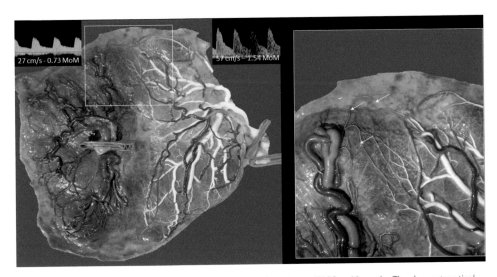

Figure 14.4 Images of a monochorionic pair with TTTS and coexistent TAPS at 28 weeks. The deepest vertical pocket was 11 cm in the receptor and 1.3 cm in the donor. At 28 weeks, we coagulated a visible artery-to-vein anastomosis and three tiny, unspecified anastomoses. We could not draw a Solomon line on the placenta because of intra-amniotic bleeding. After the surgery, TTTS disappeared but TAPS persisted. At 29 weeks, we gave an intrauterine transfusion to the donor for a haemoglobin of 6 g/dL and a partial exchange transfusion of the recipient for a haemoglobin of 21 g/dL. She was delivered electively at 32 weeks. The placenta showed minuscule, residual artery-to-vein anastomoses from the donor (2 clamps) to the receptor (1 clamp).

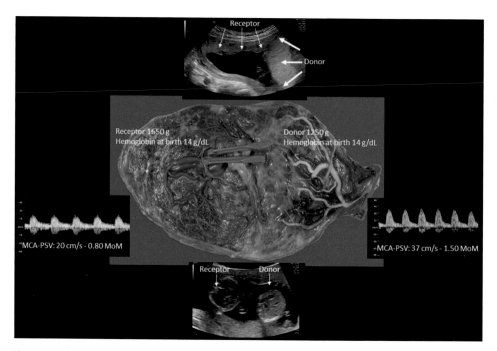

Figure 14.6 Ultrasound image of twin anemia-polycythemia at 15 weeks. The donor had the thick white part of the placenta, whereas the receptor had the thin, dark part. The receptor had a starry sky aspect of the liver. The pregnancy was managed expectantly. The MCA-PSV discordance improved spontaneously, and by 20 weeks, the MCA-PSV was concordant. She delivered at 31 weeks after spontaneous rupture of the membranes. The placenta did not show any anastomoses, as if we had performed a laser coagulation of all the anastomoses.

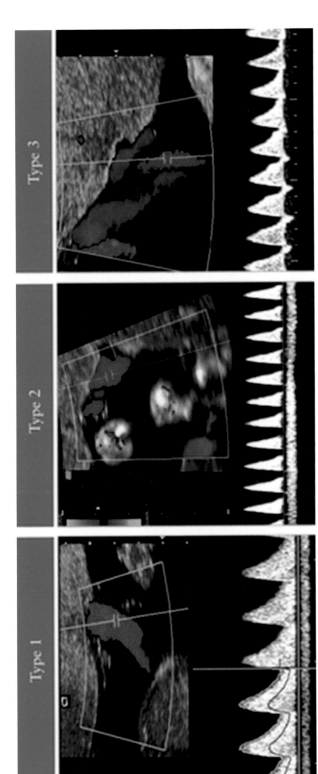

Figure 16.3 Gratacos et al. classification system for sFGR in twin pregnancies. In type I, the umbilical artery Doppler waveform has positive end-diastolic flow, while in type II, there is absent or reversed end-diastolic flow (AREDF). In type III, there is a cyclical/intermittent pattern of AREDF.[7]

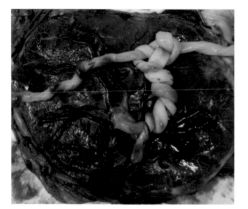

Figure 17.2 Proximate cord insertions and cord entanglement in a monoamniotic twin pregnancy

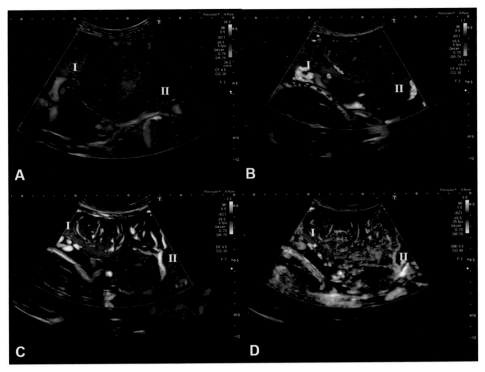

Figure 29.1 Comparison of colour Doppler imaging modalities to identify placental vasculature

The ultrasound images were taken from a monochorionic twin pregnancy with no features of twin–twin transfusion syndrome at 25+6 weeks' gestational age using:

(A) conventional colour Doppler with default obstetric mode settings (scale −34.2–34.2 cm.s^{-1}). Here the umbilical cord insertions (denoted as I and II) can be seen at the placental-amniotic interface; however, little colour signal is visible within the placental tissue.

(B) conventional colour Doppler with scale reduced to capture low flow (scale −1.7–1.7 cm.s^{-1}). In this image there is aliasing at the sites of the umbilical cord insertion into the placenta (denoted as I and II) and more vessels are seen within the placental tissue. However, the quality of the image is greatly reduced by motion artefact and signal noise and detail of the placental angio-architecture cannot be ascertained.

(C) Advanced dynamic flow with default settings (scale −3.3–3.3 cm.s^{-1}). Here the umbilical cord insertions are again seen at the placental-amniotic interface (denoted as I and II). However, in this image the branching vessels within the placenta can be seen in continuity from the cord insertions towards the materno-fetal interface, with minimal motion artefact or signal noise.

(D) Superb microvascular imaging with default settings (scale −0.8–0.8 cm.s^{-1}). Here the umbilical cord insertions can again be defined by colour signal intensity (denoted I and II) and there is an appearance of branching vessels from the cord insertions towards the materno-fetal interface, with many more and smaller vessels seen compared to ADF. In this instance there is significant motion artefact despite the relatively high frame rate.

Ultrasound images were obtained using a 1.8–6.2 MHz convex probe (i8C1, Aplio i900, Canon Medical Systems) and are reproduced here with written consent from the patient.

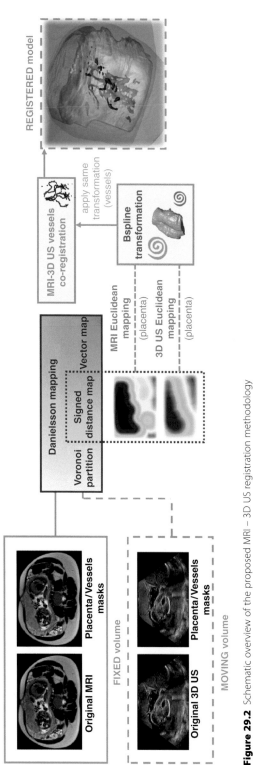

Figure 29.2 Schematic overview of the proposed MRI – 3D US registration methodology

Source: Torrents-Barrena et al. 2019 (13). TTTS-GPS: Patient-specific preoperative planning and simulation platform for twin-to-twin transfusion syndrome fetal surgery. Computer Methods and Programs in Biomedicine, 179, 104993 (Reuse licence 4784840550036)

Management of Monoamniotic Twins

Vagisha Pruthi, Shiri Shinar, Johannes Keunen, Greg Ryan and Tim van Mieghem

The Facts

Definition and Epidemiology

In monochorionic-monoamniotic twin pregnancies, two fetuses share a single placenta and a single amniotic cavity. This specific anatomic configuration is rare (8 per 100,000 pregnancies) and is the result of the late splitting of a single embryo between 8 and 13 days after fertilisation.[1] As such, monoamniotic twins are always monozygotic. Conjoined twins are a specific subtype of monoamniotic twins in whom the splitting of the embryos occurs even later in pregnancy. Monochorionic and monoamniotic twins are more common after assisted reproduction. The reason for this is unclear, but some think assisted hatching and embryo manipulation play a role.[2] Occasionally, monoamniotic twins can be the result of spontaneous or iatrogenic (amniocentesis, fetal surgery) tearing of the inter-twin amniotic membrane in diamniotic twins.

Diagnosis

It is important to determine chorionicity and amnionicity in the first trimester of pregnancy as this is the most accurate time period in which to do so. Moreover, correct determination of the number of placentas and inter-twin membranes in the first trimester is critical to counsel parents about possible pregnancy complications and to outline a plan for pregnancy surveillance. Monoamniotic twins are at significantly higher risk of adverse pregnancy outcomes than monochorionic-diamniotic or dichorionic twins. Monoamnionicity is diagnosed when no intervening membranes between two fetuses can be visualised with ultrasound (Figure 17.1). Amnionicity can be difficult to determine before 10 weeks as the inter-twin membrane in monochorionic-diamniotic twins is often very thin at that time. Transvaginal ultrasound with a high-frequency probe can help in that situation. Other ultrasound findings that may be helpful in determining amnionicity include the presence of cord entanglement, which is pathognomonic for monoamniotic twins, and the number of yolk sacs. Of note, however, is that only 68% of monoamniotic twins will have a single yolk sac and 32% will have two sacs.[3] If chorionicity and amnionicity cannot be determined by 12 weeks of gestation, referral to an expert centre is recommended.

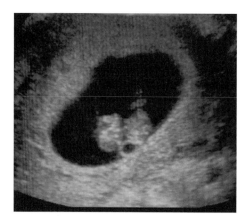

Figure 17.1 Ultrasound image of monoamniotic twin pregnancy at 7 weeks of gestation. Note the single yolk sac and the lack of intervening membrane.

Complications

Congenital Anomalies

In monoamniotic twins, the risk of birth defects is as high as 15–25%.[4,5] Usually, only one fetus is affected, and if both fetuses are affected, anomalies are often discordant. The high incidence of structural anomalies is explained by the delayed cleavage of the embryo and likely also by important blood volume shifts through large artery-to-artery anastomoses at the level of the placenta.[6] As a consequence, heart defects are the most common anomaly in monoamniotic twins (up to 30% of all anomalies). Acardiac twinning, also called twin-reversed arterial perfusion (TRAP) sequence, is a type of cardiac anomaly specific to monochorionic twins and can also occur in monoamniotic pregnancies. In this condition, which is described in more detail in Chapter 15, the acardiac mass does not have a circulation of its own and is perfused by the pump twin through placental anastomoses. The acardiac mass is never viable and compromises the healthy co-twin through cardiac failure (polyhydramnios, hydrops, fetal death) and mass effect (preterm birth). Only 4% of structural defects in monoamniotic twins have an underlying genetic aetiology, which is much less than in monochorionic-diamniotic twins (15%) or dichorionic twins (25%).

Birth defects and pregnancy terminations as a consequence of birth defects explain about half of the mortalities observed in monoamniotic twins. The management of discordant anomalies is similar to that in monochorionic-diamniotic twins except that, in case of selective reduction, cord transection should be performed after the cord flow is interrupted to prevent further cord accidents. Given the frequency and impact of birth defects in this population, we perform earlier anatomy assessment and echocardiography in these pregnancies.

Twin–Twin Transfusion Syndrome

Twin–twin transfusion syndrome (TTTS), which complicates 10–15% of monochorionic-diamniotic twins, is only seen in 2–4% of monoamniotic pregnancies.[1] This lower incidence is explained by the proximate cord insertions and large bidirectional artery-to-artery anastomoses which compensate for unidirectional flow through arterio-venous anastomoses.[6] As there is no inter-twin membrane to delineate the fetus with oligohydramnios from the fetus with polyhydramnios, TTTS is harder to diagnose in monoamniotic twins and stage I TTTS (amniotic fluid discordance) cannot be diagnosed. More advanced stages of TTTS are suspected if polyuric polyhydramnios (large bladder in one twin) is noted in combination with an empty bladder in the other twin and/or Doppler changes characteristic of TTTS. Despite the rarity of TTTS, we follow these pregnancies with biweekly ultrasounds from 16 weeks of gestation onwards.

A recent systematic review and meta-analysis documents the outcomes of TTTS in monoamniotic twins.[7] Among 890 monoamniotic twin pregnancies, only 46 developed TTTS. Expectantly managed cases miscarried in 10.7% of cases. The incidence of intrauterine, neonatal and perinatal deaths was 24.3%, 13.5% and 32.4%, respectively. Fetoscopic laser ablation of placental anastomoses did not seem to improve outcomes significantly, and this is likely due to the fact that occlusion of large inter-twin anastomoses in the presence of proximate cord insertions is often lethal for both fetuses. Although the number of cases reviewed in the paper was too low to provide strong evidence regarding the outcomes of selective cord occlusion, this strategy seemed to be associated with the best survival rates. Of note, after cord occlusion in monoamniotic twins, one should transect the cord of the dead fetus to prevent further cord accidents.

Selective Fetal Growth Restriction

Growth **restriction** is three times more common in monoamniotic twins than in singletons. Almost 40% of cases are born with a birthweight below the 10th centile[10] and 10% weigh less than the 3rd centile.[5] The incidence of selective fetal growth restriction, where only one fetus is small, is lower than in monochorionic-diamniotic twin pregnancies due to the proximate cord insertions and large placental vascular anastomoses. The average birthweight discordance in monoamniotic twins is 10%[5] compared with ~15% in diamniotic twins, and a birthweight difference of more than 25% is only seen in 3% of cases.[8] Important inter-twin weight differences increase the risk of fetal death in monoamniotic twins.

Intrauterine Fetal Death

Although the perinatal mortality of monoamniotic twins has decreased over the past three decades, still only 62–70% of monoamniotic twins diagnosed in the first trimester of pregnancy survive.[9,10] As discussed earlier, about half of the fetal losses are explained by congenital anomalies or pregnancy termination. The remaining fetal deaths are explained by cord accidents (tight entanglement) (Figure 17.2) and/or rapid inter-twin transfusion imbalances. Prevention by maternal administration of Sulindac, which reduces the fetal urinary output, the amniotic fluid volume and fetal movements, has never found widespread uptake.

The Issues

Once monoamniotic fetuses have reached a gestational age at which delivery becomes an option, prevention of stillbirth could be initiated by urgent delivery if signs of fetal distress are noted. Most centres will therefore initiate close surveillance after viability. Unfortunately, level 1 evidence on the best method, frequency and setting of surveillance is still lacking. Moreover, experts still disagree on the timing of delivery and to a lesser extent on mode of delivery. The controversy is mainly due to the rarity of these pregnancies, precluding large trials. The evidence and guidance presented in the next section mainly relies on outcomes reported in retrospective (multicentre) observational studies. Despite

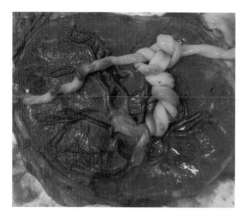

Figure 17.2 Proximate cord insertions and cord entanglement in a monoamniotic twin pregnancy (A black and white version of this figure will appear in some formats. For the colour version, please refer to the plate section.)

the fact that interventional and prospective trials are lacking, more recent studies present better outcomes than older studies, suggesting that current surveillance strategies, in combination with advances in neonatal care, have made a positive difference for these pregnancies. Additionally, a few observational studies seem to show that monoamniotic pregnancies undergoing close surveillance have better outcomes than those that do not.

The Management Options

Method of Surveillance

At our centre, we intensify fetal surveillance after 'viability'. We offer a consultation with our neonatology team to all couples expecting monoamniotic twins around 24 weeks of gestation to discuss the outcomes of preterm birth. After this discussion, the timing of variability is set, typically between 24 and 28 weeks, depending on patient preferences. At 'viability', steroids are administered for fetal pulmonary maturation. The best surveillance method for monitoring monoamniotic twin pregnancies is still unclear. Most centres initiate both ultrasound surveillance (to assess long-term well-being by assessing growth and amniotic fluid volume) in combination with fetal heart rate monitoring (to assess short-term well-being by looking for heart rate decelerations or prolonged episodes of fetal tachycardia). On Doppler ultrasound, diastolic notching in the umbilical artery or absent and reversed end-diastolic flow suggest the presence of cord compression, but these flow patterns are extremely common and often transient. As such, we don't use these indicators as triggers for delivery. Management of monoamniotic twins in expert centres is recommended given that clinician experience plays an important role in recognising triggers for delivery, but also to avoid unwarranted preterm delivery based on benign findings.

Frequency and Setting of Surveillance

Evidence is lacking on the optimal frequency of surveillance after viability, but most will recommend daily to alternate day fetal heart rate monitoring in combination with ultrasound one to three times per week.[5,11,12] Continuous fetal heart rate monitoring is impractical and only feasible in about 50% of cases and is therefore not recommended. Even with very close surveillance, fetal deaths have been reported just hours after a reassuring test, suggesting that fetal deaths are not all preventable and most large centres report fetal death rates of 2–5%, despite close surveillance.

Specialists still disagree on the optimal setting of surveillance (inpatient vs outpatient), and this has been the topic of heated debates. Unfortunately, when critically analysing the literature, most studies are confounded by the fact that location of surveillance (inpatient vs outpatient) is often linked with method and frequency of surveillance with less or no surveillance going on in outpatients and surveillance starting later in pregnancy.[10,11,12] Careful analysis of all studies, however, suggests that the risk of fetal death becomes very low once surveillance is initiated, be it in an inpatient or outpatient setting (< 5%).[5,8,10,13] At our centre, we therefore offer patients the choice, taking all risks and benefits into consideration. Of note, we discuss the risks of inpatient surveillance including an increased risk of venous thromboembolism, the economic and societal costs, the disruption to family life and an increased risk of psychiatric distress with higher rates of hopelessness and despair (42% vs 24%), thoughts of self-harm or suicide (4% vs 0%) and post-partum depression (12% vs 4%) in inpatients.[14] This should obviously be balanced with access to care and geographic constraints.

Timing of Birth

As mentioned earlier, some fetal deaths remain unpredictable, despite close surveillance. Therefore, most experts will recommend delivery when the risk of pregnancy continuation outweighs neonatal risks. A retrospective multicentre study of nearly 200 monoamniotic twin pairs showed that this balance was reached around between 32 and 33 weeks of gestation.[5] At that point, the risk of a severe, non-respiratory neonatal complication (death before discharge from the NICU, culture-proven sepsis, necrotising enterocolitis, retinopathy of prematurity more than grade II, intraventricular haemorrhage more than grade I or cystic periventricular leukomalacia) is lower than the prospective risk of fetal death (3.1%).[5] At our centre, we therefore deliver uncomplicated monoamniotic twins from 33 weeks of gestation, even though in some units, longer expectant management is offered.[15]

Mode of Delivery

Most experts will deliver monoamniotic twins by elective caesarean section given the risk of acute occlusion of cord knots during labour and delivery. Moreover, there is a risk of entanglement of the first twin in the umbilical cord of the second twin, mandating transection of that cord to allow for delivery of the first twin. This scenario creates an acute emergency and possible asphyxia of the second twin. Despite this, it is important to mention that some obstetricians still advocate for vaginal delivery of monoamniotic twins.[15]

Key Points

- Adverse pregnancy outcomes are increased in MCMA twin pregnancies.
- Highest risk of pregnancy loss is before 20 weeks' gestation.
- Increased fetal surveillance is advocated in all MCMA twins after 24 weeks' gestation – in either the inpatient or the outpatient setting.
- Elective birth is advocated from 33 weeks' gestation.

Video 17.1 Dating ultrasound at 9 weeks of gestation. Transabdominal ultrasound showing a monoamniotic twin gestation with a single yolk sac and a single amniotic cavity.

Video 17.2 First-trimester ultrasound at 12 weeks of gestation. Transabdominal ultrasound showing a monoamniotic twin gestation. Note the presence of cord entanglement and the absence of a dividing inter-twin membrane.

References

1. Glinianaia SV, Rankin J, Khalil A et al. Prevalence, antenatal management and perinatal outcome of monochorionic monoamniotic twin pregnancy: a collaborative multicenter study in England, 2000–2013. Ultrasound Obstet Gynecol 2019;**53**:184–92.

2. Knopman JM, Krey LC, Oh C, Lee J, McCaffrey C, Noyes N. What makes them split? Identifying risk factors that lead to monozygotic twins after in vitro fertilization. Fertil Steril 2014 Jul;**102**(1):82–9.

3. Fenton C, Reidy K, Demyanenko M, Palma-Dias R, Cole S, Umstad MP. The significance of yolk sac number in monoamniotic twins. Fetal Diagn Ther 2019;**46**(3):193–9.

4. Allen VM, Windrim R, Barrett J, Ohlsson A. Management of monoamniotic twin pregnancies: a case series and systematic review of the literature. BJOG 2001 Sep;**108**(9):931–6.

5. Van Mieghem T, De Heus R, Lewi L et al. Prenatal management of monoamniotic twin pregnancies. Obstet Gynecol 2014 Sep;**124**(3):498–506.

6. Hack KE, Van Gemert MJ, Lopriore E et al. Placental characteristics of monoamniotic twin pregnancies in relation to perinatal outcome. Placenta 2009 Jan;**30**(1):62–5.

7. Murgano D, Khalil A, Prefumo F et al. Outcome of twin-to-twin transfusion syndrome in monochorionic monoamniotic twin pregnancies: a systematic review and meta-analysis. Ultrasound Obstet Gynecol 2019 Oct 8. https://doi.org/10.1002/uog.21889

8. Saccone G, Khalil A, Thilaganathan B et al. Weight discordance and perinatal mortality in monoamniotic twin pregnancies: analysis of the MONOMONO, NorSTAMP and STORK multiple pregnancy cohorts. Ultrasound Obstet Gynecol 2020 March 27;**55**(3):332–8.

9. Litwinska E, Syngelaki A, Cimpoca B, Frei L, Nicolaides KH. Outcome of twin pregnancies with two live fetuses at 11–13 weeks' gestation. Ultrasound Obstet Gynecol 2019 Oct 15. https://doi.org/10.1002/uog.21892

10. Madsen C, Søgaard K, Zingenberg H et al. Outcomes of monoamniotic twin pregnancies managed primarily in outpatient care: a Danish multicenter study. Acta Obstet Gynecol Scand 2019 Apr;**98**(4):479–86. https://doi.org/10.1111/aogs.13509

11. Heyborne KD, Porreco RP, Garite TJ, Phair K, Abril D, Obstetrix/Pediatrix Research Study Group. Improved perinatal survival of monoamniotic twins with intensive inpatient monitoring. Am J Obstet Gynecol 2005;**192**:96–101.

12. MONOMONO Working Group. Inpatient vs outpatient management and timing of delivery of uncomplicated monochorionic monoamniotic twin pregnancy: the MONOMONO study. Ultrasound Obstet Gynecol 2019 Feb;**53**(2):175–83.

13. Van Mieghem T, Shub A. Management of monoamniotic twins: the question is not 'where?', but 'how?' Ultrasound Obstet Gynecol 2019 Feb;**53**(2):151–2.

14. Winkler SS, Mustian MN, Mertz HL. The psychosocial impact of inpatient management of monoamniotic twin gestations. J Matern Fetal Neonatal Med 2016;29:1877–80.

15. Anselem O, Mephon A, Le Ray C, Marcellin L, Cabrol D, Goffinet F. Continued pregnancy and vaginal delivery after 32 weeks of gestation for monoamniotic twins. Eur J Obstet Gynecol Reprod Biol 2015 Nov;194:194–8.

Chapter 18

Maternal Complications in Multiple Pregnancy

Sarah Rae Easter and Mike Foley

The Facts

Maternal Morbidity in Multiple Pregnancy

Considering the prevalence of fetal and prematurity-associated complications in multifetal gestations, clinicians dedicate a tremendous amount of resources to optimise neonatal outcomes in these high-risk pregnancies. From use of ultrasound to screen for placental complications to assessments for risk of preterm birth, the majority of guidelines in the management of twin and higher-order multiple pregnancies centre on the fetus.[1] A well-known but less overtly considered set of complications of multifetal pregnancies are those related to maternal health. The increased association between multifetal pregnancies and adverse maternal outcomes relative to singleton pregnancies is not only intuitive, but is also well described in the literature. Yet we lack specific guidelines or screening protocols to monitor for the well-known maternal complications of multifetal pregnancies.

The complexity of addressing maternal complications of multifetal pregnancies is underscored by evolutionary and societal imperative – the unspoken acknowledgement that mothers of multiples assume more risk for the potential reward of more offspring. This biologic truth coupled with the confounded epidemiology of multifetal pregnancy in the era of assisted reproductive technology (ART) challenges any attempt to systematically improve maternal outcomes in this population.[2] The exclusion of multifetal pregnancies in many clinical trials coupled with the knowledge of differential impact of obstetric interventions in twin compared to singleton populations can further challenge the development of an evidence-based strategy. In the absence of evidence-based guidelines, the obstetric care provider must adopt a uniform approach to prevention and management of maternal complications of multifetal pregnancies characterised by a high index of suspicion rooted in an understanding of epidemiology and pathophysiology. The tenets of this strategy include universal maternal risk assessment to provide risk-appropriate antenatal care, avoidance of severe maternal morbidity (SMM) at the time of delivery and comprehensive post-partum follow-up aimed at early detection and prevention (Figure 18.1).

Patient-Level Pathophysiology

Multifetal pregnancies carry an increased risk of a range of maternal complications. The clinical impact of some complications such as hyperemesis, gestational diabetes or anaemia may be minimal in the context of an otherwise high-risk pregnancy. Other diagnoses such as hypertension, haemorrhage and caesarean delivery may be causal on the pathway to SMM. Though the severity of these maternal complications may vary, their increased prevalence in

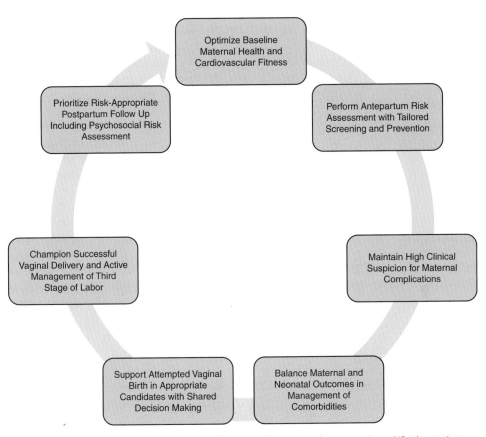

Figure 18.1 Framework for standardised approach to optimising maternal outcomes in multifetal gestations

multifetal pregnancies relative to singleton pregnancies underscores the extreme aberrations in physiology required to support two or more fetuses and their accompanying placentas.

The role of the placenta in hallmark diseases of pregnancy such as pre-eclampsia, gestational diabetes and hyperemesis is well described. Reason coupled with evidence suggests that the increase in placental mass accompanying multifetal pregnancies would increase the risk of these complications arising from the placental milieu. Observational data demonstrating a 6.5% prevalence of pre-eclampsia in singleton pregnancies and a rate of 12.7% in twins and 20.0% in triplets lend support to this notion. The known association between ART, pre-eclampsia and twins and higher-order multiples further confounds the relationship between placental pathophysiology and multifetal gestations. A review of cardiovascular physiology highlights the contribution of maternal haemodynamics to the hallmark diseases affecting multifetal pregnancies and may help explain the increased prevalence of more severe maternal outcomes in this population.

Contemporary studies underscore the importance of the maternal cardiovascular adaptation to pregnancy in the pathogenesis of comorbidities thought to arise from the placenta, including pre-eclampsia or fetal growth restriction. If an increase in cardiac output (CO) is the hallmark physiologic adaptation of pregnancy, clinical intuition would suggest the increase in this parameter is more dramatic in multiple pregnancies. Echocardiographic studies support this increase in CO accompanied by a decrease in total vascular resistance (TVR).[3] Longitudinal data demonstrate that patients with twin pregnancies complicated by placental insufficiency or pre-eclampsia show a decrease in CO and an increase in TVR compared to those without complication (Table 18.1).[4] These studies parallel findings from the singleton literature supporting the association between aberrant maternal haemodynamics and adverse fetal and obstetric outcomes (Table 18.1).

Echocardiographic assessment of cardiac function during twin pregnancies highlights the importance of diastolic function. Diastolic function refers to the ability of the heart to relax during ventricular filling and, in the context of pregnancy, accommodate the increased plasma volume requisite to increase stroke volume and CO. Echocardiographic studies of uncomplicated twin pregnancies demonstrate a progressive decrease in diastolic function across trimesters supporting the toll of this subacute state of volume overload on the maternal heart. Post-partum assessment of diastolic function demonstrates impaired ventricular relaxation relative to first trimester values. Physiologically these findings can be considered evidence of the early adaptations in diastolic function in twin pregnancies or support the long-term impact of this exaggerated cardiovascular demand. The aforementioned changes in both systolic and diastolic function in twin pregnancies highlight the extreme adaptation required to support a multifetal pregnancy and perfuse the associated placentas.

Population-Level Data

A deeper understanding of the hallmark cardiovascular adaptations to pregnancy helps underscore some of the pathophysiology of pregnancy-associated comorbidities, like pre-eclampsia,

Table 18.1 Changes in haemodynamic parameters in uncomplicated twin compared to other pregnancies

Parameter	Change across Uncomplicated Twin Pregnancy	Twin vs Singleton Pregnancy	Complicated* vs Uncomplicated Twin Pregnancy	Change across Complicated* Twin Pregnancy
Heart Rate	Increase	None	None	None
Stroke Volume	None	Higher	Higher	None
Cardiac Output	Increase	Higher	Lower	None
Systolic Blood Pressure	Increase	None	None	None
Diastolic Blood Pressure	Increase	None	None	None
Mean Arterial Pressure	Increase	None	None	None
Total Vascular Resistance	Decrease	Lower	Lower	None

* Complicated twin pregnancy is defined as pre-eclampsia or gestational hypertension or birthweight of one or both twins less than the 5th percentile for gestational age.

found in multifetal pregnancies. At the other end of the scientific spectrum, changes in haemodynamics can also inform the interpretation of studies exploring the epidemiology of extreme adverse outcomes including severe maternal morbidity or mortality. Studies from the Centers for Disease Control and World Health Organization independently report a threefold increase in the risk of all causes of maternal mortality for multifetal pregnancies compared to singleton pregnancies.[2] These epidemiologic associations between multifetal pregnancy and SMM are remarkably consistent across a large time span in a variety of practice settings. The relative contribution of maternal comorbidities and available resources to improve maternal outcomes undoubtedly varies according to clinical environment. But the relative stability of the risk factors and their magnitude of effect underscores the obvious – there is something fundamentally different about multifetal pregnancy compared to singleton pregnancies.

For the physiologist, the aforementioned findings offer fascinating insight into the maternal cardiovascular adaptation to twin pregnancy. For the epidemiologist, the adverse maternal outcomes suggest potential public health interventions to improve outcomes. For the clinician, these physiologic and epidemiology studies considered in tandem offer important background to help contextualise the downstream maternal complications associated with multifetal gestations. Cardiovascular maladaptation may be a risk factor for developing pregnancy-specific comorbidities, but it also contributes to the maternal response to the physiologic challenge of pregnancy, labour and delivery.

The Issues

Addressing Maternal Risk

Simply stating a patient is at an increased risk of adverse outcomes relative to a singleton pregnancy without identifying a modifiable risk factor or intervention is of little use to the clinician charged with managing the patient at the bedside. Conversely, an understanding of the increased maternal risks associated with multifetal pregnancy compared to singleton pregnancy is helpful to both raise clinical suspicion for adverse maternal outcomes and offer background context on the limited physiologic reserve that may accompany this extreme haemodynamic state. A broad overview of the maternal risks associated with multifetal pregnancy is a key part of counselling to encourage awareness of symptoms. National guidelines support offering non-directive patient counselling about the risks associated with higher-order multifetal pregnancies including the option of multifetal pregnancy reduction of one or more fetuses. The majority of evidence on multifetal pregnancy reduction centres on optimising neonatal outcomes but patient counselling should incorporate the maternal medical risks of multifetal pregnancy situated in the context of pre-existing maternal comorbidities.

Quantifying an individual's risk of severe maternal morbidity is challenging, but evidence-based scoring systems or algorithms exist. Using data from a French multicentre study of twin pregnancies, Korb and colleagues developed two algorithms to quantify maternal risk incorporating characteristics known at the onset of pregnancy and developing across the course of gestation.[5] Key early risk factors for severe maternal morbidity included a pregnancy conceived by in vitro fertilisation (IVF), nulliparity and maternal country of birth. These risk factors evolved later in pregnancy to include the presence of pre-eclampsia, placenta praevia and fetal macrosomia. This type of individualised risk assessment presented to patients as absolute and not relative risk is more clinically useful than the aforementioned studies comparing women with multifetal gestations to women with singleton gestations.

First-Trimester Clinical Complaints

After appropriate counselling, attention should be directed towards available strategies for maternal risk reduction. National guidelines support the use of low-dose aspirin beginning at 12 weeks for all patients with multifetal pregnancies to reduce the risk of pre-eclampsia. Contemporary meta-analyses demonstrate a relative risk for preterm pre-eclampsia of 0.62 (95% CI 0.45–0.87).[6] Subsequent stratified analyses demonstrate this reduction in preterm pre-eclampsia was confined to trials where aspirin was initiated prior to 16 weeks at a dose at or above 100 mg. The inclusion of twin and multifetal pregnancies in studies examining the impact of aspirin on pre-eclampsia is variable. Most guidelines continue to endorse administration of 81 mg of aspirin. The evidence supporting the efficacy of a slightly higher dose coupled with the increased volume of distribution and clearance in multifetal pregnancy could support a role for higher doses of 100–150 mg in this population.

Management of other first-trimester maternal issues such as nausea and vomiting of pregnancy or hyperemesis gravidarum parallels recommendations for singleton pregnancies. Multifetal pregnancies carry with them an increased metabolic demand warranting dedicated anticipatory guidance and tailored consideration in addressing complications. The Institute of Medicine (IOM) recommends a gestational weight gain of 37–54 pounds for women of normal weight, 31–50 pounds for overweight women and 25–42 pounds for those with comorbid obesity.[7] The increased metabolic demand and higher nutritional requirement of multifetal pregnancies may lower the threshold for initiation of supplemental nutrition. The reported tolerance of enteral nutrition coupled with known complications of total parenteral nutrition including line-associated sepsis and thromboembolic disease make enteral nutrition via nasogastric tube the preferred approach. The IOM recommendations are derived from studies demonstrating decreased rates of preterm birth and larger neonatal birthweights in women achieving the set thresholds, but the impact of this weight gain on maternal outcomes is unknown.[7] Monitoring for excessive weight gain is equally important to optimise pregnancy outcomes and long-term maternal health.

Physical activity in pregnancy plays an important role in avoiding excessive weight gain. Authorities acknowledge the benefits of physical activity and encourage aerobic and strength-conditioning exercises for women with uncomplicated pregnancies. However, they go on to list multiple gestation at risk of premature labour as an absolute contraindication to aerobic exercise during pregnancy without quantifying this level of risk for the clinician. If improving cardiopulmonary reserve is a benefit of physical activity and patients with multifetal gestations are subject to complications rooted in failure to compensate to haemodynamic demands, reason would suggest that women with multifetal pregnancies may derive additional benefits from exercise. With this in mind, reinforcing the recommendation of 150 minutes per week of moderate-intensity aerobic activity equivalent to brisk walking in women with multifetal pregnancies seems warranted. The ability of physical activity to improve obstetric outcomes in women with multifetal gestation is unknown, but early encouragement of physical activity is a low-risk intervention with the potential short- and long-term benefits to a woman's health.

Third-Trimester Clinical Conundrums

After this initial anticipatory guidance, the majority of antenatal care for women with multifetal gestations is dedicated to the prevention and early detection of complications arising in the late second and third trimester such as spontaneous preterm birth, fetal growth restriction or pre-eclampsia (Table 18.2). Many guidelines support screening, diagnosis and management for pregnancy complications in a similar way as singleton pregnancies. However, close attention to the rationale and evidence informing these recommendations in singletons and how they may (or may not) be applicable to multifetal pregnancies is warranted. For example, gestational diabetes mellitus (GDM) can be considered another placentally mediated adaptation or complication of multifetal pregnancies associated with the aforementioned increased metabolic demand. The rationale for universal screening for GDM is derived from randomised controlled trial and meta-analysis data demonstrating a reduction in rates of shoulder dystocia, macrosomia and pre-eclampsia with treatment. Though macrosomia and shoulder dystocia seem less relevant for multifetal pregnancies, the pooled relative risk reduction for pre-eclampsia is estimated at 0.66 (95% CI 0.48–0.90), highlighting the importance of glycaemic control for maternal indications.

Given the baseline complexity of multifetal pregnancies and the higher prevalence of adverse outcomes, management of comorbidities may often occur in the inpatient setting to which underscores the importance of prevention of venous thromboembolism (VTE). A key principle of VTE prophylaxis is encouraging physical activity. There is no evidence to support bed rest in the management of obstetric conditions with the most robust data supporting its lack of efficacy or even potential harm. Activity restriction may offer the benefit of lowering blood pressure in cases of pre-eclampsia, but ambulation should still be encouraged in this population to both reduce the risk of VTE and prevent deconditioning.[9] In addition to activity, contemporary guidelines support the use of pharmacologic VTE prophylaxis in patients hospitalised for at least 72 hours who are not at high risk for bleeding or imminent childbirth.[10] The main drawback for pharmacologic prophylaxis is the possibility that recent medication administration may be a contraindication to neuraxial analgesia. Guidelines recommend waiting 4–6 hours since the last prophylactic dose of unfractionated heparin and 12 hours since the last dose of prophylactic low-molecular-weight heparin before proceeding with neuraxial analgesia. Balancing the need for VTE prophylaxis in this high-risk population with a similarly elevated risk of imminent delivery suggests that a pharmacologic approach centred on unfractionated heparin seems reasonable. From a practical standpoint, if a patient is too unstable to wait the 4 hours between unfractionated heparin administration and neuraxial analgesia for delivery, then it is possible her clinical condition may also be unstable enough to warrant general anaesthesia at delivery.

Management Options

Balancing Maternal Risks with Neonatal Outcomes

Despite the best efforts at prevention, complications of multifetal pregnancy are inevitable and when they arise, general recommendations are to manage them as you would a singleton pregnancy. Developing guidelines specific to twin or higher-order multiple pregnancies would be challenging if not impossible both due to the tremendous effort required and the paucity of evidence supporting management strategies specific to this population.[8] Managing multifetal pregnancies in a similar approach to singleton

Table 18.2 Contributing factors and proposed management strategies for common causes of severe maternal morbidity in multifetal pregnancies

Type of Morbidity	Contributing Factors	Management Strategies
Haemorrhage	Uterine atony	Active management of 3rd-stage early uterotonic administration Delivery in operating room Dedicated anaesthesia support
	Abnormalities of placentation	High index of suspicion Early surgical intervention Experienced surgeon available
	Exaggerated anaemia	Consideration of IV iron Ensure availability of blood
	Caesarean delivery	Encourage vaginal birth Prepare for breech extraction
Hypertensive Disorders	Increased placental mass	Universal low-dose aspirin Multifetal reduction counselling
	Maternal cardiovascular health	Support single embryo transfer Encourage physical activity
	Atypical presentations common	Low index of suspicion Close clinical follow-up
	Preterm presentations common	Closely monitor maternal status Balance with fetal outcomes
Cardiopulmonary Events	Extreme haemodynamic demand	Screening echocardiography Consider in delivery timing
	Antepartum deconditioning	Encourage physical activity Consider physical therapy
	Complications of transfusion	Cross-matched blood available Earlier surgical intervention
Venous Thromboembolism	Activity restriction	Explicitly prohibit bed rest and encourage physical activity
	More inpatient hospitalisations	Pharmacologic prophylaxis Support inpatient activity
	Complex clinical presentation	Low threshold for diagnostics Consider empiric anticoagulation

pregnancies makes practical sense but fails to account for the unique considerations affecting both maternal and neonatal outcomes (Figure 18.2).

Consider a case of pre-eclampsia. Expectant management of pre-eclampsia with severe features is advocated prior to 34 weeks in appropriately selected populations to improve neonatal outcomes without increasing maternal risk. The benefit of prolonging pregnancy for two or more neonates must be balanced with the higher risk of adverse maternal outcomes and limited ability to compensate haemodynamically to the demands of pregnancy. Patients with multifetal pregnancies are more likely to present with atypical features of the disease demanding more frequent laboratory surveillance and a lower threshold to explore seemingly unrelated subjective complaints. Though ambulatory monitoring of pre-eclampsia can be considered in the absence of severe features, the need for increased maternal and fetal surveillance in twins relative to singletons makes inpatient management an appealing option. Keeping anticipated maternal outcomes and the resources and personnel available to address these at a given centre is of paramount importance and somewhat independent of neonatal needs.[11] With the complexities of balancing maternal risk with neonatal outcomes in mind, patients with maternal or obstetric comorbidities may benefit from the presence of a clinician with experience caring for complicated multifetal pregnancies.

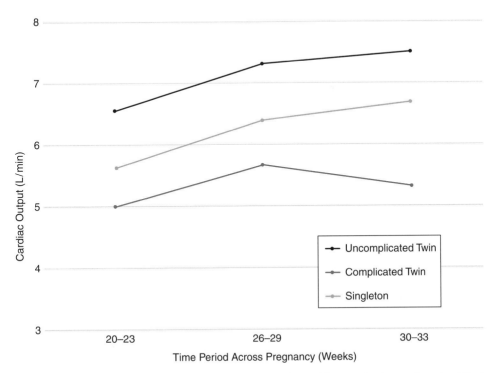

Figure 18.2 Balancing maternal and fetal outcomes when considering delivery timing in complicated multifetal gestations

Ensuring a Safe and Successful Vaginal Birth

Whether spontaneous or indicated, delivery timing is only one consideration in the conversation on maternal outcomes for multifetal pregnancy. For twin pregnancies in particular, the decision to attempt a trial of labour in hopes of vaginal birth or to pursue an elective caesarean delivery is an evolving clinical question. Despite a wealth of research focusing on the interaction between neonatal outcomes and mode of delivery, few studies have explored this question for maternal morbidity and mode of delivery.

The publication of a landmark randomised controlled trial – the Twin Birth Study – supported the neonatal safety of attempted twin vaginal birth when the presenting fetus is cephalic.[12] Their composite maternal outcome including death and serious maternal morbidity was 7.3% in the planned caesarean delivery group and 8.5% in the planned vaginal birth group (odds ratio 0.86, 95% CI 0.65–1.13). Current guidelines aimed at preventing primary caesarean delivery encourage an attempted vaginal delivery for twins when the presenting fetus is cephalic.

These recommendations rely on the data of Barrett and colleagues and apply the known short and long-term morbidity associated with caesarean delivery from the singleton population. Using French data, Madar and colleagues attributed 20.6% (95% CI 12.9–28.2) of SMM to caesarean delivery, highlighting attempted vaginal delivery as a maternal risk reduction strategy. But observational data from the United States show a higher odds of haemorrhage for women attempting vaginal delivery compared to those electing for caesarean delivery. The need for operative vaginal or caesarean delivery of one or both twins during the course of labour may account for some of the conflicting findings in the literature. The increased rates of operative vaginal and intra-partum caesarean delivery in twin pregnancies coupled with variable provider experience in twin vaginal birth and breech extraction highlight that an attempted vaginal birth carries unique considerations in this population.

Guidelines encouraging attempted vaginal birth for twins fail to elaborate on the accompanying anticipatory counselling and proactive intra-partum management requisite to optimise patient outcomes and satisfaction. The concept of breech extraction, the safety data supporting its use and how this differs from a singleton breech vaginal delivery should be discussed. The possibility of intra-partum presentation change from cephalic to noncephalic presentation as well as the potential role of internal podalic version and breech extraction to expedite delivery of the unengaged cephalic second twin would suggest all patients – even those with cephalic second twins at the onset of labour – be prepared for this possibility. External cephalic version of the non-vertex second twin increases the odds of caesarean delivery of the second twin compared to breech extraction, suggesting its practice should be limited if not abandoned. Ideally, all providers performing twin vaginal deliveries should have a baseline comfort with breech extraction to optimise maternal outcomes. Whether or not a patient with a cephalic second twin should be encouraged to elect caesarean delivery if a provider with this skill set is unavailable is unclear. Clinicians should prioritise shared decision-making, taking into account patient preference, obstetric history and future fertility goals when counselling patients about mode of delivery for twins.

Mitigating Maternal Risk at Delivery

Regardless of mode of delivery, the third stage is a time of increased risk for twins and higher-order multiples. Though uterine atony is most classically associated with multifetal pregnancy, abnormalities of placentation such as placenta praevia and placenta accreta spectrum are more prevalent in this population. As with many obstetric comorbidities, the management of post-partum haemorrhage independent of aetiology parallels that of single-ton pregnancy. But the high risk of post-partum haemorrhage and peri-partum hysterec-tomy in multifetal pregnancies coupled with concerns about increased downstream morbidity warrants a proactive approach predating the patient's arrival on labour and delivery.[14]

Optimising maternal status in anticipation of delivery is a key component of antenatal care. Early workup and aggressive management of the anaemia of pregnancy, including the use of intravenous iron, is central. Patients with underlying cardiovascular risk factors, including increasing maternal age, chronic hypertension, pre-eclampsia, pre-gestational diabetes or mater-nal cardiovascular disease, may benefit from transthoracic echocardiography in the third trimester to assess ventricular systolic and diastolic function.[3,4] The diagnosis of overt systolic failure in the absence of cardiopulmonary complaints is unlikely, but impaired ventricular relaxation may limit the patient's ability to tolerate large volume transfusion, putting the patient at risk of transfusion-associated circulatory overload (Table 18.3). Concerns for limited haemo-dynamic reserve may impact clinical decision-making for the provider tasked with managing a haemorrhage, prompting earlier decision to proceed with uterine artery embolisation or definitive surgical management with hysterectomy.

Being prepared for a potential haemorrhage is important for any delivery, but even more so for those involving multifetal pregnancies.[14] Active management of the third stage, early medical management with uterotonics and tranexamic acid and availability of blood products are the mainstays of avoiding haemorrhage-associated SMM in this population. National guidelines support delivery of term twin gestations in basic care centres – some of which may have limited blood bank availability or surgical support.[11] For patients with multifetal gestation with other haemorrhage risk factors or compounding maternal comor-bidities, consideration should be given to the appropriate delivery setting to ensure the patient has the adequate resources and personnel available to address her anticipated intra-partum needs. For some centres, this may involve ensuring additional blood products or anaesthesia care providers are available. For others, this may prompt discussion of transfer of care to optimise maternal outcomes. Regardless of the exact circumstances, a proactive

Table 18.3 Distinguishing transfusion-associated acute lung injury (TRALI) from transfusion-associated circu-latory overload (TACO) in haemorrhage-associated pulmonary oedema

Feature	TRALI	TACO
Oedema Pathophysiology	Exudate	Transudate
Blood Component	Typically plasma or platelets	Any
Blood Pressure	Hypotension	Hypertension
Temperature	Elevated	Normal
White Blood Cell Count	Leukopenia	Unchanged
BNP	Low	Elevated
Echocardiogram	Normal ejection fraction	Decreased ejection fraction
Diuretics	Worsen	Improve
Fluid Response	Improve	Worsen

approach incorporating maternal comorbidities to prepare for anticipated needs will optimise maternal outcomes at the time of delivery.

Optimising Post-partum Maternal Care

Delivery certainly poses a high-risk time for mothers of multifetal gestations, but the psychosocial complexities of parenting multiples highlights the post-partum period as a vulnerable time.[15] Rates of depression and anxiety are higher in parents of multiples with preterm infants requiring admission to the neonatal intensive care unit, conferring additional risk. This coupled with the challenges of breastfeeding, the financial impact and social considerations make the need for increased post-partum support self-evident (Figure 18.3). This need is perhaps even greater for parents suffering from a loss of one or more fetuses during their pregnancy. Close-interval follow-up at the two-week post-partum mark either via phone or in person offers an opportunity for early detection and intervention for post-partum mood disorders. The need for reliable contraception should be emphasised at the six-week visit and throughout post-partum care independent of comorbid diagnoses of infertility or subfertility.

Patients with prolonged hospitalisations or traumatic birth experiences may benefit from a dedicated visit 3–6 months post partum to review the circumstances of delivery and screen for evidence of childbirth-associated post-traumatic stress disorder. This may be particularly important for patients transferred to referral centres for delivery who may have an otherwise limited ability to access information about the circumstances of their deliveries as a part of post-partum care. This extended post-partum follow-up also affords providers the opportunity to discuss the impact of pregnancy-associated complications on not only future pregnancies, but also on long-term health. Regardless of the approach to post-partum care, dedicated attention to the maternal psychosocial state is an essential component of optimising maternal outcomes in multifetal pregnancies.

Prioritising maternal outcomes in multifetal pregnancies isn't easy. The healthcare system, available scientific evidence and even the patient often focus on the fetal

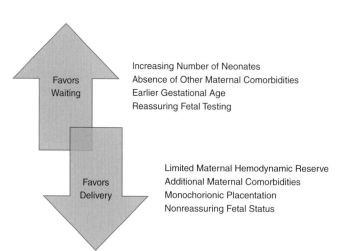

Favors Waiting

Increasing Number of Neonates
Absence of Other Maternal Comorbidities
Earlier Gestational Age
Reassuring Fetal Testing

Favors Delivery

Limited Maternal Hemodynamic Reserve
Additional Maternal Comorbidities
Monochorionic Placentation
Nonreassuring Fetal Status

Figure 18.3 Algorithm for clinical decision about delivery timing

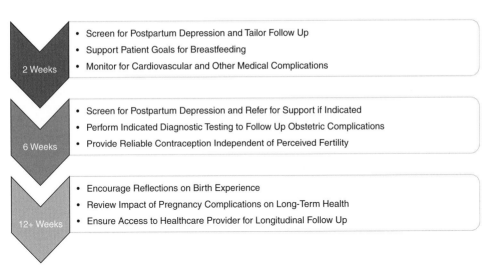

Figure 18.4 Outline for postpartum follow-up

component of this high-risk state. The obstetric care provider may be the first and sometimes only line of defence against adverse maternal outcomes. A uniform approach to management followed by tailored risk-appropriate care as clinical complexities arise is paramount. As decreasing severe maternal morbidity and mortality climbs towards the top of the public health agenda, one must hope that studies and guidelines dedicated to minimising the maternal complications of multifetal pregnancies will follow. Until that time, the obstetric care provider must be the champion for maternal health in multifetal pregnancies.

Key Points

- An increase in placental mass, exaggerated physiologic needs and complexities in clinical management contribute to higher rates of maternal morbidity in multiple pregnancies.
- Hallmark haemodynamic changes of multiple pregnancy include an increased CO with exaggerated plasma volume expansion.
- Failure to meet these physiologic demands contribute to the pathophysiology of obstetric and fetal processes such as growth restriction and pre-eclampsia.
- Administration of low-dose aspirin and attention to optimising nutrition are key tenets of risk reduction in the first trimester.
- Instruct patients to avoid bed rest and engage in physical activity to minimise risk of venous thromboembolism and maximise cardiopulmonary fitness.
- Balancing maternal risk and fetal benefit in multiple pregnancy should incorporate a model of shared decision-making between the patient and her provider.
- Encourage attempted vaginal delivery in patients with a cephalic presenting first twin and ensure support is available to facilitate a safe and successful vaginal birth of the second, independent of presentation.

- Actively manage the third stage of labour, keeping in mind the comparatively limited cardiopulmonary reserve to manage large volume transfusion.
- Ensure dedicated post-partum follow-up acknowledging the psychosocial impact of multiple pregnancy – particularly those with a complex antenatal course.
- Refer patients with comorbidities complicating multiple pregnancy to hospitals with the resources and personnel to address maternal, not just neonatal needs.

References

1. Committee on Practice Bulletins – Obstetrics, Society for Maternal–Fetal Medicine. ACOG Practice Bulletin No. 169: Multifetal gestations: twin, triplet and higher-order multifetal pregnancies. Obstet Gynecol 2016 Oct;**128**(4):e131–e146.

2. Santana DS, Cecatti JG, Surita FG et al. Twin pregnancy and severe maternal outcomes: the World Health Organization multi-country survey on maternal and newborn health. Obstet Gynecol 2016;**127**(4):631–41.

3. Ghi T, Kuleva M, Youssef A et al. Maternal cardiac function in complicated twin pregnancy: a longitudinal study. Ultrasound Obstet Gynecol 2011;**38**:581–5.

4. Ghi T, Esposti D, Montaguti E et al. Maternal cardiac evaluation during uncomplicated twin pregnancy with emphasis on the diastolic function. Am J Obstet Gynecol 2015;**213**(3):375.e1–e8.

5. Korb D, Schmitz T, Seco A et al. Risk factors and high-risk subgroups of severe acute maternal morbidity in twin pregnancy: A population-based study. PLoS One 2020;**15**(2):e0229612.

6. Roberge S, Bujold E, Nicolaides KH. Aspirin for the prevention of preterm and term preeclampsia: systematic review and metaanalysis. Am J Obstet Gynecol 2018;**218**(3):287–93.

7. Fox NS, Rebarber A, Roman AS, Klauser CK, Peress D, Saltzman DH. Weight gain in twin pregnancies and adverse outcomes: examining the 2009 IOM guidelines. Obstet Gynecol 2010;**116**(1):100–6.

8. SMFM Research Committee, Grantz KL, Kawakita T et al. SMFM special statement: state of the science on multifetal gestations: unique considerations and importance. Am J Obstet Gynecol 2019 Aug;**221**(2):B2–B12.

9. Crowther CA, Han S. Hospitalisation and bed rest for multiple pregnancy. Cochrane Database Syst Rev 2010 (7). Art. No.: CD000110. https://doi.org/10.1002/146518 58.CD000110.pub2

10. D'Alton ME, Friedman Am, Smiley RM et al. National Partnership for Maternal Safety: consensus bundle on venous thromboembolism. Obstet Gynecol 2016;**128**(4):688–98.

11. American Association of Birth Centers; Association of Women's Health, Obstetric and Neonatal Nurses; American College of Obstetricians and Gynecologists et al. Obstetric Care Consensus #9: Levels of Maternal Care. Am J Obstet Gynecol 2019;**221**(6):B19–B30.

12. Hutton EK, Hanna ME, Ross S et al. Maternal outcomes at 3 months after planned caesarean section versus planned vaginal birth for twin pregnancies in the Twin Birth Study: a randomized controlled trial. BJOG 2015;**122**(12):1653–62.

13. Easter SR, Robinson JN, Lieberman E, Carusi D. Association of intended route of delivery and maternal morbidity in twin pregnancy. Obstet Gynecol 2017;**129**(2):305–10.

14. Main EK, Goffman D, Scavone BM et al. National Partnership for Maternal Safety: consensus bundle on obstetric hemorrhage. Obstet Gynecol 2015 Jul;**126**(1):155–62.

15. American College of Obstetricians and Gynecologists. ACOG Committee Opinion No. 736: optimizing postpartum care. Obstet Gynecol 2018;**131**(5):e140–e150.

Risk Assessment and Screening for Preterm Birth in Multiple Pregnancy

Amanda Roman, Alexandra Ramirez, Guillermo Gurza and Vincenzo Berghella

Introduction

Preterm birth (PTB) is defined as delivery before 37 completed weeks of gestation, with extreme PTB defined as occurring at less than 28 weeks, very preterm delivery occurring between 28 and 32 weeks and moderate-to-late PTB occurring from 32 to 36 weeks.[1] Worldwide, about 15 million babies are born preterm each year, and PTB accounts for 1 million neonatal deaths and an additional 125,000 deaths in children before five years of age, representing the leading cause of both neonatal and childhood mortality.[2,3] Prematurity is associated with increased perinatal morbidity and long-term neurodevelopmental impairment. Survival and neurological prognoses improve with advancing gestational age. In the United States, the rate of twin births in 2018 was 32.6 per 1,000 births, but they accounted for 20% of all PTB, with 60.3% delivering before 37 weeks, 19.5% delivering before 34 weeks and 10.7% delivering before 32 weeks. Of singleton pregnancies, 8.2% delivered before 37 weeks, 2.1% delivered before 34 weeks and 1.2% delivered before 32 weeks.[4] Twins are also at increased risk for low birthweight (LBW) and have a five times higher risk of early neonatal and infant death and complications related to prematurity and LBW.[4]

Pathophysiology

The increased incidence of PTB among twin/multiple pregnancies is probably associated with different pathophysiology: maternal complications associated with physiological changes (cardiovascular and endocrine adaptation to multiple pregnancy), fetal complications unique to multiple pregnancy and directly associated with chorionicity, uterine over-distension, cervical insufficiency, intrauterine infection or inflammation, hormonal disorders, placental insufficiency and uterine hypoxia. It is therefore important to individualise the risk factors associated with PTB among asymptomatic and symptomatic twin pregnancies.

Prevention of Multiple Pregnancy

Avoidance of Multiple Pregnancy

The best practice to prevent PTB is to avoid multiple pregnancy. Diverse societies have recommended a single embryo transfer during in vitro fertilisation (IVF) to avoid multiple pregnancy. However, the twin pregnancy rate remains high among women undergoing artificial reproductive techniques (ART). Approximately 30.4% of ART-conceived infants are twins and 1.1% are triplets and higher-order multiples. The number of fetuses correlates directly with the number of embryos, zygotes or oocytes transferred following reproductive techniques. In a systematic review and meta-analysis, the risk for monozygotic twin (MZT) and monochorionic twin (MCT) pregnancies after IVF is increased with blastocyst transfer (prolonged embryo culture) compared with cleavage-stage embryo transfer (23 studies, OR 2.16, 95% CI, 1.74–2.68, I2 = 78%).[5] Conventional IVF compared with intra-cytoplasmic sperm injection (ICSI) and assisted hatching was associated with a statistically significant increased risk of MZT pregnancy (9 studies, OR 1.19, 95% CI, 1.04–1.35, I2 = 0; 16 studies, OR 1.17, 95% CI, 1.09–1.27, I2 = 29%, respectively). Embryo biopsy for pre-implantation genetics, embryo cryopreservation and oocytes donation were not associated with MZT pregnancies after IVF. Prevention of spontaneous conception is not possible, and medical ovarian stimulation and intrauterine sperm transfer still offer a great risk of twins and multiple pregnancy. A single embryo transfer offers the best practice to prevent twins or multiple pregnancy.

Multifetal Reduction and Selective Fetal Termination

Another method to decrease the risk of PTB and neonatal complications in multiple pregnancy is multifetal reduction. A systematic review evaluated embryonic reduction at 8–14 weeks of gestation in both trichorionic-triamniotic (TCTA) and dichorionic-triamniotic (DCTA) pregnancies compared with expectant management (this review included eight studies with a total of 249 DCTA and 1,167 TCTA pregnancies).[6] In TCTA pregnancies, there were lower risks (17.3% vs 50.2%) of PTB < 34 weeks (RR = 0.36, 95% CI: 0.28–0.48), whereas the risk of miscarriage < 24 weeks (8.1% vs 7.4%) did not significantly increase (RR = 1.08, 95% CI: 0.58–1.98). The embryonic reduction to twins in DCTA triplets, either of the fetus with a separate placenta or one of the MC pair, was significantly associated neither with an increased risk of miscarriage (8.5 vs 13.3%, P = 0.628 and RR = 1.22, 95% CI: 0.38–3.95, respectively) nor with a lower risk of PTB (51.9 vs 46.2%, P = 0.778 and RR = 0.5, 95% CI: 0.04–5.7, respectively).

Fetal reduction of DCDA twins to a singleton pregnancy before 14 weeks is associated with a lower risk of PTB < 34 weeks (1.6% vs 11.7%) and < 37 weeks (9.5% vs 56.7%). There were also improvement in rates of miscarriage of one twin (0% vs 4.8%) and early pregnancy loss < 24 weeks of gestation, while gestational diabetes (11.1% vs 10%), hypertensive diseases of pregnancy (6.3% vs 15%) and intrauterine growth restriction (0% vs 3.3%) were not significantly different. Early fetal reductions (11–14 weeks) have better outcomes than later fetal reductions (15–23 weeks): preterm delivery < 37 weeks (14% vs 28%, p = 0.004), < 34 weeks (1.8% vs 12%, p = 0.001), < 32 weeks (1.8% vs 8%, p = 0.012) and decreased composite neonatal morbidity (2.9% vs 10.7%, p = 0.025).[6]

Therefore, fetal reduction should be considered in certain cases of twin and multiple order pregnancy where the risk for adverse outcome seems exceptionally high. The benefit of fetal reduction not only includes lower frequencies of pregnancy loss, PTB and LBW infants, but it also may decrease antenatal complications, caesarean delivery and neonatal deaths.

Chorionicity is an important factor associated with the incidence of PTB and perinatal outcomes in twin pregnancies. Monochorionic-diamniotic (MCDA) twin pregnancies are at higher risk of PTB associated with maternal and fetal complications compared with DCDA twin pregnancies. In a retrospective cohort of 175 (30.2%) MCDA twin pregnancies and 405 (69.8%) DCDA pregnancies, the incidence of PTB < 34 weeks was significantly increased in the MCDA pregnancies: 61 (34.9%) versus 93 (23.0%), respectively with OR 1.80 (1.22–2.65). the increase was seen both for the medically indicated (fetal reasons) PTB: 22 (12.6%) versus 20 (4.9%) with OR 2.49 (1.34–5.63) and spontaneous PTB (SPTB): 108 (61.7%) versus 195 (48.1%) with OR 1.74 (1.21–2.49), while maternal indication of PTB was not different: 30 (17.1%) versus 65 (16.1%) with OR: 1.05 (0.55–1.70).[7]

Fetal Complications As a Cause of Preterm Birth

Twin–Twin Transfusion Syndrome (TTTS)

A unique complication of MCDA pregnancies is twin–twin transfusion syndrome (TTTS). Twin–twin transfusion syndrome complicates 8–10% of MCDA pregnancies. The prevalence of TTTS is approximately 1–3 per 10,000 births. Twin–twin transfusion syndrome contributes highly to the fetal indications of PTB; a systematic review including 26 studies (2,699 twin pregnancies) showed that the pooled proportions of PTB < 32 weeks of gestation among MCDA pregnancies affected by TTTS classified by Quintero stages were increased as the severity of TTTS progressed. Quintero stage I: two studies (9/34); 27.1% (13.9–42.8) stage II, three studies (20/47); 42.8% (29.4–56.9) stage III, three studies (32/58); 53.3% (36,1–70.2) and stage IV: three studies (11/18) 59.9% (37.9–80). There are also differences in perinatal outcomes according to TTTS treatment modality. Overall PTB occurred in 74.1% (95% confidence interval 36.9–97.8) of pregnancies managed expectantly, 43.5% (26.5–51.3) treated with laser and 65.3% (45.8–80.7) managed with amnioreduction.[8] However, data on PTB outcomes were limited by the small sample size.

Other Fetal Complications

Other MCDA-specific complications affecting prematurity rates include selective intrauterine growth restriction (sIUGR) and twin anaemia polycythaemia sequence (TAPS). The gestational age at delivery in 134 MCDA twin pregnancies diagnosed with sIUGR between 18 and 26 weeks was 35.4 (16–38) weeks if umbilical artery (UA) Doppler with positive diastolic flow, and 30.7 (27–40) weeks if persistent absent or reversed end-diastolic flow. In women affected by TAPS, the rate of preterm premature rupture of the membranes (PPROM) was 44.4% in the treated TAPS group versus 18.2% in the non-treated TAPS group, and the mean gestational age at delivery was 33.4 ± 3 weeks and 30.4 ± 5.7 weeks, respectively.[9]

Single Intrauterine Death in Twin and Preterm Births

Single intrauterine death (sIUD) in twin pregnancy is associated with a significant risk of co-twin demise and PTB, especially in MC twins. The risk of PTB in twin pregnancy after sIUD according to the gestational age at death was evaluated among 3,013 twin gestations (2,469 DC and 544 MC). Median gestational age at birth was lower in the pregnancies complicated by sIUD compared with those that were not (32 weeks: interquartile range (IQR), 29–34.3 weeks vs 36.7 weeks: IQR, 35–37.6; P < 0.001), and this difference persisted when stratifying the data according to chorionicity (P < 0.0001 for both MC and DC pregnancies). The overall risk was higher in pregnancies complicated by sIUD compared with those which did not experience fetal loss. Preterm birth at < 34 weeks was 66.1% (41/62) versus 15.5%

(457/2,948), RR 4.27 (3.5–5.2); PTB < 32 weeks 48.4% (30/62) versus 7.9% (233/2,948), RR 6.12 (4.6–8.1); and PTB < 28 weeks 19.4% (12/62) versus 1.6% (46/2948), RR 12.40 (6.9–22.2). This association was observed both in MC and DC twin gestations. The risk of PTB at < 34 weeks of gestation was higher when the sIUD occurred at a later gestational age (chi-square test for trend, P < 0.001).[10] In summary, monochorionicity is a strong risk factor for PTB compared to dichorionicity in twins due to the inherited unique complications such as TTTS, TAPS, single IUFD and selective IUGR.

Maternal Indications for Preterm Birth

History of Previous Preterm Birth

The incidence of history of PTB and subsequent twin pregnancies is about 10% in most studies.[7] Several retrospective cohorts have shown an increased risk of PTB in twin pregnancy with history of singleton PTB. The preterm prediction study in twins showed an increased risk of recurrent PTB < 37 weeks (80% vs 50%; RR 1.6. 95% CI 1.18–2.17, p = 0.03) (n = 147). Three retrospective studies in the United States showed an increased risk of recurrent PTB < 37 weeks in subsequent twin pregnancy (73.9% vs 44.4%; OR: 3.5, 95% CI 1.4–9.37), recurrent spontaneous PTB < 35 weeks (37.7% vs 23.0%; OR 2.0, 95%CI 1.41–2.9, P < 0.001) and recurrent PTB < 32 weeks (26% vs 3.5%; OR 9.7, 95%CI 2.95–32.4, P<0.001) when comparing prior PTB with prior term delivery.[11] In summary, history of PTB of a singleton or a twin gestation is a strong risk factor for recurrent PTB in subsequent twin pregnancies.

Smoking during Pregnancy

There are few studies assessing smoking in twin pregnancies. In a retrospective study of 401 twin pregnancies, 276 (69%) women were non-smokers and 125 (31%) were smokers.[12] The rate of PTB < 37 weeks was significantly increased (1.4 (1–2)] in women who smoked 10 or more cigarettes per day. The gestational age decreased with the number of cigarettes smoked per day in primiparus and multiparus. Women who stopped smoking prior to 16 weeks had similar outcomes to those of non-smokers.

Pre-eclampsia

Pre-eclampsia complicates 5–8% of all pregnancies and is highly associated with preterm delivery (spontaneous or medically indicated). In a large cohort that included 86,765 live births in a single institution, 4,672 (4%) singletons and 1,399 (43%) twins were born < 37 weeks. Preterm severe pre-eclampsia was more common in twin pregnancies (79 (2.4%) vs 352 (0.4%), p < 0.001, RR 5.70 (95% CI 4.47–7.26)). This remained significantly different for preterm severe pre-eclampsia from 24 0/7 to 31 6/7 weeks [54 (0.8%) vs 214 (0.2%), p < 0.001] and 32 0/7 to 36 6/7 weeks [25 (1.7%) vs 138 (0.3%), p < 0.001]. Among the 1,905 infants born between 24 0/7 and 31 6/7 weeks of gestation, delivery for severe pre-eclampsia was equally common between singleton and twin gestations (9% vs 8%, p = 0.53). However, when evaluating those delivered between 32 0/7 and 36 6/7 weeks of gestation, the rate of PTB for severe pre-eclampsia was greater for singletons than twins (7% vs 5%, p = 0.031). The rates of hemolysis, elevated liver enzymes and low platelets (HELLP), abruption, eclampsia and fetal criteria for delivery were similar between singleton and twin gestations. Women with a twin gestation were more likely to be diagnosed with severe pre-eclampsia based on lab abnormalities alone (12% vs. 3%, p = 0.002). All other categories of diagnostic criteria were similar between twins and singletons.[13]

The American College of Obstetricians and Gynecologists recommends daily low-dose aspirin beginning before 16 weeks of pregnancy, including multiple pregnancy, for women at risk of pre-eclampsia in order to reduce the risk of premature and severe pre-eclampsia, thus reducing prematurity caused by this process.

Mode of Conception: Spontaneous versus Reproductive Technologies

A prospective cohort study compared all DC twin pregnancies in nulliparous women following fresh in vitro fertilisation/intra-cytoplasmic sperm injection (ICSI) or ICSI cycles (n = 320) with spontaneously conceived DC twin pregnancies in nulliparous women (n = 170). After adjusting for confounders (maternal age and body mass index), the risks of very PTB (OR 5.2, 95% CI 2.1–12.9), extremely low birthweight (OR 2.2, 95% CI 1–3.9), admission to a neonatal intensive care unit (OR 2.0, 95% CI 1.2–3.2) and perinatal mortality (OR 2.3, 95% CI 1.2–4.0) were significantly higher in the ART group.[14]

Race/Ethnicity

Some studies showed higher prematurity rates in pregnant women who are black, younger and with a low-educational level.[13] Smoking and primiparity also seem to be related to shorter gestational age at birth in twin pregnancy.[8]

Cervical Length Measurement in Asymptomatic Women

In 1996, a preterm prediction study evaluated the risk factors for PTB in twin gestations.[15] Multiple variables were evaluated in 147 women with twin pregnancy at 24 and 28 weeks, including maternal demographics, obstetric history, biochemical markers and transvaginal ultrasound at 24 and 28 weeks. A transvaginal ultrasound cervical length (TVUCL) ≤ 25 mm at 24 weeks was the best predictor of SPTB at < 32, < 35 and < 37 weeks. Since then, multiple prospective studies evaluating TVUCL in twins have been published. A systematic review including 16 studies in asymptomatic women with twin pregnancies (n = 3213) showed that TVUCL ≤ 20 mm at 20–24 weeks was the most accurate tool in predicting PTB < 32 and < 34 weeks of gestation (pooled sensitivities, specificities and positive and negative likelihood ratios of 39% and 29%, 96% and 97%, 10.1 and 9.0, and 0.64 and 0.74, respectively). A TVUCL ≤ 25 mm at 20–24 weeks of gestation had a pooled positive likelihood ratio of 9.6 to predict PTB < 28 weeks of gestation. The predictive accuracy of TVUCL for PTB was low in symptomatic women. Despite large variation in gestational age at TVUCL and different cut-off points for cervical length and definitions of PTB, the summary receiver operating characteristic (ROC) curve indicated a good predictive capacity of short cervical length for PTB. Sensitivity and specificity for PTB < 34 weeks gestation were 78% and 66%, respectively, for 35 mm, 41% and 87% for 30 mm, 36% and 94% for 25 mm, and 30% and 94% for 20 mm.

A recent individual patient-level meta-analysis evaluated the effect of gestational age and cervical length measurements in the prediction of SPTB in twin pregnancies.[16] A total of 6,188 TVUCL measurements were performed on 4,409 twin pregnancies in 12 studies. Multinomial logistic regression analysis determined probabilities for birth at ≤ 28, 28–32,

32–36 and ≥ 36 weeks as a function of gestational age (GA) at screening and CL measurements. Both GA at screening and TVUCL had a significant and non-linear effect on GA at birth. The best prediction of PTB ≤ 28 weeks was provided by screening at ≤ 18 weeks (P < 0.001) whereas the best prediction of birth between 28 and 36 weeks was provided by screening at ≥ 24 weeks (P < 0.001).

In summary, all these studies established that TVUCL before 24 weeks is the best predictor of PTB in twin pregnancy, and the shorter the TVUCL and the earlier GA at presentation, the higher the risk of PTB at any given gestation. While TVUCL is currently the best tool available to screen for PTB in twin pregnancy, independent of other risk factors, the ACOG and the SMFM still recommend against TVUCL in twins as there are no current proven therapies to offer and TVUCL should be reserved for randomised controlled studies.

Amniotic Fluid Sludge

Amniotic fluid (AF) was described in 2005 as a dense aggregate of particulate matter seen in close proximity to the internal cervical os and having imaging characteristics similar to gallbladder sludge seen by ultrasound. Sludge has been proposed as an additional ultrasound marker for preterm delivery.

In a large cohort including 635 twin pregnancies with TVUCL from 22 0/7 to 25 6/7 weeks, sludge was present in 61 (9.6%) of them. The risk of PTB < 35 weeks in women with sludge was 36.8% versus 16.5% (OR: 2.11; 95% CI: 1.04–4.27). Sludge constitutes the third marker associated with PTB after TVUCL < 25 mm and fetal fibronectin.[17] In summary, amniotic fluid sludge is an independent marker of PTB; however, its presence has not been used to select a better candidate in clinical practice.

Cervical Examination

This study evaluated the risk of antepartum cervical examination at every prenatal visit in twin pregnancy from 1988 through 1991. Eighty-nine women received extensive PTB prevention education and routine cervical examination at each clinic visit (7.6 ± 3.2 cervical examinations per patient) versus 288 women who received cervical examination for obstetric indications only. There were no significant differences in PTB < 37 weeks 77.3% versus 66.7%, p = 0.07, medical complications or infectious morbidity. There were significantly less PPROM among the patients attending the Twin Clinic (12.4% vs 23.6%, P = 0.03).[18] Larger studies will be needed to assess this finding. In summary, routine manual cervical examinations for prediction or prevention of PTB in twin pregnancies cannot be recommended.

Uterine Activity Evaluation

In 1995, a meta-analysis of six randomised trials involving 260 twin pregnancies compared daily home uterine activity monitoring (HUAM) versus abdominal palpation. This study did not find any difference in the incidence of PTB (RR: 1.01; 95% CI: 0.79–1.30; p = 0.95). However, when women with twin pregnancy and cervical dilation > 2 cm were evaluated, the incidence of preterm labour was significantly decreased by 56%; RR 0.44 (0.25–0.78, p = 0.005).[19] In summary, HUAM cannot be recommended for twin pregnancies.

Fetal Fibronectin

A recent systematic review showed that positive fetal fibronectin (fFN) was associated with a significantly increased risk of PTB among women with twin pregnancies who are either asymptomatic or symptomatic for PTB.[20] Among symptomatic women, positive fFN was predictive of PTB < 28 weeks (OR 12.06, 95% CI 4.90–29.70, I2 = 0%), PTB <32 weeks (OR 10.03, 95% CI 6.11–16.47, I2 = 0%), PTB <34 weeks (OR 6.26, 95% CI 3.85–10.17, I2 = 30%), PTB <37 weeks (OR 5.34, 95% CI 3.68–7.76, I2 = 15%) and delivery within 14 days of testing (OR 13.95, 95% CI 4.33–44.98, I2 = 0%) were significantly increased in women with a positive fFN. An fFN level of ≥50 ng/mL was considered positive in most studies. However, gestation at measurement varied from any time during pregnancy from 22 to 34 weeks. The systematic review considered that cervicovaginal fFN demonstrated limited and inconclusive accuracy in predicting sPTB among asymptomatic and symptomatic women with twin pregnancies. A negative fFN test is more valuable as it could be useful in identifying women who are not at risk of delivery within seven days of testing. In summary, cervicovaginal fFN alone has low to moderate accuracy in predicting SPTB in asymptomatic twin gestations with a higher negative predictive value.

Screening for Bacterial Vaginosis

Prospective studies found no association between the presence of untreated bacterial vaginosis at 24 and 28 weeks of gestation and SPTB at < 32, < 35 and < 37 weeks of gestation.[15]

Table 19.1 Summary of recommendations

Intervention	Recommendation
Prevention of multiple pregnancies	Limit to one embryo transfer Consider fetal reduction
Fertility treatment	IVF increases the risk of preterm birth
Chorionicity	Monochorionic twins have higher risk of spontaneous labour and fetal indications for delivery
History of previous preterm birth	Either previous singleton or twin preterm delivery increase the risk of PTB
Cervical length measurement in asymptomatic women	Cervical length < 25 mm before 24 weeks. The shorter the TVUCL, the higher the risk of PTB
Amniotic fluid sludge	Increased risk of preterm delivery
Routine cervical examination	Not recommended
Fetal fibronectin	Negative fFN test is more valuable
Maternal activity restriction	Not recommended
Tocolysis	Not recommended
Home uterine activity evaluation	Not recommended
Bacterial vaginosis	Not associated with preterm delivery

Key Points

- Twin pregnancies have an increased risk of pregnancy loss, PTB and adverse neonatal outcomes.
- The best practice to prevent PTB is to avoid multiple pregnancies. Fetal reduction should be considered in certain cases of twin and higher-order pregnancies where the risk for adverse outcome seems exceptionally high.
- Determining chorionicity during the first trimester is very important in counselling about risk of PTB and perinatal outcomes in twin pregnancies.
- Fetal complications unique to twin pregnancy (TTTS, selective intrauterine sIUGR, TAPS and sIUD) are important indications for PTB.
- Spontaneous labour is the most common cause of preterm delivery. Transvaginal cervical length before 24 weeks is the best tool to predict spontaneous PTB, independent of other risk factors.
- Maternal indications for PTB include pre-eclampsia, gestational diabetes, smoking, age and race.

References

1. Blencowe H, Cousens S, Oestergaard MZ et al. National, regional, and worldwide estimates of preterm birth rates in the year 2010 with time trends since 1990 for selected countries: a systematic analysis and implications. Lancet 2012 Jun 9;**379** (9832):2162–72. PubMed PMID: 22682464.

2. Nour NM. Premature delivery and the millennium development goal. Rev Obstet and Gynecol 2012;5(2):100–5. PubMed PMID: 22866189. Pubmed Central PMCID: 3410509.

3. Liu L, Oza S, Hogan D et al. Global, regional, and national causes of under-5 mortality in 2000–15: an updated systematic analysis with implications for the Sustainable Development Goals. Lancet 2016 Dec 17;**388** (10063):3027–35. PubMed PMID: 27839855. Pubmed Central PMCID: 5161777.

4. Martin JA, Hamilton BE, Osterman MJK. Births in the United States, 2018. NCHS data brief. 2019 Jul(346):1–8. PubMed PMID: 31442195.

5. Busnelli A, Dallagiovanna C, Reschini M, Paffoni A, Fedele L, Somigliana E. Risk factors for monozygotic twinning after in vitro fertilization: a systematic review and meta-analysis. Fertil Steril 2019 Feb;**111**(2):302–17. PubMed PMID: 30691632.

6. Anthoulakis C, Dagklis T, Mamopoulos A, Athanasiadis A. Risks of miscarriage or preterm delivery in trichorionic and dichorionic triplet pregnancies with embryo reduction versus expectant management: a systematic review and meta-analysis. Hum Repr. 2017 Jun 1;**32** (6):1351–9. PubMed PMID: 28444191.

7. Roman A, Saccone G, Dude CM et al. Midtrimester transvaginal ultrasound cervical length screening for spontaneous preterm birth in diamniotic twin pregnancies according to chorionicity. Eur J Obstet Gynecol Reprod Biol 2018 Oct;229:57–63. PubMed PMID: 30107361.

8. D'Antonio F, Benlioglu C, Sileo FG et al. Perinatal outcomes of twin pregnancies affected by early twin–twin transfusion syndrome: A systematic review and meta-analysis. Acta obstetricia et gynecologica Scandinavica 2020 Mar 11. PubMed PMID: 32162305.

9. Gratacos E, Lewi L, Munoz B et al. A classification system for selective intrauterine growth restriction in monochorionic pregnancies according to umbilical artery Doppler flow in the smaller twin. Ultrasound Obstet Gynecol 2007 Jul;**30**(1):28–34. PubMed PMID: 17542039.

10. D'Antonio F, Thilaganathan B, Dias T, Khalil A, Southwest Thames Obstetric

Research Center. Influence of chorionicity and gestational age at single fetal loss on risk of preterm birth in twin pregnancy: analysis of STORK multiple pregnancy cohort. Ultrasound Obstet Gynecol 2017 Dec;50(6):723–7. PubMed PMID: 28150444.

11. Tarter JG, Khoury A, Barton JR, Jacques DL, Sibai BM. Demographic and obstetric factors influencing pregnancy outcome in twin gestations. Am J Obstet Gynecol 2002 May;186(5):910–12. PubMed PMID: 12015510.

12. Wisborg K, Henriksen TB, Secher NJ. Maternal smoking and gestational age in twin pregnancies. Acta obstetricia et gynecologica Scandinavica 2001 Oct;80 (10):926–30. PubMed PMID: 11580737.

13. Henry DE, McElrath TF, Smith NA. Preterm severe preeclampsia in singleton and twin pregnancies. J Perinatol 2013 Feb;33(2):94–7. PubMed PMID: 22678139.

14. Moini A, Shiva M, Arabipoor A, Hosseini R, Chehrazi M, Sadeghi M. Obstetric and neonatal outcomes of twin pregnancies conceived by assisted reproductive technology compared with twin pregnancies conceived spontaneously: a prospective follow-up study. Eur J Obstet Gynecol Reprod Biol 2012 Nov;165 (1):29–32. PubMed PMID: 22884795.

15. Goldenberg RL, Iams JD, Miodovnik M et al. The preterm prediction study: risk factors in twin gestations. National Institute of Child Health and Human Development Maternal–Fetal Medicine Units Network.Am J Obstet Gynecol 1996 Oct;175 (4 Pt 1):1047–53. PubMed PMID: 8885774.

16. Kindinger LM, Poon LC, Cacciatore S et al. The effect of gestational age and cervical length measurements in the prediction of spontaneous preterm birth in twin pregnancies: an individual patient level meta-analysis. BJOG 2016 May;123(6):877–84. PubMed PMID: 26333191.

17. Spiegelman J, Booker W, Gupta S et al. The independent association of a short cervix, positive fetal fibronectin, amniotic fluid sludge, and cervical funneling with spontaneous preterm birth in twin pregnancies. Am J Perinatol 2016 Oct;33 (12):1159–64. PubMed PMID: 27434692.

18. Bivins HA Jr, Newman RB, Ellings JM, Hulsey TC, Keenan A. Risks of antepartum cervical examination in multifetal gestations. Am J Obstet Gynecol 1993 Jul;169(1):22–5. PubMed PMID: 8333461.

19. Colton T, Kayne HL, Zhang Y, Heeren T. A metaanalysis of home uterine activity monitoring. Am J Obstet Gynecol 1995 Nov;173(5):1499–1505. PubMed PMID: 7503191.

20. Marleen S, Dias C, MacGregor R et al. Biochemical predictors of preterm birth in twin pregnancies: a systematic review involving 6077 twin pregnancies. Eur J Obstet Gynecol Reprod Biol 2020 May 5;250:130–42. PubMed PMID: 32446146.

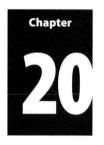

Prevention of Preterm Birth in Multiple Pregnancies

Abdallah Adra

Introduction

Twin pregnancies are associated with an increased risk of perinatal morbidity and mortality, primarily due to spontaneous preterm deliveries. A number of strategies regarding secondary prevention of preterm birth (PTB) have been proposed, including oral tocolytics, bed rest, hospitalisation, home uterine activity monitoring, use of progesterone, cerclage and, most recently, cervical pessary. There is much heterogeneity among health care providers when it comes to obstetric care of twin gestations,[1] and although twins have been well represented in many studies of PTB, these studies have failed to identify adequate predictive tests (short cervical length established more than two decades ago remains the single best predictor) and to establish effective interventions.[2]

Our current armamentarium to prevent PTB is limited, particularly in multiple gestations. The objective of this chapter is to review the evidence and efficacy of the different interventions used in contemporary obstetric practice to reduce PTB in multiple pregnancy. Given the paucity of literature for triplet and higher-order pregnancies, the chapter concentrates mainly on twin pregnancy.

Routine Hospitalisation and Bed Rest

Bed rest with or without hospitalisation has been commonly recommended to women with multifetal gestations. However, a Cochrane review demonstrated no benefit from routine hospitalisation or bed rest for women with an uncomplicated twin pregnancy. No reduction in the risk of preterm birth or perinatal death was evident, although there is a suggestion that fetal growth may be improved.[3] Until further evidence is available, bed rest with or without hospitalisation in women with multiple pregnancies is not recommended because of the lack of benefit and the risk of thrombosis and deconditioning associated with prolonged bed rest.

Prophylactic Tocolytics

Based on available evidence, there is no role for the prophylactic use of any tocolytic agent in women with multifetal gestations, including the prolonged use of betamimetics for this indication. The use of tocolytics to inhibit preterm labour in multifetal gestations has been associated with a greater risk of maternal complications such as pulmonary oedema. The administration of oral betamimetics specifically did not reduce the incidence of preterm birth, low-birthweight newborns or neonatal mortality in women with multifetal gestations when compared with placebo, and it has been associated with increased maternal and fetal cardiac stress and gestational diabetes mellitus.[4]

Cervical Cerclage

While widely accepted in singleton pregnancies, the use of cervical cerclage has been a source of great controversy in twin pregnancies. There are four clinical scenarios where cervical cerclage has been used for the argument of preventing or reducing PTB in multiple gestations: multiples-only indication, history-indicated, ultrasound-indicated and physical-exam indicated cerclage (or rescue cerclage).

Many obstetricians are hesitant to offer cerclage in women with twins regardless of sonographic or physical exam findings, in accordance with several current practice guidelines recommending against cerclage in multiple gestations, largely based on meta-analyses demonstrating lack of benefit in reducing PTB and improving neonatal outcomes, and even a potential harm with cerclage in twins. However, these meta-analyses should be interpreted with caution, as data were obtained from small trials with varying selection criteria and management protocols for mostly history-indicated and ultrasound-indicated cerclage in twins.

Multiples-Only-Indicated Cerclage

Studies suggest no benefit and a possible detrimental effect of elective cerclage performed at the end of the first trimester routinely in twin pregnancy without a known history of cervical insufficiency. One of the earliest studies assessing the efficiency of elective cerclage in preventing PTB and reducing neonatal mortality followed a group of 50 twin pregnancies occurring after ovulation induction, half of which were non-randomly selected to undergo elective cerclage. The rate of PTB and neonatal mortality was not significantly different between the study and the control group managed expectantly. Hence, the use of prophylactic cerclage to reduce spontaneous PTB for the sole indication of twin pregnancy has not been shown to be beneficial and is not recommended.[5]

History-Indicated Cerclage

History-indicated cervical cerclage is performed early in pregnancy based on poor obstetric or gynaecologic history. However, the targeted population in which history-indicated cerclage is recommended and most likely to be beneficial has still not been well established based on different professional society guidelines. Moreover, these guidelines pertain to women with a current singleton pregnancy whereas no recommendations exist regarding history-indicated cerclage in twin pregnancy owing to a lack of relevant data.

A recent small retrospective case-control study looked at 41 women with a twin pregnancy who had undergone a first-trimester history-indicated cerclage during an 11-year period at a single centre, comparing them to a control group of 41 women who were managed expectantly. Gestational age at delivery was higher in the cerclage group than in those managed expectantly (median 35 vs 30 weeks; P < 0.0001). Rates of spontaneous PTB before 24, 28, 32 and 34 weeks were significantly lower in the cerclage group than in the control group. Median birthweight was higher in the cerclage group, with lower rates of low birthweight (< 2,500 g) and very low birthweight (< 1,500 g) than in the group managed expectantly. Rates were also lower in the cerclage group for stillbirth, admission to the neonatal intensive care unit and composite adverse neonatal outcome.[6] In contrast, other retrospective cohort studies of history indicated cerclage have not shown efficacy suggesting the need for adequate randomised trials on cerclage placement in this subset of women.

Ultrasound-Indicated Cerclage

A Cochrane review found that when performed in twin pregnancies, ultrasound-indicated cervical cerclage was correlated with an increased incidence of adverse perinatal outcomes including higher rates of perinatal death, low birthweight and respiratory distress syndrome, and it had no benefit in terms of the prevention of PTB.[7] This has led to the SMFM recommendations in the 'Choosing Wisely' programme advocating against the use of cerclage in twin pregnancy with a short cervix owing to the lack of appropriate studies. Of note, the five trials included in the Cochrane review did not study twin pregnancy exclusively (i.e. they included singleton pregnancies), and in fact ultrasound-indicated cerclage in twins has not been studied in a dedicated randomised controlled trial.

Two retrospective cohort studies compared the perinatal outcomes in 222 twin pregnancies with short cervical length (CL ≤ 25 mm at 16–24 weeks) and who were managed with either ultrasound-indicated cerclage (n = 100) or no cerclage (n = 122). After adjusting for gestational age on presentation, there were no differences in the rate of PTB at 28, 32 and 35 weeks between the two groups. However, in the pre-planned subgroup analysis of twin pregnancies with CL ≤ 15 mm before 24 weeks, cerclage placement was associated with a significant prolongation of pregnancy by almost four more weeks, significantly decreased spontaneous PTB at less than 34 weeks by 49% and admission to the neonatal intensive care unit by 58% compared to controls.[8,9]

These two retrospective cohort studies provide evidence that the use of cervical cerclage in twin gestations with short cervix, mostly in those with CL ≤ 15 mm, can potentially reduce the risk of spontaneous PTB at less than 34 weeks of gestation. Ultimately, the results require confirmation in randomised controlled trials.

Physical Examination-Indicated Cerclage (PEIC)/Rescue Cerclage

The first and only randomised controlled trial evaluating physical examination-indicated cerclage (PEIC) in twins was recently published. It was a multicentre (eight centres) randomised controlled trial of women with twin pregnancy and asymptomatic cervical dilatation from 1–5 cm between 16 to 23 6/7 weeks. The primary outcome was the incidence of PTB < 34 weeks. The Data Safety Monitoring Board recommended stopping the trial due to significant decrease of perinatal mortality in the cerclage group. Thirteen women were eventually enrolled in each group (cerclage versus no cerclage). The mean gestational age at delivery was 29.1 weeks (cerclage group) versus 22.5 weeks (no cerclage) (p < 0.01). Perinatal mortality was also significantly reduced in the cerclage group. The authors concluded that, despite the small sample size as the enrolment did not reach the intended 52 cases, they were able to show a significant benefit to physical exam indicated cerclage in twin gestation.[10]

Based on this trial and findings of other retrospective cohort studies and case series that have reported on outcomes of mid-trimester emergency cerclage in twin pregnancies, it seems reasonable to conclude that PEIC/rescue cerclage may prolong gestation, reduce PTB at less than 34 weeks and lower neonatal morbidity and mortality.

Results of Meta-analysis/Systematic Review

A recent systematic review and meta-analysis eloquently summarises these findings. It included a total of 16 randomised controlled trials and cohort studies with 1,211 women, comparing the efficacy of cerclage with no cerclage for women with twin pregnancies.[11] Outcomes indicated that cerclage placement for twin pregnancies with a cervical length of < 15 mm was associated with significant prolongation of pregnancy by a mean difference of 3.89 weeks of gestation and a reduction of PTB at less than 37, 34 and 32 weeks of gestation, compared with those pregnancies in the control group. For women with a dilated cervix of > 10 mm, cerclage placement was associated with significant prolongation of pregnancy by a mean difference of 6.78 weeks of gestation; a reduction of PTB at less than 34, 32, 28 and 24 weeks of gestation and improvement of perinatal outcomes compared with those in the control group. However, for twin pregnancies with a normal cervical length (cerclage for an indication for women with a history of PTB or twin alone), the efficacy of cerclage placement was less certain because of the limited data.

Management Options

The use of cervical cerclage for PTB in twin pregnancy is somewhat limited to the following scenarios:

- When the cervix is dilated 1–4 cm at 16–24 weeks of gestation (physical examination indicated, rescue or emergency cerclage).
- In asymptomatic women without cervical dilatation before 24 weeks but with a short cervix detected incidentally by transvaginal ultrasound (TVUS) and only when ≤ 15 mm in length (ultrasound-indicated cerclage).

Cervical Pessaries

A cervical pessary is a silicone ring with a small diameter to be fitted around the cervix and a larger diameter to fix the device against the pelvic floor. This effectively rotates the cervix toward the posterior vaginal wall and corrects the cervical angle.

The unequivocal benefits of using the cervical pessary in the prevention of PTB in twin pregnancies have not been established. The results of different clinical trials are not only contradictory, but two of the most recent meta-analyses have yielded conflicting conclusions.

Two randomised clinical trials published in the year 2016 yielded conflicting results.[12,13] The first was a multicentre (10 centres, eight countries), randomised clinical trial in unselected twin pregnancies of cervical pessary placement from 20 to 24 weeks of gestation until elective removal or delivery versus expectant management. A total of 1,180 (56.0%) of the 2,107 eligible women agreed to take part in the trial; 590 received cervical pessary and 590 had expectant management. There were no significant differences between the pessary and control groups in rates of spontaneous birth < 34 weeks (primary outcome), perinatal death, adverse neonatal outcome or neonatal therapy. A post hoc subgroup analysis of 214 women with short cervix (≤ 25 mm) also showed no benefit from the insertion of a cervical pessary.[12]

The second was a prospective, open-label, multicentre, randomised clinical trial conducted in five hospitals in Spain (PECEP-Twins). The objective was to test whether a cervical pessary reduces PTB in twin pregnancies with a sonographic short cervix. Cervical length was measured in 2,287 women; 137 pregnant women with a sonographic cervical length ≤ 25 mm were randomly assigned to receive a cervical pessary or expectant management. Spontaneous PTB < 34 weeks of gestation (primary outcome) was significantly less frequent in the pessary group than in the expectant management group. Pessary use was associated with a significant reduction in the rate of birthweight < 2,500 grams. No significant differences were observed in composite neonatal morbidity outcome or neonatal mortality (none) between the groups. No serious adverse effects associated with the use of a cervical pessary were observed.[13]

More recently the STOPPIT2 trial was published. In the STOPPIT 2 open label multicentre randomised controlled trial (57 centres), 503 twin pregnancies with cervical length </= 35mm between 18–10+6 weeks gestation were randomized (253 to standard care and 250 to cervical pessary). The trial concluded that the cervical pessary is ineffective for the prevention of preterm birth in women with a twin pregnancy and a short cervix and should not be used for this purpose.[14]

Results of Meta-analyses/Systematic Review

There are several meta-analyses and systematic reviews, published in the past three years, on the use of cervical pessary for the secondary prevention of PTB in both singleton and twin pregnancies, with conflicting results.

The most recently published meta-analysis included 12 studies involving both singleton (7) and twin (5) pregnancies (8 evaluated pessary vs no pessary in women with a short cervix; 2 assessed pessary versus no pessary in unselected multiple gestations; 2 compared pessary vs vaginal progesterone in women with a short cervix). The placement of a cervical pessary did not reduce the risk of PTB (< 37, < 34, < 32, and < 28 weeks of gestation) or adverse perinatal outcome in women with (a) an unselected twin gestation, (b) a twin gestation and a cervical length < 38 mm or (c) a twin gestation and a cervical length ≤ 25 mm. In addition, there were no significant differences in the risk of SPTB < 34 weeks of gestation between pessary and vaginal progesterone in women with a twin gestation and a cervical length < 38 mm; however, in a pre-specified subgroup analysis of women with cervical length of 28 mm or less (25th percentile), the pessary significantly reduced the PTB rate at less than 34 weeks of gestation from 46% (16/35) to 21% (10/47) (RR 0.47, 95% CI 0.24–0.90) and significantly improved the composite of poor perinatal outcomes (19% versus 50%, $p < 0.001$).[15] Addition of the STOPPIT trial data to these meta-analyses may change these findings.

Management Options

Despite current uncertainty about the role of the cervical pessary in preventing PTB in women with twin gestations, it is reasonable to conclude the following:

- Although the cervical pessary is widely used in clinical practice, no guidelines for management and use of cervical pessary during pregnancy have been clearly formulated.
- There is no role for the prophylactic pessary to reduce PTB in unselected twin pregnancies.
- There is possible value in the use of the pessary in reducing PTB and adverse neonatal outcome in asymptomatic twin pregnancies with short cervix identified by transvaginal sonography, but the cut-off value for a short cervix in twin pregnancies has yet to be agreed on.

Progesterone

Progesterone is produced naturally in the body and has a role in maintaining pregnancy. It is not known whether giving progesterone (by injection, orally or by vaginal suppositories or gels) to women with multiple pregnancy during pregnancy is beneficial or harmful to the woman and her babies.

Unselected Twins

17-alpha-hydroxyprogesterone caproate (17-OHPC)

There are three well-powered randomised controlled trials, all included in a meta-analysis on the effectiveness of intramuscular progestogens to improve perinatal outcome in twin pregnancies, that have studied the role of 17-OHPC in prevention of SPTB in twin pregnancies, two conducted in the USA and one in Lebanon.[16]

The three trials involved a total of 1,183 women with twin gestation, randomised to receive either weekly injections of 17-OHPC (n = 679) or matching placebo (n = 504) starting at 16–24 weeks and ending at 34–36 weeks of gestation. There were no significant differences in the rate of PTB before 28, 32 and 35 weeks or mean gestational age at delivery. While composite neonatal morbidity occurred with similar frequency in the 17-OHPC and placebo groups in the two US trials, respiratory distress syndrome and culture-confirmed sepsis was significantly lower in the 17-OHPC group, when compared to placebo, in the Lebanon trial.

Vaginal Micronised Progesterone

Five randomised controlled trials (1,503 women) involving the use of vaginal micronised progesterone for the prevention of PTB in unselected twin gestations are included in the Cochrane review of 'Prenatal administration of progestogens for preventing spontaneous preterm birth in women with a multiple pregnancy'.[17] There was no difference in the incidence of PTB before 34 weeks, perinatal death rates or any of the other maternal or infant outcomes. No studies reported neurodevelopmental disability at childhood follow-up.

A very recently published randomised controlled trial conducted at 22 hospitals in Europe and involving 1,169 women with unselected twin pregnancies revealed that universal early administration of vaginal progesterone at a dose of 600 mg per day from 11 to 14 weeks of gestation, as compared to placebo, did not reduce the incidence of spontaneous birth between 24 and 34 weeks of gestation. Post hoc time to event analysis led to the suggestion that progesterone may reduce the risk of spontaneous birth < 32 weeks in women with cervical length < 30 mm and it may increase the risk for those with cervical length ≥ 30 mm.[18]

Twins with Short Cervix

17-alpha-hydroxyprogesterone caproate (17-OHPC)

Two trials studied the use of 17-OHPC in reducing the risk of PTB in twin gestations with a short cervix identified by a transvaginal ultrasound examination in the second half of the pregnancy.

A secondary analysis of a double-blind, placebo-controlled randomised controlled trial of 221 women categorised by cervical length (CL) and randomised to receive 250 mg 17-OHPC IM weekly injections versus placebo showed no reduction in the rate of PTB before 35 weeks, neither in women with CL 25th centile (64.3% vs 45.8%, P = 0.18) nor in those with CL > 75th centile (38.1% vs 35.5%, P = 0.85).[19]

A randomised controlled trial of 165 women, conducted in France and involving asymptomatic women with twin gestation between 24 and 31 (6/7) weeks with CL ≤ 25 mm by

TVUS, who were randomised to receive either placebo or 500 mg IM injections of 17-OHPC, repeated twice weekly until 36 weeks or delivery found there was no significant difference in median time to delivery (45 vs 51 days) and treatment with 17-OHPC was associated with a significant increase in rate of preterm delivery before 32 weeks.[20]

Vaginal micronised progesterone

Two randomised controlled trials have evaluated the effectiveness of vaginal micronised progesterone in reducing the risk of preterm birth in twin gestations with a short cervix identified by a transvaginal ultrasound examination.

A PREDICT trial secondary analysis of a sub-population of high-risk twin pregnancies, including those with CL ≤ 10th centile at 20–24 weeks' gestation, history of spontaneous preterm delivery before 34 weeks and miscarriage after 12 weeks found no significant difference in the mean gestational age at delivery between the progesterone and placebo group either in patients with a short cervix or in those with a history of PTD or late miscarriage. Similarly, there were no significant differences between the treatment groups in maternal or neonatal complications and mean ASQ score at 6 and 18 months of age.[21]

A randomised controlled trial in asymptomatic women with twins and a CL 20–25 mm at 20–24 weeks (250 women included; 77% had short cervix out of 322 women with dichorionic twin pregnancy!) found a significant reduction in PTB < 34 weeks and in both neonatal morbidity and early neonatal death.[22]

Individual Participant Data Meta-analyses of Progesterone for Prevention of Preterm Birth in Twin Gestations

The first individual participant data meta-analysis published in 2015 involved 13 trials including 3,768 women with twin pregnancy and 7,536 babies. Neither 17-OHPC IM nor vaginal micronised progesterone reduced the incidence of adverse perinatal outcome in unselected women with an uncomplicated twin gestation. In a subgroup of women with a cervical length (CL) ≤ 25 mm, vaginal progesterone reduced adverse perinatal outcome when cervical length was measured at randomisation or before 24 weeks of gestation. The authors concluded that vaginal progesterone may be effective in reducing PTB and neonatal morbidity in women with CL of ≤ 25 mm, but further research is warranted to confirm this finding.[16]

The second updated meta-analysis of individual patient data, of vaginal progesterone for the secondary prevention of SPTB in women with a twin gestation and a short cervix published in 2017, included six trials. It involved 303 women and 606 infants; 144 women received no treatment or placebo and 159 women received vaginal progesterone. Vaginal progesterone reduced PTB at < 33 weeks (43% in placebo group vs 31% in progesterone group, p = 0.01). Vaginal progesterone significantly reduced respiratory distress syndrome by 30% (RR = 0.7; 95% CI:0.56–0.89), birthweight < 1,500 grams by 47% (RR = 0.53; 95% CI: 0.35–0.80), mechanical ventilation by 46% (RR = 0.54; 95% CI: 0.36–0.81), neonatal death by 47% (RR = 0.53; 95% CI: 0.35–0.81). In a subgroup analysis, it was found that the reduction in the rate of PTB at less than 33 weeks and in neonatal mortality was similar, irrespective of degree of cervical shortening, dose of progesterone and prior history of SPTB.[23]

Management Options

For unselected twin gestations, based on the literature reviewed, progesterone treatment, whether weekly intra-muscular injections of 17-OHPC or vaginal micronised progesterone, does not reduce the incidence of SPTB and therefore is not recommended.[24]

For twin gestations with short cervix (< 25 mm) diagnosed at < 24 weeks gestation, it is also fair to conclude that the preventive administration of 17-OHPC has shown no benefits for prolonging pregnancy or reducing perinatal risk. It is thus not recommended in this context. The daily administration of vaginal progesterone may, however, be effective in reducing perinatal risk in women with short cervix (< 25 mm), but results remain conflicting and most international guidelines are still not recommending this intervention outright.[24,25]

Prevention of Spontaneous Preterm Labour and Birth in Triplets and Higher-Order Pregnancy

The evidence base for interventions to reduce spontaneous preterm labour and birth in triplets and higher-order pregnancy is poor. There are no established proven effective interventions. Given the conflicting evidence for twin gestations, it is reasonable to assume that the few potential preventative interventions for twins are likely to be less effective in triplets and higher-order multiple pregnancy.

Key Points (See Table 20.1)

- The most common cause of perinatal morbidity and mortality in multiple pregnancy is spontaneous preterm labour and delivery.
- Routine bed rest with or without hospitalisation and oral tocolytics have not been shown to be effective in prevention of SPTB in multiple pregnancy.
- Cervical cerclage for the sole indication of multiple pregnancy or if there is a previous history of spontaneous preterm delivery and/or mid-trimester loss has not been shown to be effective.
- Physical examination indicated or rescue cerclage when the cervix is dilated between 1 cm and 4 cm at 16–24 weeks of gestation has some merit in reducing adverse outcomes and can be considered.
- Ultrasound-indicated cerclage when the cervix is ≤ 15 mm and not dilated on transvaginal ultrasound before 24 weeks of gestation in asymptomatic women may reduce PTB and improve neonatal outcomes.
- Cervical pessary in unselected twin gestations for prevention of preterm labour and delivery is not recommended.
- Cervical pessary in women with short cervix on transvaginal ultrasound may reduce PTB and adverse neonatal outcome, but the exact cervical length threshold to intervene is not clear.
- 17-alpha-hydroxyprogesterone caproate (17-OHPC) given intramuscularly weekly has not been shown to be effective in twin gestation for reducing SPTB in unselected twin pregnancy or twin pregnancy where the cervix is short.
- Daily vaginal micronised progesterone has not been shown to be effective in reducing SPTB in unselected twin gestation.
- Daily vaginal micronised progesterone may be effective in reducing SPTB and its consequences in twin gestation where the cervix is short (< 25 mm) before 24 weeks of gestation, but results are conflicting and current international guidelines do not go as far as to recommend its use.

Table 20.1 Summary of management options for prevention of spontaneous preterm delivery in multiple pregnancy

	Unselected multiple pregnancy	History indicated	Physical examination indicated	US indicated (i.e. short cervix)	Triplets or higher-order pregnancies
Bed rest with or without hospitalisation	No	No	No studies	No studies	No
Oral Tocolytics	No	No	No studies	No studies	No
Cervical Cerclage	No	No	Rescue cerclage if Cx 1–4 cm dilated between 16 and 24 weeks	Cerclage if TVUS CL $\leq$ 15 mm < 24 weeks of gestation	?
Cervical pessary	No	No	No	May be effective, but CL cut-off unclear	?
Progesterone: 17-OHPC	No	No	No studies	No	?
Progesterone: vaginal micronised	No	No	No studies	May be effective if CL $\leq$ 25 mm < 24 weeks of gestation	?

US = ultrasound; Cx = cervix, TVUS = transvaginal ultrasound; CL = cervical length; 17-OHPC = 17-alpha-hydroxyprogesterone caproate

- There is little published evidence to guide recommendations for any intervention to reduce SPTB in triplet or higher-order multiple pregnancy.

Acknowledgements

The author would like to acknowledge Nour Adra, medical student at the American University of Beirut, for her valuable contribution to the content of this chapter, notably through her assistance in finding the relevant literature and organising the list of references.

References

1. Adra A, Khalife D, Usta I et al. Practice patterns of obstetric care in twin gestation: the value of MFM consultation. J Matern Fetal Neonatal Med September 2020;20 (9): 1–7.

2. SMFM Research Committee, Grantz K, Kawakita T et al. SMFM special statement: State of the science on multifetal gestations: unique consideration and importance. Am J Obstet Gynecol 2019;221(2):B2–B12. https://doi.org/10.1016/j.ajog.2019.04.013

3. Crowther CA, Han S. Hospitalization and bed rest for multiple pregnancy. Cochrane Database Syst Rev 2010, issue 7 Art. No: CD000110.

4. Ashworth MF, Spooner SF, Verkyul DA, Waterman R, Ashurst HM. Failure to prevent preterm labor and delivery in twin pregnancy using prophylactic oral salbutamol. BJOG 1990;97:878–82.

5. American College of Obstetricians and Gynecologists. Multifetal gestations: twin, triplet and higher-order multifetal pregnancies. Practice Bulletin Number 169. Obstet Gynecol 2016;128:e131–e146.

6. Rottenstreich A, Levin G, Kleinstern G et al. History-indicated cervical cerclage in management of twin pregnancy. Ultrasound Obstet Gynecol 2019;54:517–23.

7. Rafael TJ, Berghella V, Alfirevic Z. Cervical stitch (cerclage) for preventing preterm birth in multiple pregnancy. Cochrane Database Syst Rev 2014;9:CD009166.

8. Roman A, Rochelson B, Fox NS et al. Efficacy of ultrasound-indicated cerclage in twin pregnancies. Am J Obstet Gynecol 2015;212(788):e1–e6.

9. Adams TM, Rafael TJ, Kunzier NB, Mishra S, Calixte R, Vintzileos AM. Does cervical cerclage decrease preterm birth in twin pregnancies with a short cervix? J Matern Fetal Neonatal Med 2018;31(8):1–7.

10. Roman A, Zork N, Haeri S et al. Physical exam indicated cerclage in twin pregnancy: A randomized controlled trial. Am J Obstet Gynecol 2020;223(6):902.e1–902.e11. https://doi.org/10.1016/j.ajog.2020.06.047

11. Li C, Shen J, Hua K et al. Cerclage for women with twin pregnancies: a systematic review and meta-analysis. Am J Obstet Gynecol 2019;6:543–557.

12. Nicolaides K, Syngelaki A, Poon L et al. Cervical pessary for prevention of preterm birth in unselected twin pregnancies: a randomized controlled trial. Am J Obstet Gynecol 2016;214:3.e1–e9.

13. Goya M, De la Calle M, Pratcorona L et al. Cervical pessary to prevent preterm birth in women with twin gestation and sonographic short cervix: a multicenter randomized controlled trial (PECEP-TWINS). Am J Obstet Gynecol February 2016;214(2):145–52. https://doi.org/10.1016/j.ajog.2015.11.012

14. Norman JE, Norrie J, MacLennan G et al. The Arabin pessary to prevent preterm birth in women with a twin pregnancy and a short cervix: the STOPPIT 2 RCT. Health Technol Assess. 2021 Jul;25(44):1–66. https//:doi.org/10.3310/hta25440

15. Conde-Agudelo A, Romero R, Nicolaides K. Cervical pessary to prevent preterm birth in asymptomatic high-risk women: a systematic review and meta-analysis. Am J Obstet Gynecol July

2020;**223**(1):42–65.e2. https://doi.org/10.1016/j.ajog.2019.12.266

16. Schuit E, Stock C, Rode L et al. Effectiveness of progestogens to improve perinatal outcome in twin pregnancies: an individual participant data meta-analysis. BJOG 2015 January;**122**(1):27–37.

17. Dodd JM, Grivell RM, Obrien CM, Dowswell T, Deussen AR. Prenatal administration of progestogens for preventing spontaneous preterm birth in women with a multiple pregnancy (review). Cochrane Database *Syst Rev* 2019 (11). Art. No: CD 012024.

18. Rehal A, Benkő Z, Matallana C et al. Early vaginal progesterone versus placebo in twin pregnancies for prevention of spontaneous preterm birth (EVENTS): a randomised double-blind trial. Am J Obstet Gynecol 2021;**224**(1):86.e1–86.e19. https//:doi.org/10.1016/j.ajog.2020.06.050

19. Durnwald C, Momirova V, Peaceman A et al. Second trimester cervical length and risk of preterm birth in women with twin gestations treated with 17 alpha hydroxyprogesterone caproate. J Matern Fetal Neonatal Med 2010;**23**(12):1360–4.

20. Senat M, Porcher R, Winer N et al. Prevention of preterm delivery by 17 alpha-hydroxyprogesterone caproate in asymptomatic twin pregnancies with a short cervix: a randomized controlled trial. Am J Obstet Gynecol 2013;**208**(194):e1–e8.

21. Klein K, Rode L, Nicolaides K, Krampl-Bettelheim E, Tabor A for the PREDICT Group. Vaginal micronized progesterone and risk of preterm delivery in high-risk twin pregnancies: secondary analysis of a placebo-controlled randomized trial and meta-analysis.Ultrasound Obstet Gynecol 2011;**38**:281–7.

22. El-refaie W, Abdelhafez MS, Badawy A. Vaginal progesterone for prevention of preterm labor in asymptomatic twin pregnancies with sonographic short cervix: a randomized clinical trial of efficacy and safety. Arch Gynecol Obstet 2016;**293**:61–7.

23. Romero R, Conde-Agudelo A, El-Refaie W et al. Vaginal progesterone decreases preterm birth and neonatal morbidity and mortality in women with a twin gestation and a short cervix: an updated meta-analysis of individual patient data. Ultrasound Obstet Gynecol 2017;**49**:303–14.

24. Sentilhes L, Senat MV, Ancel PY et al. Prevention of spontaneous preterm birth: Guidelines for clinical practice from the French College of Gynecologists and Obstetricians (CNGOF). Eur J Obstet Gynecol Reprod Biol 2017(210):217–24.

25. National Institute for Health and Care Excellence. Multiple Pregnancy: Antenatal Care for Twin and Triplet Pregnancies. Clinical Guideline no. 129. London: National Institute for Health and Care Excellence, 2011.

Optimal Antenatal Care in Multiple Pregnancy

Leanne Bricker

Introduction

Women with multiple pregnancy are at higher risk of almost all maternal complications in pregnancy. Maternal mortality is more than double that of singleton gestations and this is often overshadowed by fetal considerations, reflected in the literature with few published studies from the developed world addressing maternal risks. For fetuses or babies of multiple pregnancies, premature birth is the main cause of adverse outcome, but there are important contributions from fetal growth pathology, fetal abnormality and complications of shared placentation. Cerebral palsy is also increased amongst twins and even more so amongst triplets and higher-order multiples with aetiologies not entirely restricted to prematurity. Given the higher risk of complications, there are a number of additional elements of care, which necessitates more monitoring and increased contact with the healthcare team. Additionally, the increased risk may have a psychosocial and economic impact on women and their families and may heighten anxiety, resulting in a specific need for more information and support in pregnancy. This chapter summarises the additional elements of antenatal care required to identify complications and optimise outcomes in multiple pregnancy, but it does not address how to manage these complications once detected and diagnosed.

Existing Guidelines and the Case for Following Them

There are a number of national/international guidelines relating to various aspects of care of multiple pregnancy. The most comprehensive guideline is the United Kingdom's (UK) National Institute for Health and Care Excellence (NICE) guideline.[1] In the UK, the stillbirth rate in twins nearly halved between 2014 and 2016 and there was also a reduction in neonatal mortality, and this is thought to be partly due to publication and subsequent uptake of the NICE guideline in 2011.[2] This view is further supported by an audit undertaken of 30 maternity units in the UK where reduction in stillbirths, neonatal unit admission and neonatal mortality was directly linked to uptake and implementation of NICE quality standards derived from the NICE guideline.[3]

Early Pregnancy

The use of obstetric sonography in early pregnancy is widespread and is known to improve gestational dating, thus reducing induction of labour for post-mature pregnancy, and it also ensures early detection of multiple pregnancy. Accurate dating and amnionicity and chorionicity determination are key to planning and providing optimal antenatal care, including discussion about screening for aneuploidy and other fetal complications (fetal abnormality, fetal growth restriction and complications of shared placentation). Furthermore, it allows labelling of each fetus and timely discussion about the risks of higher-order multiple pregnancy and also consideration of multifetal pregnancy reduction in settings where this is possible. If chorionicity and amnionicity cannot be determined, the woman should be referred for specialist evaluation for clarification. If still undetermined, the pregnancy should be treated as monochorionic until proven otherwise.

With regard to labelling fetuses, if the fetus closest to the cervix in early pregnancy is labelled fetus 1 and further numbering is assigned to the other fetuses, it does not accurately determine which will be the leading fetus as pregnancy progresses, or indeed birth order. The presenting twin will change between left and right fetus in 8.5% of cases and the birth order will change from the last scan in 5.9% delivered vaginally versus 20.3% delivered by caesarean section.[4] Correct orientation labelling in relation to the mother as maternal left and maternal right in laterally orientated fetuses or upper and lower in vertically orientated fetuses allows consistency with longitudinal biometric assessment, accuracy in interpreting screening results and undertaking invasive diagnostic tests when necessary, and it avoids confusion about birth order, ensuring the parents and paediatric team are aware of the possibility of peri-partum switch (i.e. change in birth order).

Screening for Fetal Complications

Down's syndrome and other aneuploidies (see Table 21.1)

Down's syndrome and other aneuploidy screening in multiple pregnancy is complex as (1) there is a higher risk of aneuploidy, (2) the detection rate (sensitivity) of screening tests is lower compared with screening in singleton pregnancy, (3) the false positive rate is higher, (4) the likelihood of being offered invasive diagnostic testing and the risk of complications of the testing is higher and (5) if there is an affected fetus, the management is complex because of the risks to the surviving normal fetus or fetuses. Women need to be fully informed about these issues before the screening test and also afterwards in the event of a positive result.

The options include nuchal translucency screening with or without additional elements (maternal age, other maternal factors and serum screening), second-trimester serum screening or cell-free DNA (cfDNA) non-invasive prenatal testing (NIPT). In the first trimester for twin pregnancy combined screening (nuchal translucency (NT), maternal age, other maternal factors, and serum screening – beta-human chorionic gonadotropin and pregnancy-associated plasma protein-A) can be offered. For dichorionic (DC) twin pregnancies, risks should be calculated for each fetus. For monochorionic (MC) twin pregnancies, each fetus has the same risk of Down's syndrome or other aneuploidy, and the overall risk is the same as in a singleton pregnancy. Therefore, the NT measurement should be averaged and used to calculate a pregnancy-specific risk. For triplets, there are no normograms for serum screening, and therefore NT and maternal age are the only available screening methods.[1] If the woman presents too late for first-trimester screening, the NICE guideline recommends offering second-trimester serum screening for twins. For triplet pregnancy there are no second-trimester screening options.[1]

Non-invasive prenatal testing is commercially available for screening for trisomies 21, 18 and 13 with high levels of accuracy and low false positive and false negative rates in singleton pregnancy. A published study including a meta-analysis of seven other studies found that

Table 21.1 Down's syndrome screening test options in multiple pregnancy

Type of Multiple Pregnancy	First Trimester	Second Trimester
Dichorionic twins	Combined NT test (Calculate fetus-specific risk) OR NIPT	Serum screening (Calculate pregnancy-specific risk) OR NIPT
Monochorionic twins	Combined NT test (Calculate pregnancy-specific risk by using average NT) OR NIPT	Serum screening (Calculate pregnancy-specific risk) OR NIPT
Triplets or higher-order	NT and maternal age alone	No available test
Vanishing twin	Combined NT test OR NIPT But note not as accurate	Serum screening OR NIPT But note not as accurate

NT = nuchal translucency; NIPT = non-invasive prenatal testing

the performance of NIPT for trisomy 21 in twin pregnancy is similar to that for singleton pregnancy and significantly better than first-trimester combined or second-trimester serum biochemical testing.[5] However, accuracy for trisomies 18 and 13 remains unclear due to the small numbers of cases.

It is important to note that in multiple pregnancy where chromosomal abnormality is likely to be discordant (particularly if there is dizygosity or polyzygosity), where it is not obvious (i.e. no visible structural features aiding identification of the affected fetus) invasive testing will be required to identify and confirm diagnosis of an affected fetus. If the woman opts for invasive diagnostic testing, this should be performed by a specialist who has the expertise to subsequently perform selective termination of pregnancy if required.[6]

Structural Abnormalities

Structural abnormalities are more common in twin, triplet and higher-order pregnancies, mainly because of the higher incidence in monozygotic twins (due to cleavage of the conceptus) compared with dizygotic twins. The management is complex when one fetus has an abnormality. Timely diagnosis allows more choice, preparation time, optimal fetal surveillance depending on the anomaly, involvement of the multidisciplinary team (e.g. genetics team, paediatric surgeons) and appropriate birth planning (place, timing and mode), including access to intrauterine therapy where relevant. Ultrasound assessment will take longer and visualisation may be limited by fetal positions, but mid-trimester ultrasound is expected to be as effective in multiple pregnancy as it is in singleton pregnancy with similar detection rates. Therefore, as in singleton pregnancy, routine anomaly screening by ultrasound between 18 and 20+6 weeks of gestation is recommended.

Abnormalities specific to monozygotic twins are usually midline, such as holoprosencephaly and neural tube defects and cardiac abnormalities. For this reason, the value of fetal echocardiography in addition to routine anatomy scan is debated. Not all monozygotic twins are MC twins, however; therefore this would need to be applied to all twins irrespective of chorionicity unless discordant-sex twins are excluded, which can complicate the situation if the couple do not want to know the gender of the babies. Guidance on this subject advocate that the anomaly scan should include extended heart views but formal fetal echocardiography is not necessary if there is no other risk factor.[1,7,8]

Fetal Growth Pathology

Fetuses of multiple pregnancies are at increased risk of being small for gestational age (SGA) and if there is placental dysfunction, of fetal growth restriction (FGR). Both SGA and FGR fetuses and babies have poorer perinatal outcomes and therefore identifying growth problems is important. The pathophysiology of growth pathology in MC and DC pregnancies differs. In DC twins the pathophysiology is similar to singleton growth problems whereas in MC twins it is often related to unequal sharing of the single placenta and does not always follow the same pattern in evolution and deterioration as singleton pregnancy. Symphysis-fundal height measurement is not effective in identifying growth problems in twin pregnancy and serial ultrasound scans are required to identify both small babies and a significant size difference between the fetuses. The frequency of ultrasound scan assessment depends on the chorionicity.

It is well described that fetal growth in twins is different to that in singletons with reduction in growth velocity in the third trimester, and this is more marked in MC twins.[9] There is a current debate amongst experts about whether specific growth charts for twins should be used to monitor fetal growth. Proponents of twin charts argue that use of such charts would (1) result in more accurate diagnosis of twin growth pathology, (2) identify those at risk of increased morbidity and mortality and (3) result in avoiding overdiagnosis of twin growth pathology and therefore unnecessary intervention and preterm delivery. The opposing argument is that (1) the charts have not been validated clinically in prospective research, (2) such charts are not in use for other high-risk obstetric conditions associated with fetal growth pathology (e.g. diabetes), (3) multiple pregnancy is a high-risk situation and using specific charts may hide that risk and (4) we should not rely on fetal size alone anyway in evaluating fetal growth pathology – that is, fetal well-being evaluation includes evaluating growth velocity and Dopplers.

Historically there has been inconsistency in defining growth restriction in multiple pregnancy. Recently a panel of experts using the Delphi process defined selective fetal growth restriction (sFGR) for both MC and DC pregnancy.[10] See Table 21.2 for diagnostic criteria. The formula for calculating the estimated fetal weight (EFW) discordance percentage is: EFW larger fetus – EFW smaller fetus / EFW larger fetus x 100 (e.g. 700 g – 540 g / 700 g x 100 = 23%). Growth pathology in DC twin pregnancy is managed very similarly to growth pathology in singleton pregnancy. In MC twin pregnancy, however, it is classified according to the type of abnormality in the umbilical artery Doppler of the smaller fetus and management depends on severity and type.

Table 21.2 Diagnostic criteria for selective growth restriction in twin pregnancy (Delphi method consensus adapted from Khalil et al.[10])

	Monochorionic twin pregnancy	Dichorionic twin pregnancy
Solitary parameter	EFW of one twin < 3rd centile	
Contributory parameters	At least 2 of the following: EFW of one twin < 10th centile AC of one twin < 10th centile EFW discordance >/= 25% Smaller twin UA PI > 95th centile	At least 2 of the following: EFW of one twin < 10th centile EFW discordance >/= 25% Smaller twin UA PI > 95th centile

EFW = estimated fetal weight, AC = abdominal circumference, UA PI = Umbilical artery pulsatility index

Complications of Shared Placenta

Twin–Twin Transfusion Syndrome (TTTS)

Ten to fifteen per cent of MC pregnancies develop twin–twin transfusion syndrome (TTTS) and in severe cases the outcome is significantly improved if treated with fetoscopic laser ablation. Given that there is available treatment it is essential to screen for TTTS to allow timely access to therapy. It usually presents between 16 and 24 weeks of gestation and therefore earlier screening would need to be very effective to advocate its use. There are several studies evaluating first-trimester parameters for TTTS screening – namely NT and/or crown–rump length (CRL) discordance and/or ductus venosus Doppler blood flow – but they all show low sensitivity and variable specificity, and there is potential to cause unnecessary anxiety. First-trimester screening for this complication is therefore not advised.[1,7] The recommendation for screening is scan every two weeks from 16 weeks of gestation until delivery but a step up to weekly scans if there are concerning features such as inter-twin membrane folding or liquor discordance.[1,7]

Twin Anaemia-Polycythaemia Sequence (TAPS)

Twin anaemia-polycythaemia sequence (TAPs) is an uncommon complication unique to monochorionic placentation whereby there is a severe inter-twin haemoglobin discordance, apparently due to chronic transfer of blood via miniscule placental arterial-venous anastomoses. It can occur at any gestation and is relatively rare – 2–3% of MC twin pregnancies – but in complicated MC pregnancies with sFGR, or after laser treatment for TTTS, it occurs more commonly. It can be detected by measuring middle cerebral artery peak systolic velocity (MCA-PSV) whereby the donor has an MCA-PSV > 1.5 multiple of the median (MoM) (due to fetal anaemia) and the recipient has an MCA PSV < 1.0 MoM (due to polycythaemia). Unlike TTTS on ultrasound examination, there is no significant polyhydramnios-oligohydramnios sequence, but there can be a difference in the echogenicity and thickness of the two placental territories. The recipient may have cardiomegaly and the donor may have a 'starry sky' appearance in the fetal liver. It is associated with increased risk of adverse outcome for both fetuses.

Management options include expectant management, fetoscopic laser ablation, intrauterine transfusion of the donor and partial exchange transfusion of the recipient or selective reduction. There are no prospective controlled trials of these management options and currently the best treatment/approach is not known. Experts individualise treatment according to gestation, severity and personal preference/experience. Some advocate screening all MC pregnancies for TAPs, but most international guidelines recommend screening only in MC pregnancies complicated by TTTS which has been treated or sFGR.[1,7,8] Universal screening may be advised when the best management approach is known.

Other Shared Placenta Complications

See other chapters for details about diagnosis and management of monoamnioticity, twin-reversed arterial perfusion (TRAP) sequence and conjoined twinning.

Screening for Maternal Complications

Hypertensive Disorders of Pregnancy

Women with multiple pregnancy have much higher risk of developing gestational hypertension, pre-eclampsia or eclampsia. Additionally, such disorders are more likely to occur earlier and be more severe. The UK NICE guideline for 'Hypertension in Pregnancy' recommends that women with one high-risk factor or at least two moderate-risk factors take oral low-dose aspirin (75–150 mg daily) from 12 weeks of gestation until birth.[11] Multiple pregnancy is considered a moderate risk factor. As with singleton pregnancy, to detect hypertensive disorders it is recommended that a woman's blood pressure is measured and urine tested for protein at each antenatal contact.

Gestational Diabetes

Gestational diabetes is due to a relative insulin insufficiency secondary to the diabetogenic effect of placental hormones (human placental lactogen, progesterone and cortisol). In multiple pregnancy there is a larger placental mass, which increases the amount of placental hormones and therefore theoretically the risk of developing gestational diabetes. In practice, however, there is conflicting evidence about whether the occurrence of gestational diabetes is increased in multiple pregnancy and whether it is advisable to screen for, and this area warrants further research.

Anaemia

There is a higher incidence of maternal anaemia in multiple pregnancy. This coupled with the higher risk of post-partum haemorrhage and the demands of breastfeeding more than one baby after birth makes it imperative to optimise maternal haemoglobin level antenatally. Routine iron and folic acid supplementation for this purpose is not necessary, but the NICE guideline recommends checking the full blood count at 20–24 weeks and 28 weeks of gestation (cf. singleton pregnancy where it is advised at 28 weeks of gestation only) to identify women who may need iron and folic acid supplementation in time to effectively treat anaemia.[1]

Other Maternal Complications

In multiple pregnancy there is an increased risk of almost all other complications of pregnancy, such as placenta praevia, obstetric cholestasis and antepartum haemorrhage. Additionally, all minor ailments of pregnancy are worse. The management of these complications and ailments is no different compared with management in singleton pregnancies.

Prediction and Prevention of Preterm Labour

Prediction

To predict spontaneous preterm birth (SPTB) in twin and triplet pregnancy, the diagnostic accuracy of several factors/tests has been studied – ultrasonographic cervical length (CL) measurement, fetal fibronectin test (FFT), home uterine activity monitoring, digital cervical examination, screening for bacterial vaginosis, past obstetric history of preterm birth and composites of these approaches. Both a previous history of SPTB and abnormal CL measurements have been shown to be predictors of preterm birth in multiple pregnancy. The NICE guideline concluded that a CL of < 25 mm at 18–24 weeks of gestation is a good predictor of SPTB in twin pregnancy and a CL measurement of < 25 mm at 14–20 weeks of gestation is a good predictor of spontaneous preterm birth in triplet pregnancy.[1]

Prevention

Interventions that have been studied to prevent spontaneous preterm labour in twin and triplet pregnancy include bed rest, oral tocolytics, progesterone (intramuscular or vaginal), cervical cerclage and cervical pessary. None of these interventions have been found effective, but much interest remains in progesterone treatment in particular and there is large body of published literature in this regard. It must be noted that in the recent update of the NICE guideline, the expert panel withheld recommendations about whether to use progesterone as they were 'aware that new evidence would be emerging about the use of vaginal progesterone in subgroups of women with a shot cervix which may change conclusions about its effectiveness'.[1] At the time of writing this chapter, the situation is unchanged and therefore the current advice remains that in the absence of an effective intervention routine, screening to predict preterm delivery is not recommended in twin and triplet pregnancy and the use of progesterone (either vaginal or intramuscular) has not been proven effective.

Use of Corticosteroids

Giving timely antenatal corticosteroids reduces neonatal complications in preterm babies, albeit it is thought that they are less effective in multiple pregnancy. Given the substantial risk of preterm delivery in multiple pregnancy, the question arises about whether giving an untargeted course of steroids routinely at a given gestation or whether giving multiple courses at regular intervals may be beneficial. However, a single course remote from delivery dampens its effect and multiple courses compared with a single course do not improve outcomes but are associated with potential harm – that is, lower birthweight and head circumference.[12] It is therefore better to avoid untargeted routine single or multiple courses of steroids and to advocate targeted steroids when indicated – that is, when preterm labour or birth is imminent – and therefore to shift the focus towards informing all women with twin and triplet pregnancy of the increased risk of preterm birth and the benefits of targeted steroids and to provide information about symptoms and signs to be aware of so they can present in a timely manner.[1]

A second question does arise – if a woman is given a targeted course of steroids but preterm labour is arrested and she does not deliver, should a further course be given if she presents at a later preterm gestation with signs or symptoms of threatened preterm labour or if iatrogenic preterm delivery is planned? A recent individual patient data meta-analysis of 11 trials found that repeat prenatal steroids given to women at ongoing risk of preterm birth after an initial course is beneficial for the neonate but to provide clinical benefit with the least effect on fetal growth, the number of repeat treatments and total dose should be limited.[13]

Planning Delivery

In addition to discussing risks of spontaneous preterm labour and delivery and preparing women for this possibility, many multiple pregnancies will progress uncomplicated, and an important aspect of optimal antenatal care is to ensure an informed discussion occurs about place, timing and mode of delivery. While in triplet and higher-order pregnancies caesarean delivery is advocated, discussions in twin pregnancy should include details of the risks and benefits of vaginal delivery versus caesarean section and pain relief options if vaginal delivery is planned. Discussions should also include who will be present at the delivery (more personnel than in singleton pregnancy) and the potential for the need for specialist neonatal care even if delivery is not preterm.

Other Aspects of Care

Information and Emotional Support

In current times women and their families have access to a wide range of information sources, some of which may be misleading or poor. The high-risk nature of multiple pregnancy and additional care requirements may lead to anxiety and stress for the woman and her family and it is important to ensure women are supported with good information, are guided to reliable sources of further information and can clarify issues of concern. They should be encouraged to think about socio-economic aspects of raising more than one child. This process of information sharing and provision of information can take place via a number of formats.

Nutritional Supplements, Diet and Lifestyle Advice

It has been suggested in multiple pregnancy that as the metabolic needs of the mother are greater than in singleton pregnancy, a high-calorie diet may help with her nutritional state. However, boosting weight gain might not be advantageous. There are no randomised clinical trials to provide guidance. The NICE guideline group reviewed the limited literature and concluded that the few published studies were of very low quality and there was no evidence to give different advice to that given in singleton pregnancy.[1] They did, however, recommend that the woman is referred to a dietician if necessary.

How and Where to Deliver Care

Given the extra elements required to deliver optimal antenatal care in multiple pregnancy it seems logical that this should be provided in a dedicated service whether it be in a clinic staffed by a dedicated multidisciplinary team or delivered by a core team in a specialised model. A Cochrane systematic review found only one small randomised controlled trial (RCT) (162 women) of specialised antenatal care in multiple pregnancy and the intervention was extra midwifery support (not specialist obstetric care).[14] There was no difference in incidence of postnatal depression (this was the primary outcome), perinatal mortality, stillbirth, neonatal mortality and breastfeeding. The intervention group members were more likely to have caesarean delivery. From other studies, all conducted in the USA, there is some evidence of improved outcomes, but it is conflicting and limited for the following reasons: (1) there is a potential for bias (e.g. women at lower risk may have had better access to this care for financial, educational or other reasons), (2) it is not clear whether it is the actual elements of care (and if so which elements) or the continuity and specialist knowledge of the caregivers that makes the difference and (3) as the evidence comes from one healthcare setting (i.e. the USA) where in particular there is little midwifery input, it may not be reproducible in other settings.[15] What does, however, appear to be clear is that continuity and consistency of care by the same experienced and knowledgeable professionals contributes to better outcomes. For this reason, the NICE guideline recommends that 'clinical care for women with twin and triplet pregnancies should be provided by a nominated multidisciplinary team consisting of a core team of named specialist obstetricians, specialist midwives and ultrasonographers, all of whom have experience and knowledge of managing twin and triplet pregnancies'. This team should have access to refer to an enhanced team including a perinatal mental health professional, a women's health physiotherapist and infant feeding specialist and a dietician.[1]

The NICE guideline also specifies a schedule of appointments which includes timing of ultrasound scans according to whether the pregnancy is twins or triplets and based on chorionicity and amnionicity, and it also details recommended timing of delivery.[1] The International Society of Ultrasound in Obstetrics and Gynecology (ISUOG) guideline specifies what elements should be measured and evaluated at each scan.[7] These schedules provide guidance for the minimal requirements and recognises that if there are comorbidities or complications there may be a need to deviate from the schedule. See Table 21.3.

Indication for Referral to Tertiary-Level Fetal Medicine Services

Easy access to care is important and therefore the principle of care close to home and local expertise is important. But there are complications of multiple pregnancy which require specific expertise. When these complications occur, clinical decisions and choices can be complex and it is crucial to recognise this and refer to specialist fetal medicine services with appropriate expertise. The NICE guideline identified complications which would fit this criterion as follows: a high-risk aneuploidy screening result, monoamnionicity, any triplet pregnancy with a shared placenta, or pregnancies complicated by discordant fetal growth, fetal anomaly, discordant fetal death, TTTS, conjoined fetuses, TRAP or suspected TAPs.[1]

Key Points

- Twin and triplet pregnancies are high risk for both mother and babies and require additional elements of care to identify and manage complications effectively and to optimise outcomes.
- In managing multiple pregnancy, it is proven that uptake and implementation of evidence-based guidelines improves outcomes.

Table 21.3 Recommended schedule of antenatal appointments and ultrasound scans for uncomplicated twin and triplet pregnancy according to chorionicity and amnionicity (adapted from NICE guidelines and the ISUOG Practice Guideline)[1,7]

Dichorionic-diamniotic twins (DCDA)	Offer women with uncomplicated dichorionic twin pregnancies at least eight antenatal appointments with a healthcare professional from the core team. At least two of these appointments should be with the specialist obstetrician. Combine appointments with scans when crown–rump length measures from 45 mm to 84 mm (at approximately 11 weeks 0 days to 13 weeks 6 days) and then at estimated gestations of 20, 24, 28, 32 and 36 weeks. At the 11–13 week scan confirm dating, labelling, chorionicity and amnionicity, and screen for trisomy 21 if desired. At the 20 week scan evaluate detailed anatomy, biometry, DVP, CL. At each scan from 24 weeks onwards assess fetal growth, DVP, UA-PI. Offer additional appointments without scans at 16 and 34 weeks. Offer delivery from 37 weeks of gestation.
Monochorionic-diamniotic twins (MCDA)	Offer women with uncomplicated monochorionic-diamniotic twin pregnancies at least nine antenatal appointments with a healthcare professional from the core team. At least two of these appointments should be with the specialist obstetrician. Combine appointments with scans when crown–rump length measures from 45 mm to 84 mm (at approximately 11 weeks 0 days to 13 weeks 6 days) and then at estimated gestations of 16, 18, 20, 22, 24, 28, 32 and 34 weeks. At the 11–13 week scan confirm dating, labelling, chorionicity and amnionicity, and screen for trisomy 21 if desired. At the 16 week scan evaluate fetal growth and DVP. At the 20 week scan evaluate detailed anatomy, biometry, DVP, CL, UA-PI and MCA-PSV, EFW discordance. At each scan from 22 weeks onwards assess fetal growth, DVP, UA-PI, MCA-PSV, EFW discordance. Offer delivery from 36 weeks of gestation.
Trichorionic-triamniotic triplets (TCTA)	Offer women with uncomplicated trichorionic-triamniotic triplet pregnancies at least seven antenatal appointments with a healthcare professional from the core team. At least two of these appointments should be with the specialist obstetrician. Combine appointments with scans when crown–rump length measures from 45 mm to 84 mm (at approximately 11 weeks 0 days to 13 weeks 6 days) and then at estimated gestations of 20, 24, 28, 32 and 34 weeks. Ultrasound evaluation elements are the same as for DCDA twins Offer an additional appointment without a scan at 16 weeks. Offer delivery from 35 weeks of gestation.

Table 21.3 (cont.)

Monochorionic-triamniotic (MCTA) and dichorionic-triamniotic triplets (DCTA)	Offer women with uncomplicated monochorionic-triamniotic and dichorionic-triamniotic triplet pregnancies at least 11 antenatal appointments with a healthcare professional from the core team. At least two of these appointments should be with the specialist obstetrician. Combine appointments with scans when crown–rump length measures from 45 mm to 84 mm (at approximately 11 weeks 0 days to 13 weeks 6 days) and then at estimated gestations of 16, 18, 20, 22, 24, 26, 28, 30, 32 and 34 weeks. Ultrasound evaluation elements are the same as for MCDA twins. Offer delivery from 35 weeks of gestation.
Any twin or triplet pregnancy where there is a shared amnion	Women with twin and triplet pregnancies involving a shared amnion should be offered individualised care from a consultant in a tertiary-level fetal medicine service.

DVP = deepest vertical pocket, CL = cervical length, UA-PI = umbilical artery pulsatility index, MCA-PSV = middle cerebral artery peak systolic velocity, EFW = estimated fetal weight. For monoamnionicity refer to Chapter 17.

- Care needs to be delivered by healthcare professionals with specific knowledge and expertise ensuring consistency and continuity, and this may be best delivered in the context of a specialist clinic or service.
- Early pregnancy care should include a scan to accurately date the pregnancy, label fetuses and determine chorionicity and amnionicity.
- An individualised care schedule should be followed based on chorionicity, amnionicity and other risk factors specific to the woman.
- Screening for fetal complications should be offered along with specific information about the complex clinical issues and decisions that may result from such screening.
- Later care should focus on presentation and management of complications such as preterm labour, growth restriction and maternal complications and planning for delivery.
- Complex cases should be referred to specialists in fetal medicine.
- Emotional support and relevant reliable information should be given to mitigate the stress and anxiety associated with these high-risk pregnancies.
- Interventions for which there is no solid evidence base should be avoided.

References

1. National Institute for Health and Care Excellence (NICE), UK. Twin and Triplet Pregnancy (NG137), 2019. www.nice.org.uk/guidance/ng137

2. Kilby MD, Gibson JL, Ville Y. Falling perinatal mortality in twins in the UK: organisational success or chance? BJOG 2019;**126**(3):341–7.

3. NICE Works: Twins and Multiple Births Association Maternity Engagement Project Final Report. https://twinstrust.org/uploads/assets/afcc44b3-776e-4341-8a16e9bd990c3425/NICE-works-final-report.pdf

4. Dias T, Ladd S, Mahsud-Dornan S, Bhide A, Papageorghiou AT, Thilaganathan B. Systematic labeling of twin pregnancies on ultrasound. Ultrasound Obstet Gynecol 2011;**38**:130–3.

5. Gil MM, Galeva S, Jani J et al. Screening for trisomies by cfDNA testing of maternal blood in twin pregnancy: update of the Fetal Medicine Foundation results and meta-analysis. Ultrasound Obstet Gynecol 2019;**53**(6):734–42.

6. Royal College of Obstetricians and Gynaecologists (RCOG). Green-Top Guideline (no. 8). Amniocentesis and chorionic villus sampling. 2010. www.RCOG.org.uk

7. Royal College of Obstetricians and Gynaecologists (RCOG). Green-Top Guideline (no. 51). Management of monochorionic twin pregnancy. 2016. www.RCOG.org.uk

8. ISUOG practice guideline. Role of ultrasound in twin pregnancy. Ultrasound Obstet Gynecol 2016;**47**:247–63.

9. Stirrup OT, Khalil A, D'Antonio F, Thilaganathan B, on behalf of the Southwest Thames Obstetric Research Collaborative (STORK). Fetal growth reference ranges in twin pregnancy: analysis of the Southwest Thames Obstetric Research Collaborative (STORK) multiple pregnancy cohort. Ultrasound Obstet Gynecol 2015;**45**:301–7.

10. Khalil A, Beune I, Hecher K et al. Consensus definition and essential reporting parameters of selective fetal growth restriction in twin pregnancy: a Delphi procedure. Ultrasound Obstet Gynecol 2019 Jan;**53** (1):47–54.

11. National Institute for Health and Care Excellence (NICE), UK. Hypertension in pregnancy: diagnosis and management (NG133), 2019. www.nice.org.uk/guidance/ng133

12. Crowther CA, Harding JE. Repeat doses of prenatal corticosteroids for women at risk of preterm birth for preventing neonatal respiratory disease. *Cochrane Database Syst Rev* 2007;(3):CD003935.

13. Crowther CA, Middleton PF, Voysey M et al. Effects of repeat prenatal corticosteroids given to women at risk of preterm birth: an individual participant data meta-analysis. PLoS Med. 2019 12;**16** (4):e1002771.

14. Dodd JM, Dowswell T, Crowther CA. Specialised antenatal clinics for women with a multiple pregnancy for improving maternal and infant outcomes. Cochrane Database *Syst Rev* 2015;(11). Art. No.: CD005300. https://doi.org/10.1002/146518 58.CD005300.pub4

15. Bricker L. Optimal antenatal care for twin and triplet pregnancy: the evidence base. Best Pract Res Clin Obstet Gynaecol 2014;**28**(2):305–17. https://doi.org/10 .1016/j.bpobgyn.2013.12.006. Epub 2013 Dec 17. PMID: 244

Chapter 22

Triplet and Higher-Order Pregnancy
Special Considerations

Ann McHugh and Fergal Malone

Introduction

The rate of triplet and higher-order multiple (HOM) pregnancies increased more than 400% during the 1980s and 1990s, peaking at 193.5 per 100,000 births in 1998. The initial increased incidence has been attributed to two main factors, namely advanced maternal age at conception and the increased use of assisted reproductive technology (ART).[1] However, with improved cryopreservation techniques in ART, the reduction in the number of embryos transferred with each cycle and the increase in the number of multifetal pregnancy reduction procedures, there was a decrease in the rate of triplet and HOM pregnancies to 93 per 100,000 births in 2018. This represents an 8% decline from the 2017 rate of 101.6 per 100,000 births and a 52% fall from the peak in 1998. In summary, the incidence of HOM pregnancy is decreasing but still present, so knowledge of the facts and issues remains essential for the maternal fetal medicine specialist.

The Facts

Higher-order multiple births are naturally conceived in approximately one-fifth of cases, one- to two-thirds are a consequence of ovulation induction or superovulation and 13–44% are associated with ART.[2] Assisted reproductive technology itself does not appear to increase the risk of composite neonatal morbidity (culture-proven sepsis, respiratory distress syndrome or Apgar Score < 7 at 5 minutes) or perinatal death in triplet pregnancies,[3] despite the fact that mothers undergoing ART are older and tend to deliver at an earlier gestational age.[4] Triplet pregnancies resulting from ART are most likely to be trizygotic and therefore trichorionic. However, monochorionic placentation is more common in spontaneously conceived triplets. Multifetal pregnancies carry significant risks for both mother and fetus (Tables 22.1 and 22.2). Such pregnancies are associated with an approximately fivefold increased risk of intrauterine fetal death and a sevenfold increased risk of neonatal death when compared with singleton pregnancies. The risks of perinatal morbidity and mortality increase with the presence of each additional fetus. Maternal complications in pregnancy and the puerperium, including rates of maternal depression, increase substantially in multifetal pregnancies. Societal costs in relation to the provision of healthcare and the financial burden of HOM pregnancies on parents are tenfold higher for triplets.[5] Triplet and HOM pregnancies also pose many challenges for the obstetrician in relation to appropriate screening, prenatal care and timing of delivery.

Table 22.1 Incidence (%) of maternal complications in triplet and quadruplet pregnancies[6–9]

	Triplets	Quadruplets
PIH	35	72
PET	23–25	50–67
GDM	7–31	12
Anaemia (Hb < 104 g/L)	37	27–58
PPH (requiring blood transfusion)	9	12

PIH: pregnancy-induced hypertension; PET: preeclampsia; GDM: gestational diabetes mellitus; Hb: haemoglobin; g/L: grams per litre; PPH: post-partum haemorrhage

Table 22.2 Incidence (%) of perinatal complications in triplet and quadruplet pregnancies[1,2,10,11]

	Triplets	Quadruplets
Delivery < 37 weeks	94	98
Delivery < 32 weeks	37	65
Delivery < 28 weeks	8–14	14–30
Average GA at delivery (weeks)	32	30
Average BW (grams)	1,687	1,200
Admission to NICU	64	75
Infant mortality rate (per 1,000 live births)	53	96*

GA: gestational age; BW: birthweight; NICU: neonatal intensive care unit
*Quadruplet and quintuplet data combined

The Issues

Prenatal Care

Triplet and HOM pregnancies should be offered first-trimester ultrasonography to estimate gestational age and importantly, to determine chorionicity and amnionicity. Estimation of gestational age should be from the largest fetus to avoid underestimating gestational age due to the presence of an early growth-restricted fetus. The total number of antenatal visits women with HOM pregnancies require has not been clearly defined and therefore each patient's requirement for antenatal visits should be individualised and managed under the supervision of a specialist obstetrician.

If chorionicity cannot be determined, the pregnancy should be managed as a monochorionic pregnancy until proven otherwise due to the potential adverse effect of chorionicity on perinatal outcome.[12] A systematic review and meta-analysis of nine studies of 1,373 triplet pregnancies (1,062 trichorionic (TC), 261 dichorionic-triamniotic (DCTA) and 50 monochorionic-triamniotic (MCTA)) reported a higher risk of perinatal death (OR 3.3, 95% CI 1.3–8.0) and intrauterine demise (OR 4.6, 95% CI 1.8–11.7) in DCTA compared with TC triplet pregnancies, even when controlling for a difference in gestational age at birth between the two groups (mean difference, 1.1 weeks (95% CI −0.3 to 2.5 weeks), P = 0.12). The incidence of composite morbidity in TC and DCTA triplets was 30% (95% CI 21.1–38.9%) and 34% respectively (95% CI 22–48%), with the risk of neurological morbidity (OR 5.4, 95% CI 1.6–18.3) significantly higher in DCTA compared with TC triplets. Only one study reported on outcomes of MCTA pregnancies and therefore no formal comparison can be made with the other groups.[13]

Prenatal Screening

All women with triplet and HOM pregnancies are candidates for aneuploidy screening, regardless of maternal age. However, several limitations must be considered when screening for aneuploidy in triplet and HOM pregnancies. Serum screening tests are not useful in women with triplet gestations compared with singleton gestations because of the inability to differentiate which feto-placental unit contributed to the overall serum marker level.[1] The use of second-trimester serum screening for trisomy 21 in triplet pregnancies is no longer recommended for the same reason and also because other, more reliable options exist, such as nuchal translucency measurement.[3] While non-invasive prenatal testing (NIPT) using cell-free fetal DNA from the plasma of pregnant women is a useful screening tool for fetal aneuploidy in singleton and twin pregnancies, there are limited data on its use in women with triplet and HOM pregnancies.[1] Owing to the low fetal fraction for each fetus, NIPT for multiple pregnancies is more difficult. There is a greater likelihood of trisomies 21, 18 and 13 in triplet pregnancies and increased false positive rates with screening tests. The size ratio-based approach has been well established in estimating fetal fractions for HOMs. Fetal fraction has a positive correlation with gestational age in triplet pregnancies, and fetal sex can be determined with an accuracy of 97.6%.[14] It should be noted that higher fetal fraction thresholds for HOM must be reached for NIPT to be accurately interpretable, equating to a 9% fetal fraction required for triplet pregnancies and a 12% fetal fraction for quadruplet pregnancies.[15]

Prenatal Diagnosis

Amniocentesis and chorionic villous sampling (CVS) can be performed in women with triplet or HOM pregnancies who desire definitive testing. Amniocentesis and CVS have similar procedure-associated pregnancy loss rates of between 1.0 and 1.8%, which are slightly increased when compared to singleton pregnancies.[1] However, technical difficulties may be encountered when performing amniocentesis and CVS in women with triplet or HOM pregnancies, with a sampling error rate for CVS of approximately 1%. Sampling error can be reduced in triplet pregnancies by using both transabdominal and transcervical approaches in the same patient. The sampling error rate can be reduced with amniocentesis by using indigo carmine. Indigo carmine can be injected into the gestational sac being sampled before removing the needle. When a second needle is then inserted into the second sac the appearance of a clear sample of amniotic fluid can confirm that two separate sacs have been sampled.

Risks with Triplet and Higher-Order Multiple Pregnancies

Miscarriage

The rate of miscarriage increases with HOM pregnancy and approaches 11% for triplet pregnancies. The true rate of miscarriage in HOM pregnancy is unknown as most are not reported.

Medical Complications of Pregnancy

Medical complications of pregnancy are more common in women with triplet and HOM pregnancies than with singleton gestations. Risks include hyperemesis, gestational diabetes mellitus, hypertensive disorders, anaemia, haemorrhage, caesarean delivery and post-partum depression.[1] However, despite these risks, there have been improved maternal and neonatal outcomes in HOM pregnancy over the past two decades.[16] The incidence of hypertensive disorders associated with HOM pregnancy is proportional to the total number of fetuses, with a rate of hypertensive disorders in triplets of up to 35% (Table 22.1), and a higher rate of atypical pre-eclampsia than in singleton pregnancies.[17]

Spontaneous Preterm Birth

Women with triplet and HOM pregnancies have a higher risk of spontaneous preterm birth (PTB) compared to women with a singleton pregnancy, with up to 75% of triplet pregnancies experiencing spontaneous birth before 35 weeks of gestational age. This risk is amplified if other risk factors for preterm birth exist.[12] Fetuses that reach viability carry a significant chance of delivery at an extremely preterm gestational age (< 28 weeks). Triplet pregnancies carry an 8–14% risk of extreme preterm delivery whereas quadruplets carry a risk of up to 30% (Table 22.2). Extreme preterm delivery is associated with significant risks of neonatal morbidity and mortality.

It is not recommended that predictive tests such as fetal fibronectin testing be used to predict the risk of spontaneous PTB in triplet pregnancy. The use of progesterone, pessaries, bed rest, tocolytics and cervical cerclage for the prevention of spontaneous PTB in triplet and HOM pregnancies is not routinely recommended.[1,12] Cervical length measurement assessed in mid-gestation is a poor predictor of PTB at less than 28, 30 and 32 weeks of gestational age, respectively, in asymptomatic triplet pregnancy[18] and there is a limited predictive value for cervical length measurement before 25 + 0 weeks in triplet pregnancy.[19] In symptomatic women the positive predictive value of fetal fibronectin or short cervical length is also poor, and use of these tests is not recommended to direct management in this setting.[1] The lack of utility of such screening tests for spontaneous PTB for triplets or HOMs is likely because such pregnancies are already at such increased risk that the incremental value of an abnormal fibronectin or short cervix is minimal.

Selective Growth Restriction

Antenatal care of patients with HOM pregnancy should occur in a tertiary-level medical institution. Not uncommonly, selective fetal growth restriction can occur with HOM pregnancies. Clinically important indicators of selective growth restriction include an estimated fetal weight (EFW) discordance of 25% or more in TC pregnancies or if the EFW of any of the fetuses is below the 10th centile for gestational age.[12] Additionally, women with DCTA and MCTA triplet pregnancy should be monitored for feto-fetal transfusion syndrome. Twin anaemia-polycythaemia sequence (TAPS) is a complication affecting monochorionic pregnancies and can occur in an MC pair of a triplet or HOM pregnancy. When TAPS occurs the recipient twin develops polycythaemia and the donor twin develops anaemia, but without the polyhydramnios-oligohydramnios sequence observed in feto-fetal transfusion syndrome.[12] Although routine screening for TAPS is not recommended, regular monitoring for all other complications of monochorionicity, which can occur at any gestational age, is important.

Management Options

Expert clinical recommendations suggest that continuing an uncomplicated TC or a DCTA triplet pregnancy beyond 35+6 weeks of pregnancy is associated with an increased risk of fetal demise.[12] Therefore, some experts recommend that planned birth should be offered to uncomplicated TC and DCTA pregnancies at 35 weeks of gestational age. However, in an MCTA triplet pregnancy or a triplet pregnancy that involves a shared amnion, the timing of birth should be individualised in each case.[12] One course of antenatal corticosteroids should be administered to all patients who are between 24 and 34 weeks of gestation, provided that they have an increased risk of delivery within seven days, irrespective of the fetal number.[1] We do not recommend routine prophylactic administration of antenatal corticosteroids at an arbitrary gestational age to all asymptomatic triplet or HOM gestations in the absence of a specific added risk.

The optimal route of delivery for women with triplet pregnancy remains unknown. Although there are no absolute contraindications to vaginal birth, there is limited and very low quality evidence in this area with only retrospective cohort studies identified. Small observational studies have suggested that similar perinatal outcomes can be obtained for women undergoing a planned trial of labour compared with those who undergo a planned caesarean delivery with an uncomplicated triplet pregnancy, provided that the leading triplet is in a vertex presentation.[20,21] There were no differences in adverse maternal or neonatal outcomes by either planned delivery approach.[21] However, although case series of successful vaginal triplet delivery exist, there remains no large prospective studies to demonstrate the safety of this route. Given the practical difficulties involved in accurately monitoring each fetus with confidence in a triplet or HOM gestation throughout labour and delivery, caesarean section is the favoured mode of delivery in most centres. The optimal type of uterine incision has not been established.

Multifetal Pregnancy Reduction (MFPR)

In the first trimester a substantial number of women with HOM pregnancies undergo spontaneous reduction of one or more fetuses, commonly referred to as the 'vanishing twin'. The probability of this spontaneous reduction increases with the number of gestational sacs with a rate of 53% for triplets and 65% for quadruplets. In the second and third trimesters up to 17% of triplets experience intrauterine demise of one or more fetuses.[1]

Multifetal reduction is the practice of reducing the number of fetuses in a multifetal pregnancy. This topic is explored in detail in Chapter 4. The aim is to reduce the chances of preterm delivery and to improve the outcome for the remaining fetuses. The fetus or fetuses that are technically easiest to access are generally chosen for MFPR provided no obvious abnormalities are identified in the other remaining fetuses, such as an increased nuchal translucency. Aneuploidy testing can be performed before the reduction to assist patients in making decisions about interventions. Aneuploidy testing is recommended for the fetus(es) being retained so as to avoid the chance of retaining a genetically abnormal fetus. If there is a monochorionic pair within an HOM gestation, it is recommended that both fetuses in the MC pair are reduced, given the associated negative effects on the development of the remaining twin of an MC pair if only one is reduced.

In TC pregnancies, a meta-analysis has demonstrated that fetal reduction to twins was associated with a lower risk (17% versus 50%) of preterm birth before 34 weeks of gestational age (RR = 0.36, 95% CI 0.28–0.48), without a concomitant increase in the risk of miscarriage (8.1% vs 7.4%) (RR = 1.08, 95% CI 0.58–1.98). Expectant management of DCTA triplet pregnancies demonstrated rates of miscarriage and preterm birth of approximately 9% and 52%, respectively. While this meta-analysis was inconclusive, it did suggest that in a DCTA triplet pregnancy, fetal reduction to twins was possibly associated with a lower risk of preterm birth without an increased risk of miscarriage.[22]

A Cochrane review concluded that women who underwent pregnancy reduction from triplets to twins compared with those who continued with expectant management of a triplet pregnancy had lower frequencies of pregnancy loss, antenatal complications, preterm birth, low-birthweight infants, caesarean delivery and neonatal deaths. Post MFPR, the pregnancy outcomes were similar to those observed in women with spontaneously conceived twin gestations.[23]

Counselling patients in relation to MFPR, especially for couples who may have undertaken extensive fertility treatments to become pregnant in the first instance, can be challenging. Conveying the specific risks of a multifetal pregnancy to patients who are concerned that they may never have a child can be difficult. A multidisciplinary team approach should be adopted to support patients during their decision-making. The multidisciplinary team may include mental health professionals, social workers, neonatologists and obstetricians.

Fertility treatment and ART have contributed significantly to the numbers of multifetal pregnancies. Multifetal pregnancy reduction should not be a solution for the negative consequences of HOM pregnancies. A recent analysis of 15 years of European IVF Monitoring (EIM) Consortium activity demonstrated that the initial aims of the programme were met. These included collection and publication of regional European data on census and trends on ART utilisation, effectiveness, safety and quality. Over that period the number of triplet deliveries was reduced from 3.7% in 1997 to 0.6% in 2011 and clear trends towards transferring fewer embryos were observed.[24] The proportion of countries with a compulsory register increased over the 15 years and continued regulation in this area is crucial to reduce the number of HOM pregnancies. Appropriate standards of practice in ART and fertility treatment should be enforced to reduce the occurrence of multifetal pregnancy and the need for MFPR.

Key Points

- Triplet and higher-order multiple (HOM) pregnancies carry significant maternal and fetal risks. Women should be counselled regarding the possible complications of HOM pregnancy and offered close antenatal surveillance for such complications.
- Fetal risks in HOM pregnancy relate mainly to prematurity and intrauterine growth restriction. Monochorionicity in HOM pregnancy poses additional risks of feto-fetal transfusion syndrome or reversed arterial perfusion sequence.
- There remains limited guidance on appropriate surveillance and management of HOM pregnancies with many guidelines suggesting an individualised approach in relation to timing and mode of delivery.
- Challenges in relation to prenatal screening, sonographic assessment of growth and well-being and fetal monitoring increase with increasing fetal number.
- Multifetal pregnancy reduction (MFPR) to twins should be discussed with patients with HOM pregnancies (≥ 3). If selected, this should be performed in a specialist fetal medicine centre.

- Multifetal pregnancy reduction should not be considered as a solution for the complications and adverse outcomes of HOM pregnancies. Instead, primary prevention strategies should be followed in fertility clinics to reduce the need for MFPR.
- Long-term neurodevelopmental follow-up of survivors of HOM pregnancies, including those managed expectantly and those who have undergone MFPR, is required.

References

1. Committee on Practice B-O. Society for Maternal-Fetal M. Practice Bulletin No. 169: multifetal gestations: twin, triplet, and higher-order multifetal pregnancies. Obstet Gynecol 2016;**128**(4):e131–e146.

2. Multiple gestation associated with infertility therapy: an American Society for Reproductive Medicine Practice Committee opinion.Fertil Steril 2012;**97**(4):825–34.

3. Shah JS, Roman T, Viteri OA, Haidar ZA, Ontiveros A, Sibai BM. The relationship of assisted reproductive technology on perinatal outcomes in triplet gestations. Am J Perinatol 2018;**35**(14):1388–93.

4. Badreldin N, Peress DA, Yee LM, Battarbee AN. Neonatal outcomes of triplet pregnancies conceived via in vitro fertilization versus other methods of conception. Am J Perinatol 2021;**38**(8):810–15.

5. Collins J. Cost efficiency of reducing multiple births. Reprod Biomed Online 2007;**15**(suppl 3):35–9.

6. Malone FD, Kaufman GE, Chelmow D, Athanassiou A, Nores JA, D'Alton ME. Maternal morbidity associated with triplet pregnancy. Am J Perinatol 1998;**15**(1):73–7.

7. Ombelet W, De Sutter P, Van der Elst J, Martens G. Multiple gestation and infertility treatment: registration, reflection and reaction – the Belgian project. *Hum Reprod* 2005;**11**(1):3–14.

8. Chibber R, Fouda M, Shishtawy W et al. Maternal and neonatal outcome in triplet, quadruplet and quintuplet gestations following ART: a 11-year study. Arch Gynecol Obstet 2013;**288**(4):759–67.

9. Elliott JP. High-order multiple gestations. *Semin Perinatol* 2005;**29**(5):305–11.

10. Devine PC, Malone FD, Athanassiou A, Harvey-Wilkes K, D'Alton ME. Maternal and neonatal outcome of 100 consecutive triplet pregnancies. Am J Perinatol 2001;**18**(4):225–35.

11. Seoud MAF, Toner JP, Kruithoff C, Muasher SJ. Outcome of twin, triplet, and quadruplet in vitro fertilization pregnancies: the Norfolk experience. Presented in part at the 7th World Congress of IVF and Assisted Procreation, Paris, France, June 28 to July 3, 1991; and the 47th Annual Meeting of The American Fertility Society, Orlando, Florida, October 18 to 25, 1991. *Fertil Steril* 1992;**57**(4):825–34.

12. National Institute for Health and Care Excellence. Twin and Triplet Pregnancy. National Institute for Health and Care Excellence: Clinical Guidelines. London: National Institute for Health and Care Excellence, 2019.

13. Curado J, D'Antonio F, Papageorghiou AT, Bhide A, Thilaganathan B, Khalil A. Perinatal mortality and morbidity in triplet pregnancy according to chorionicity: systematic review and meta-analysis. Ultrasound Obstet Gynecol 2019;**54**(5):589–95.

14. Chen M, Jiang F, Guo Y et al. Validation of fetal DNA fraction estimation and its application in noninvasive prenatal testing for aneuploidy detection in multiple pregnancies. Prenat Diagn 2019;**39**(13):1273–82.

15. Chen M, Jiang F, Guo Y, Yan H, Wang J, Zhang L, et al. Validation of fetal DNA fraction estimation and its application in noninvasive prenatal testing for aneuploidy detection in multiple pregnancies. Prenatal Diagnosis. 2019;**39**(13):1273–82.

16. Kyeong KS, Shim JY, Oh SY et al. How much have the perinatal outcomes of triplet pregnancies improved over the last two decades? Obstet Gynecol Sci 2019;62 (4):224–32.

17. Hardardottir H, Kelly K, Bork MD, Cusick W, Campbell WA, Rodis JF. Atypical presentation of preeclampsia in high-order multifetal gestations. Obstet Gynecol 1996;87(3):370–4.

18. Fichera A, Pagani G, Stagnati V et al. Cervical-length measurement in mid-gestation to predict spontaneous preterm birth in asymptomatic triplet pregnancy. Ultrasound Obstet Gynecol 2018;51(5):614–20.

19. Rosen H, Hiersch L, Freeman H, Barrett J, Melamed N. The role of serial measurements of cervical length in asymptomatic women with triplet pregnancy. J Matern Fetal Neonatal Med 2018;31(6):713–19.

20. Mol BW, Bergenhenegouwen L, Velzel J et al. Perinatal outcomes according to the mode of delivery in women with a triplet pregnancy in the Netherlands. J Matern Fetal Neonatal Med 2019;32(22):3771–7.

21. Peress D, Dude A, Peaceman A, Yee LM. Maternal and neonatal outcomes in triplet gestations by trial of labor versus planned cesarean delivery. J Matern Fetal Neonatal Med 2019;32(11):1874–9.

22. Anthoulakis C, Dagklis T, Mamopoulos A, Athanasiadis A. Risks of miscarriage or preterm delivery in trichorionic and dichorionic triplet pregnancies with embryo reduction versus expectant management: a systematic review and meta-analysis. Hum Reprod 2017;32 (6):1351–9.

23. Dodd JM, Dowswell T, Crowther CA. Reduction of the number of fetuses for women with a multiple pregnancy. Cochrane Database Syst Rev. 2015(11): CD003932.

24. Ferraretti AP, Nygren K, Andersen AN et al. Trends over 15 years in ART in Europe: an analysis of 6 million cycles†. Human Reproduction Open 2017;2017(2). https://doi.org/10.1093/hropen/hox012

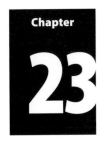

Chapter

23

Timing of Delivery in Multiple Pregnancy

Laure Noël and Basky Thilaganathan

The Facts

Importance of Dating the Pregnancy and Determining the Chorionicity

Accurate evaluation of gestational age in early pregnancy is mandatory to effect timely elective birth in both singleton and multiple pregnancies. Recommendations on the planning of delivery in multiple pregnancies also differ based on the chorionicity. The assessment of both gestational age and chorionicity are optimally carried out by ultrasound in the first trimester.[1] For in vitro fertilisation (IVF) gestations, the oocyte retrieval date or the embryonic age from fertilisation should be used to date the pregnancy.[2]

Stillbirth Rate versus Risk of Stillbirth

Twin pregnancies are known to be at increased risk of stillbirth compared to singleton pregnancies. In a retrospective study of more than 46,000 singleton and 1,500 twin pregnancies, the stillbirth rate per fetus was fivefold higher in twin (24.8/1,000 births) compared to singleton (4.6/1,000 births) pregnancies.[3] This study also demonstrated the relevance of chorionicity, as the stillbirth rates differed greatly between dichorionic-diamniotic (DCDA) and monochorionic-diamniotic (MCDA) twins at 10.8 and 58.3 per 1,000 ongoing pregnancies, respectively. However, gestation-specific by week rather than population data on stillbirth and neonatal mortality risks in multiple pregnancy are needed for clinical decisions regarding timing of birth. Here, most studies have incorrectly assumed that the stillbirth rate (fetal deaths per 1,000 total births) reflects the risk of stillbirth. Stillbirth can only occur before delivery, and therefore the risk of stillbirth is only accurately represented as a proportion of ongoing pregnancies at risk of stillbirth rather than as a stillbirth rate per 1,000 total births. When stillbirth risk is presented with the correct denominator of ongoing pregnancies, a progressive increase in this risk with advancing gestational age is evident, with this being more pronounced beyond 34 weeks of gestation (Figure 23.1).[4] Due to the higher risk of stillbirth, twin pregnancies are commonly subject to physician-scheduled elective early-term birth with a worrying trend of elective preterm in monochorionic twins due to a perceived increased risk of stillbirth and subsequent demise or severe morbidity in the co-twin.

Neonatal Mortality Rate versus Risk of Neonatal Mortality

In contrast to the risk of stillbirth, the risk of neonatal complications and subsequent death decreases with advancing gestational age and increased fetal maturity. Early recommendations pertaining to timing of birth in twins only considered stillbirth risk and did not

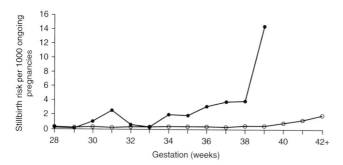

Figure 23.1 Gestation-specific risk of stillbirth per 1,000 ongoing fetuses in singletons (open circles) and twins (closed circles). Adapted from Sairam et al.[4]

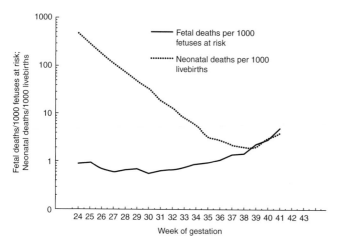

Figure 23.2 Prospective risk of stillbirth (per 1,000 ongoing gestations) and neonatal death (per 1,000 live births) in twin pregnancies. Adapted from Kahn et al.[5]

account for the higher risk of neonatal complications due to iatrogenic preterm or early-term birth. However, more recent data from large epidemiological datasets have compared the risk of stillbirth to the neonatal mortality rate with advancing gestation (Figure 23.2).[5] Neonatal mortality can only occur after birth, so one may be excused for assuming that the neonatal mortality rate expressed per 1,000 live births accurately reflects the risk of neonatal mortality at any given gestation – in contrast to the stillbirth rate versus risk. However, neonatal mortality rate data do not account for the probability of birth at any given gestation, which differs significantly in multiple gestations compared to singleton pregnancies (Figure 23.3).[6] So the accurate assessment of neonatal mortality risk needs to include the probability of birth followed by death for every week of gestation.

The Issues

Dichorionic and Monochorionic Twin Pregnancies

The optimal time for birth in uncomplicated twin pregnancies is not well established given the need to assess the prospective risk of stillbirth, the likelihood of birth and the risk of neonatal mortality for each week of gestation. The optimal timing of delivery should be

LIVE BIRTHS

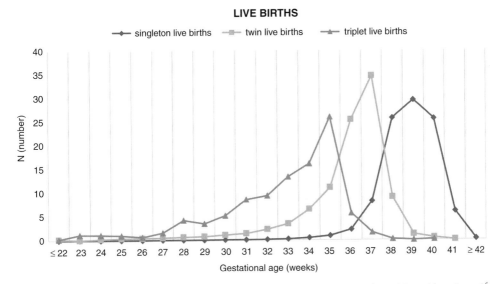

Figure 23.3 The overall distributions of singleton, twin and triplet births by gestational age. Adapted from Ko et al.[6]

based on the gestational age associated with the lowest risk of perinatal death. The assessment of the risk of stillbirth is complicated by the rarity of stillbirth, the need for very large population data sets, the lack of information on chorionicity, the inclusion of complicated pregnancies and the influence of antenatal monitoring protocols resulting in intervention bias. The latter have resulted in discrepancies between study findings and lack of generalisability of the data. As such, institutional and national recommendations for timing of birth vary between countries, from 37 to 39+6 weeks for DCDA twins, from 34 to 38+6 weeks for MCDA twins and from 32 to 35+6 weeks for monochorionic-monoamniotic (MOMO) twins (Table 23.1).

A recent individual patient data meta-analysis of 32 studies including more than 25,000 uncomplicated twin pregnancies evaluated prospective risk of stillbirth and risk of spontaneous preterm birth followed by neonatal mortality for each week beyond 34 weeks of gestation – when scheduled birth would typically be considered. The difference between risk of stillbirth and risk of neonatal death was computed to assess the benefit of expectant management versus scheduled delivery for each week of gestation (Table 23.2, Figure 23.4).[7] In dichorionic twin pregnancies, the balance of risks favoured expectant management until 37 weeks of gestation. After 37 weeks, the risk of stillbirth was significantly higher than the risk of neonatal death with a risk difference above zero (Figure 23.4a). These results support the need for scheduled birth from 37 weeks in uncomplicated dichorionic twin pregnancies to optimise fetal/neonatal outcome. In monochorionic twin pregnancies, a similar trend towards a higher risk of stillbirth was seen after 36 weeks, but this did not reach statistical significance, indicating that there is no need for elective birth before 36 weeks of gestation as has been common practice (Figure 23.4b).[7]

Table 23.1 Recommendations from various national and international guidelines for timing of birth in uncomplicated multiple pregnancies according to the number of fetuses, the chorionicity and the amnionicity

	Twins			Triplets
	Dichorionic-diamniotic	Monochorionic-diamniotic	Monochorionic-monoamniotic	
NICE (2019)	At 37 weeks	At 36 weeks	Between 32 and 33+6 weeks	At 35 weeks*
ISUOG (2016)	At 37 weeks	At 36 weeks	Between 32 and 34 weeks	-
ACOG (2019)	At 38 weeks	Between 34 and 37+6 weeks	Between 32 and 34 weeks	-
RANZCOG (2017)	-	Maximum 37 weeks	-	-
CNGOF (2009)	Between 38 and 39+6 weeks	Between 36 and 38+6 weeks	Between 32 and 35+6 weeks	-
GGOLFB (2017)	Maximum 38 weeks	Maximum 36–37 weeks	Between 32 and 34 weeks	-

* For trichorionic-triamniotic or dichorionic-triamniotic triplets
NICE: National Institute for Health and Care Excellence (UK); ISUOG: International Society of Ultrasound in Obstetrics and Gynecology; ACOG: American College of Obstetricians and Gynecologists; RANZCOG: Royal Australian and New Zealand College of Obstetricians and Gynecologists; SOGC: Society of Obstetricians and Gynaecologists of Canada; CNGOF: Collège National des Gynécologues et Obstétriciens Français; GGOLFB: Groupement des Gynécologues Obstétriciens de Langue Française de Belgique

Monochorionic-Monoamniotic Pregnancies

The rarity of MOMO twin pregnancies has resulted in a paucity of evidence on the optimal timing of birth based on risks of stillbirth and neonatal death. Perinatal mortality rates in MOMO pregnancies range between 10% and 40%, due to congenital anomalies, conjoined twinning, twin-reversed arterial perfusion (TRAP) sequence and large placental anastomoses predisposing to acute inter-twin transfusion.[8] A previous review on perinatal outcome in MOMO twin pregnancies (n = 133) showed an overall perinatal mortality rate of 23.3% with a significant rise in perinatal deaths after 32 weeks of gestation.[9] These results have been used to justify a policy of elective preterm delivery in uncomplicated MOMO twins.

In a multicentre cohort study of 193 non-anomalous MOMO twin pregnancies, the prospective risk of fetal demise decreased from 16% at 11 weeks to a minimum of 1% at 28 weeks before rising to 5% at 32–34 weeks (Figure 23.5).[8] However, no intrauterine fetal death was recorded in the 23 pregnancies that continued beyond 34 weeks. After 34 weeks, there was a dramatic drop in the overall risk of neonatal complications, including respiratory distress syndrome (Figure 23.5). The risks of fetal intrauterine death and non-respiratory neonatal complications were balanced at 32+4 weeks. The authors suggested that scheduled birth from 33 weeks of gestation was thus associated with the best fetal

Table 23.2 Prospective risks of stillbirth and neonatal death per week in singleton, dichorionic and mono-chorionic twin pregnancies from 34 weeks of gestation from individual patient data meta-analyses. Adapted from Muglu et al.[11] and Cheong-See et al.[7] Data are shown as risk per 1,000 ongoing pregnancies (stillbirths) or live births (neonatal deaths) with 95% confidence intervals in parentheses.

Gestational age (weeks)	Singleton (n = 15,124,027)	Dichorionic twins (n = 29,685)	Monochorionic twins (n = 5,486)
Stillbirth risk (per 1,000 ongoing pregnancies)			
34+0–34+6	-	1.2 (0.7 to 1.8)	0.9 (0.1 to 3.4)
35+0–35+6	-	0.8 (0.4 to 1.4)	2.8 (0.9 to 6.5)
36+0–36+6	-	1.5 (0.9 to 2.4)	4.5 (1.7 to 9.8)
37+0–37+6	0.4 (0.3–0.5)	3.4 (2.1 to 5.1)	9.6 (3.9 to 19.7)
38+0–38+6	0.5 (0.4–0.6)	10.6 (7.1 to 15.3)	7.6 (0.9 to 27.1)
39+0–39+6	0.7 (0.6–0.8)	9.3 (3.8 to 19.1)	-
40+0–40+6	1.1 (0.9–1.3)	-	-
Neonatal death risk (per 1,000 live births)			
34+0–34+6	-	6.7 (3.3 to 13.5)	12.1 (4.2 to 34.3)
35+0–35+6	-	4.6 (2.4 to 8.7)	8.1 (3.4 to 19.3)
36+0–36+6	-	3.2 (1.7 to 5.9)	5.4 (2.2 to 13.3)
37+0–37+6	0.9 (0.5–1.7)	2.2 (1.1 to 4.3)	3.6 (1.2 to 11.1)
38+0–38+6	0.4 (0.1–1.4)	1.5 (0.7 to 3.3)	2.4 (0.6 to 10.3)
39+0–39+6	0.4 (0.2–0.7)	1.1 (0.4 to 2.6)	-
40+0–40+6	0.4 (0.2–0.7)	-	-

outcome. Notably, the rate of intrauterine fetal deaths was not different between women managed as inpatients or outpatients. More recently, a systematic review of 25 studies including 1,628 non-anomalous MOMO twins after 24 weeks of gestation demonstrated rates of single and double intrauterine deaths of 2.5% and 3.8%, respectively. Of intrauterine fetal deaths, 4.3% occurred before 30 weeks, 1.0% at 31–32 weeks and 2.2% at 33–34 weeks. No intrauterine fetal death was recorded from 35 weeks of gestation.[10] The rates of neonatal death were 2.5% and 0.6% before 30 weeks and at 31–32 weeks, respectively, whereas no neonatal death was recorded from 32 weeks of gestation.

Triplet and Higher-Order Pregnancies

Evidence for timing of delivery in triplet and higher-order pregnancies is even more scarce. The National Institute for Health and Care Excellence (NICE) in the UK recommends elective delivery at 35 weeks for trichorionic-triamniotic and dichorionic-triamniotic triplets. Individual assessment is proposed for other triplets and higher-order multiples.

Management Options

The International Society of Ultrasound in Obstetrics and Gynecology (ISUOG) published up-to-date guidance on the management of twin pregnancies in 2016.[2] For uncomplicated

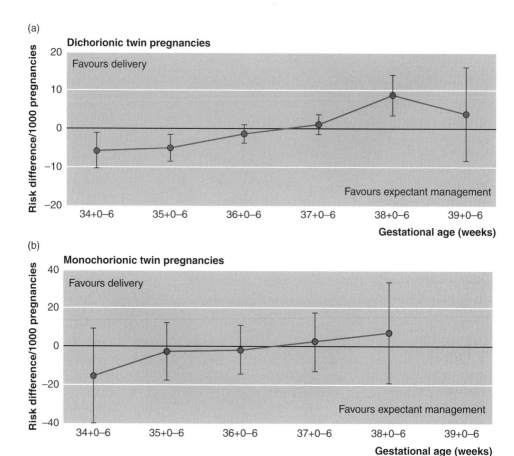

Figure 23.4 Risk difference between the prospective risk of stillbirth from expectant management and the risk of neonatal death from delivery at weekly intervals from 34 weeks of gestation in uncomplicated dichorionic (a) and monochorionic (b) twin pregnancies. Adapted from Cheong-See et al.[7]

DCDA pregnancies, ultrasound assessments are recommended in the first trimester, at around 20 weeks of gestation and then every four weeks. As long as ultrasound fetal biometry, amniotic fluid volume and umbilical artery Doppler indices remain in the normal range, scheduled birth is recommended from 37 weeks of gestation. For uncomplicated MCDA pregnancies, the ISUOG recommends ultrasound assessments in the first trimester and then every two weeks from 16 weeks onwards. At each ultrasound scan, fetal biometry, amniotic fluid volume, umbilical artery Doppler PI and middle cerebral artery peak systolic velocity should be documented. In uncomplicated MCDA pregnancies, planned delivery is recommended from 36 weeks. The management of MOMO pregnancies should take place in tertiary centres with planned delivery by caesarean section at 32–34 weeks – even though more recent evidence supports birth from 33 weeks of gestation. The antenatal surveillance strategy for uncomplicated MOMO twin pregnancies proposed by the ISUOG is similar to that of uncomplicated MCDA twin pregnancies.

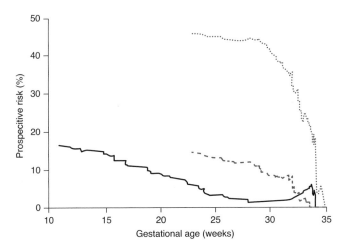

Figure 23.5 Prospective risk of stillbirth and non-respiratory neonatal complications per gestational age in 386 fetuses and 282 live-born neonates from monoamniotic twin pregnancies without major anomalies, respectively. Full bold line: risk of stillbirth. Dashed green line: risk of non-respiratory neonatal complications. Dotted red line: risk of non-respiratory neonatal complications or respiratory distress syndrome. Adapted from Van Mieghem et al.[8]

Key Points

- An accurate evaluation of the due date and the chorionicity during the first trimester is mandatory to plan further scheduled delivery.
- Multiple pregnancies are at increased risks of neonatal deaths due to spontaneous or elective preterm delivery.
- The risk of stillbirth per ongoing pregnancies increases with advancing gestational age, whereas the risk of neonatal death per live birth decreases.
- The optimal timing of delivery should be based on the risk difference between the prospective risk of stillbirth per ongoing pregnancies and the prospective risk of neonatal death at each gestational age.
- Offer planned delivery from 37 weeks for uncomplicated DCDA twin pregnancies.
- Offer planned delivery from 36 weeks for uncomplicated MCDA twin pregnancies.
- Offer planned caesarean section at 32–34 weeks for uncomplicated MOMO twin pregnancies.
- Offer planned caesarean section from 35 weeks for uncomplicated trichorionic-triamniotic and dichorionic-triamniotic triplets.

References

1. D'Antonio F, Bhide A. Early pregnancy assessment in multiple pregnancies. Best Pract Res Clin Obstet Gynaecol 2014;**28** (2):201–14.

2. Khalil A, Rodgers M, Baschat A et al. ISUOG Practice Guidelines: role of ultrasound in twin pregnancy. Ultrasound Obstet Gynecol 2016;**47**(2):247–63.

3. Russo FM et al. Stillbirths in singletons, dichorionic and monochorionic twins: a comparison of risks and causes. Eur J Obstet Gynecol Reprod Biol 2013;**170**(1):131–6.

4. Sairam S, Costeloe K, Thilaganathan B. Prospective risk of stillbirth in multiple-gestation pregnancies: a population-based analysis. Obstet Gynecol 2002;**100**(4):638–41.

5. Kahn B et al. Prospective risk of fetal death in singleton, twin, and triplet gestations: implications for practice. Obstet Gynecol 2003;**102**(4):685–92.

6. Ko HS et al. Multiple birth rates of Korea and fetal/neonatal/infant mortality in multiple gestation. PLoS One 2018;**13**(8):e0202318.

7. Cheong-See F et al. Prospective risk of stillbirth and neonatal complications in twin pregnancies: systematic review and meta-analysis. BMJ 2016;**354**:i4353.

8. Van Mieghem T et al. Prenatal management of monoamniotic twin pregnancies. Obstet Gynecol 2014;**124**(3):498–506.

9. Roque H et al. Perinatal outcomes in monoamniotic gestations. J Matern Fetal Neonatal Med 2003;**13**(6):414–21.

10. D'Antonio F et al. Perinatal mortality, timing of delivery and prenatal management of monoamniotic twin pregnancy: systematic review and meta-analysis. Ultrasound Obstet Gynecol 2019;**53**(2):166–74.

11. Muglu J et al. Risks of stillbirth and neonatal death with advancing gestation at term: a systematic review and meta-analysis of cohort studies of 15 million pregnancies. PLoS Med 2019;**16**(7)e1002838.

Mode of Delivery in Multiple Pregnancy

Amir Aviram, Jon F. R. Barret, Elad Mei-Dan and Nir Melamed

The Facts

Multiple pregnancies carry a higher risk of adverse perinatal outcomes compared with singleton gestations, mainly attributed to preterm delivery and low birthweight. Yet these are not the only perils awaiting twins. During delivery, apart from the usual indications for caesarean delivery (CD) in singleton pregnancy, delivery of the second twin may be complicated by an unexpected change in lie and presenting part, abruptio placenta following the rapid decompression of the uterus after the delivery of the first twin, prolapsed umbilical cord, changes in cervical dilatation and more. All of these may lead to a unique mode of delivery – combined delivery – in which twin A is delivered vaginally and twin B is delivered by a CD.

As such, a twin delivery remains one of the most challenging events in the daily practice of obstetricians. The perennial dilemmas that apply to any singleton delivery, such as intrapartum monitoring and operative interventions, are compounded by the presence of the second fetus. In this chapter we review the evidence concerning mode of delivery in twin gestations and address specific clinical scenarios that are often encountered in daily practice. We also briefly address triplet and higher-order pregnancies, albeit that the evidence base in this regard is limited.

The literature regarding mode of delivery in twins was limited to observational and retrospective cohort studies until the publication of the Twin Birth Study (TBS) in 2013.[1] Prior to that only one small-scale randomised controlled trial (RCT) was performed.[2] This RCT aimed to assess the management of a non-vertex twin B. Sixty women carrying twins (in all of whom twin A was cephalic and twin B was non-cephalic) were randomised to planned vaginal delivery (VD) versus planned CD. There were no significant differences between the groups in Apgar scores, birth trauma, neonatal morbidity or mortality. Yet maternal febrile morbidity was significantly higher in the CD group.

As mentioned previously, all other studies were mainly observational or retrospective in nature. A systematic review and meta-analysis published in 2011 included retrospective observational manuscripts published in the first decade of the millennium. Their results showed that while as a general rule the rate of neonatal morbidity of twin A is lower than that of twin B, it is not associated with mode of delivery or presentation of twin B. They also reported lower rates of neonatal morbidity of twin A in VD as compared with CD.[3]

In an effort to reconcile different results from different studies, the TBS, a multinational, multicentre, randomised, controlled trial, was initiated in 2003.[1] In the TBS, patients were eligible for recruitment between 32^{+0} and 38^{+6} weeks of gestation if the first twin was in the cephalic presentation and both fetuses were alive with an estimated weight between

1,500 g and 4,000 g. Exclusion criteria were monoamniotic twins, fetal reduction at 13 or more weeks of gestation, lethal fetal anomaly and contraindication to labour or VD (such as fetal compromise, twin B substantially larger than twin A, two or more previous CDs or vertical uterine incision, etc.). Women were randomised to planned VD or planned CD and delivery was planned between 37+5 and 38+6 weeks of gestation. Mothers and infants were followed up to 28 days after delivery. The primary outcome was a composite of neonatal adverse outcomes, and a composite maternal outcome was also defined.[1] Overall, data were available for a total of 1,392 women in each arm, 2,783 fetuses/infants in the planned CD arm and 2,782 fetuses/infants in the planned VD arm. Approximately 90% of women assigned to the planned CD arm had a CD, 9% had a VD of both twins and 1% had a combined delivery. In the planned VD arm, 56% patients had a VD, 40% had a CD for both twins and 4% had a combined delivery. Of this cohort approximately 75% had dichorionic-diamniotic (DCDA) and the rest had monochorionic-diamniotic (MCDA) twins.

No differences in the primary composite neonatal outcome or the composite maternal outcome were found between the groups. These results did not change in the pre-specified subgroup analyses according to parity, gestational age at randomisation, maternal age, presentation of twin B, chorionicity or the national perinatal mortality rate of the mother's country of residence. It was found, however, that the second twin was more likely than the first twin to have the primary outcome.[1] The authors of the study concluded that planned CD was not associated with better neonatal or maternal outcomes than planned VD.

While this study was the first (and will likely be the only comprehensive, large-scale RCT regarding mode of delivery in twin pregnancies), it leaves several questions unanswered. Among these questions is the significance of a weight discrepancy between the twins, the level of expertise deemed necessary of those managing multiple pregnancy births, VD of twins at less than the specified gestational age and women with previous CDs.

Interestingly, a secondary analysis of the results has shown that for pregnancies between 32+0 and 36+6 weeks of gestation, a planned VD was associated with fewer adverse outcomes compared to planned CD (OR 0.62, 95% CI 0.37–1.03). Nonetheless, at gestational ages of 37+0 weeks and above, the rate of composite perinatal outcome was 2% in the planned VD arm versus 1% in the planned CD arm (OR 2.25, 95% CI 1.06–4.77). While this may look as though CD may be favourable, we must remember that most twins are delivered well before 38 weeks. The authors of this secondary analysis concluded that 'the absolute risks at term are low and must be weighed against the increased maternal risks associated with planned CD'.[4]

Following the publication of the TBS, several sub-analyses were performed. While not sufficiently powered, they still shed light on several important questions, using the only large-scale, prospective study performed in this area. For example, a sub-analysis sought to explore the differences between planned VD and planned CD for women in the TBS cohort who presented in spontaneous labour, and concluded that in women with twins who present in spontaneous labour, planned VD compared with CD was not associated with significant differences in neonatal or maternal outcomes.[5] The same group also explored the practice of induction of labour in twin pregnancies and concluded that the need for cervical ripening by prostaglandin had no effect on the incidence of CD or adverse outcome in women with twins requiring labour induction.[6]

Neonatal outcomes at two years of age were also assessed in the TBS cohort. Overall, 4,603 children from the initial cohort of 5,565 infants (83%) were included in the study. The authors found no significant difference in the outcome of death or neurodevelopmental delay (OR 1.04, 95% CI 0.77–1.41) and concluded that planned CD had no added benefit to children at two years of age compared with planned VD in patients with characteristics similar to the TBS cohort.[7] A further paper explored whether maternal outcomes two years after delivery, such as urinary stress or faecal or flatus incontinence, were affected by planned mode of delivery in twins and found that women in the planned CD group were less likely to experience urinary stress incontinence compared with their VD group counterparts (OR 0.63, 95% CI 0.47–0.83), with no reported difference in the quality of life. No differences were found in faecal or flatus incontinence or in other maternal outcomes.[8]

Several years after the publication of the TBS, these results were further validated by the JUmeaux MODe d'Accouchement (JUMODA), a national prospective population-based cohort study in 176 maternity units in France.[9] The inclusion criteria were quite similar to those of the TBS. More than 5,900 women and their neonates were eligible for analysis, of whom roughly 25% had a CD. The authors found that the composite neonatal mortality and morbidity was increased in the planned CD arm (5.2% versus 2.2%, OR 2.38, 95% CI 1.86–2.05), but this difference was relevant only to those twins delivered prior to 37 weeks of gestation.

The Issues

Delivery of the Non-cephalic Second Twin

As mentioned earlier in this chapter, in uncomplicated DCDA or MCDA twin pregnancies after 32 weeks of gestation, if twin A is in cephalic presentation, regardless of the presentation of twin B, no differences were found in the TBS between planned VD and planned CD. Yet the delivery of twin B is at times not straightforward, especially in the era of the Term Breech Trial when manual expertise of breech deliveries declined significantly.[10] The main dilemma surrounds the optimal management of the non-cephalic twin B – whether an external cephalic version (ECV) should be attempted or whether total breech extraction should be preferred.

Several authors tried to assess the confidence level of trainees in obstetrics in VDs of twins. In one of the studies, out of a total of 417 residents only a third felt confident managing the breech second twin and 28% did not feel comfortable managing the breech second twin post-residency.[11] The solution to training gaps might be simulations, yet further studies are needed in order to determine the optimal training method for managing the second breech twin.

In 1983, a small study advocated ECV of the second non-vertex twin after delivery of the first twin in order to achieve delivery of the second twin in a vertex presentation.[12] The ECV was successful in 18/25 (72%) sets of twins after successful delivery of the first vertex twin and was not associated with increased perinatal complications.[12] Subsequent to this, other investigators published similar findings. Others, however, have reported a significantly higher incidence of VD with breech extraction (with or without internal podalic version) compared with ECV for the second non-vertex twin. Because of failed ECV or other complications, CD occurred more frequently if ECV was attempted rather than breech extraction. The TBS confirmed this observation with a 95% success rate in patients delivered by breech extraction versus 42% when ECV was attempted, and it therefore now seems conclusive that breech extraction is the optimal procedure for the non-vertex second twin.[1]

Interestingly, some have advocated that total breech extraction may even show better results than delivery of the a priori vertex twin B.

Combined Delivery

The unique entity of combined delivery should also be addressed. Several authors have published their findings through the years regarding risk factors for CD of the second twin following VD of the first. According to past reports, the rate of combined delivery is 5–10%. Most of these findings come from small-sized, retrospective studies which showed that malpresentation of the second twin is associated with higher rates of combined delivery. Combined deliveries were also associated with a higher incidence of maternal and neonatal infectious morbidity.

Recently a sub-analysis of the TBS concerning combined deliveries was published.[13] Of 842 cases where the first twin was delivered vaginally, 59 (7%) had CD for the second twin. The rate of non-cephalic presentation of twin B was more than twofold higher in the combined delivery group and the likelihood of spontaneous version of twin B (a different presentation at delivery compared to the presentation at randomisation) was also higher in the combined delivery group. In a multivariable regression model, breech presentation was not significantly associated with combined delivery (aOR 0.99, 95% CI 0.36–2.67), in contrast to transverse/oblique lie (aOR 43.74, 95% CI 15.37–124.49). Combined deliveries were more likely to be associated with fetal/neonatal death or serious neonatal morbidity (13.6% vs 2.3%, p < 0.001), five-minutes Apgar score < 7, NICU admissions, abnormal level of consciousness and prolonged ($\geq$ 24 hours) assisted ventilation. Combined delivery was also associated with fetal/neonatal death or serious neonatal morbidity (aOR 5.14, 95% CI 1.95–13.53). The authors conclude that the data can be used for counselling couples who consider trial of labour and imply that training, probably including simulation, may prove beneficial for those practising vaginal twin births.

Time Interval between Delivery of Twins

It was previously believed that the time interval between the deliveries of twins should be no longer than 30 minutes, as a prolonged interval placed the second twin at risk of asphyxia from decreased placental circulation, as well as decreased likelihood of VD. In the TBS the mean inter-twin delivery interval was 8 minutes with a range of 1 to 33 minutes.[1]

Recent studies report conflicting results. For example, one study which examined the effect of inter-twin delivery interval on neonatal outcome found that in cases where both twins were delivered vaginally (n = 151), there was no significant correlation between the inter-twin delivery interval and umbilical cord arterial pH or Apgar scores at 1, 5 and 10 minutes of twin B.[14] Another study which examined the association between inter-twin delivery interval and short-term perinatal outcomes found that a composite adverse neonatal outcome (at least one of perinatal death, admission to neonatal intensive care unit (NICU), endotracheal intubation, Apgar < 7 at five minutes and cord lactate > 4.0 mmol/L) occurred in 201/345 (58.2%) of the twins and 7 (2%) had a CD for the second twin. For the second twin delivery interval was associated with higher cord lactate, and low Apgar scores and CD were more frequent with intervals > 30 minutes. The predictors of adverse outcome were gestational age, abnormal fetal heart rate tracing and breech delivery of twin B.[15]

Most of the studies prove hard to interpret, since most of them do not correlate mode of delivery and the set-up (operating room or delivery room) with a longer twin-to-twin interval. Naturally, if there is an abnormal fetal heart rate tracing and an urgent CD is necessary, the inter-twin delivery interval will be longer than an uncomplicated VD, if only because of the need to transfer to the operating room, administer anaesthesia and so forth. As such, a longer interval may be associated with poorer outcomes, but this association is mainly confounded by the primary indication to intervene rather than the longer time that was the result of an intervention. It is safe to assume that there is probably some association between the inter-twin delivery interval and deterioration of Apgar scores and umbilical cord pH, yet a clear threshold is hard to establish and the correlation is probably weak. The UK National Institute for Health and Care Excellence (NICE) guideline uses a 20-minute interval as a cut-off for delivery of the second twin if there is an abnormal (suspicious or pathological) fetal heart rate tracing.[16]

Breech-Presenting Twin (Twin A)

The literature regarding the recommended mode of delivery of a non-cephalic twin A is scarce. First, singleton vaginal breech deliveries have been a matter of debate until the publication of the Term Breech Trial. Another concern with a breech twin A and a cephalic twin B is the potential rare complication of locked twins. This complication is uncommon with an estimated frequency of 1:500–1:800, but the mortality associated with fetal entanglement is extremely high.

A systematic review of 1 small RCT (60 twin pairs) and 16 observational studies (3,167 twin pairs) did not find significant differences between non-cephalic twin As delivered via CD or VD. Nonetheless, the authors only compared the rates of neonatal mortality and five-minute Apgar scores < 7, and for the purpose of non-cephalic twins A included only 8 low-quality observational studies. The authors concluded that 'No final conclusion can be drawn due to the small sample sizes and statistical limitations of the included studies.'[17]

The Term Breech Trial was published in 2000 and changed obstetrical practices around the world.[10] In this multinational, multicentre study, 2,088 women with singleton gestation in breech presentation were randomised to planned VD versus planned CD. The authors found that perinatal mortality, neonatal mortality or serious neonatal morbidity were lower in the planned CD group (1.6% versus 5.0%, p <0.001, RR 0.33, 95% CI 0.19–0.56). While not without controversy, these results were extrapolated to twins as well and resulted in general agreement that twins in which twin A is in breech presentation should be delivered by CD.

Currently several national guidelines specifically recommend CD for non-cephalic twin A[16] while others state that the same indications for CD in singleton gestations (such as breech presentation, placenta previa etc.) should be applied for twins.[18] Other guidelines such as the American College of Obstetricians and Gynecologists (ACOG) practice bulletin do not address a non-cephalic first twin altogether, and one can only assume that it is implied that non-cephalic twin A should be managed in the same way as a non-cephalic singleton – that is, a CD should be offered.[19]

Monochorionic-Monoamniotic Twins

The NICE guidelines, as well as the ACOG and the Society of Obstetricians and Gynaecologists of Canada (SOGC) guidelines, are unified in their recommendation that

CD should be preferred in the case of MCMA twins.[16,18,19] The main reason for this recommendation is the concern for cord complications.

Monochorionic-Diamniotic Twins

Monochorionic-diamniotic (MCDA) twin gestation may be associated with multiple ante-partum complications such as twin–twin transfusion syndrome, twin anaemia-polycythaemia sequence, twin-reversed arterial perfusion and selective fetal growth restriction. Even in the absence of recognisable monochorionic-specific complications, monochorionic twins usually experience a higher rate of adverse neonatal outcomes.

Several studies have attempted to address the issue of mode of delivery of MCDA twins, usually through retrospective analysis. Most studies compared delivery outcomes of MCDA twins with those of DCDA twins, and most did not find significant differences between these groups. Nonetheless these studies were retrospective, with various sample sizes. Most importantly, these studies do not provide practical information and tools that can be used in clinical practice to counsel couples regarding the optimal mode of delivery based on multiple factors, including chorionicity.

In the TBS 23–25% of women had monochorionic twins and approximately 2% had unknown chorionicity. While the analysis considered chorionicity as a co-factor in the primary outcome, no direct analysis was performed of the impact of mode of delivery in monochorionic twins.[1] Recently a sub-analysis of the data regarding MCDA twin was completed.[20] The authors found no differences between planned VD and planned CD for MCDA twins.

Preterm Birth and Low Birthweight

The published literature on mode of delivery for preterm and/or low-birthweight twins is very conflicting with some studies of preterm twins showing adverse outcomes associated with VD while others do not.

A systematic review and meta-analysis of the safest mode of delivery for preterm twins when twin B is in non-cephalic presentation found no difference between twins delivered by VD or CD in cephalic/non-cephalic twin pairs at 24+° to 27+6 weeks. Nonetheless, the confidence intervals were wide due to the small sample size, and the 24+° to 27+6 weeks sample was quite large, indicating significant heterogeneity and variety between the studies.[21]

Another systematic review and meta-analysis included 15 studies with more than 12,000 infants. Caesarean delivery was associated with a 41% decrease in odds of death between 23+° and 27+6 weeks (OR 0.59, 95% CI 0.36–0.95, NNT 8), especially under 24+6 weeks of gestation (OR 0.58, 95% CI 0.44–0.75, NNT 7). The odd ratios for 25+° weeks and above were not significant. Caesarean delivery was also protective with regards to severe intraventricular haemorrhage between 23+° and 27+6 weeks, yet this effect, as for mortality, was mainly visible in lower gestational ages.[22]

The NICE guidelines suggest offering CD for preterm twin deliveries between 26 and 32 weeks when twin A is in a non-cephalic presentation. Prior to 26 weeks, their recommendation is that the decision should be individualised.[16] The SOGC guidelines recommend VD of both twins as long as their individual weights exceed 1,500 grams and twin A is in a cephalic presentation. Between 500 and 1,500 grams there is no recommendation, as the writers acknowledge the lack of good-quality literature.[18]

To conclude, neonatal outcomes in twin deliveries are highly variable and depend not only on mode of delivery, but also on neonatal weight, presentations, level of neonatal care and advances in neonatal resuscitation through the years. With current knowledge, clear gestational age and birthweight thresholds are difficult to determine.

Previous Caesarean Section (Twin VBAC)

While the risks and potential adverse outcomes of trial of labour after a previous CD (TOLAC) were extensively studied for singleton gestations, data for women with twin gestation and a history of CD are less clear.

Two meta-analyses recently published have addressed twin TOLAC. In the first one, the authors included 10 studies for a total of 2,336 trials of labour and 5,736 CDs. They reported that the pooled rate for successful TOLAC was 72.2% (95% CI 59.7–83.2%) and the risk for uterine rupture during TOLAC was 0.87% (95% CI 0.51–1.31%). They found TOLAC was associated with higher risk of neonatal death (RR 3.02, 95% CI 1.07–8.54). The risks of uterine dehiscence, blood transfusions and hysterectomy were comparable, though the risk of infectious morbidity was higher in the CD group. The authors concluded that twin TOLAC is associated with a high success rate and a low rate of uterine rupture, and that the higher neonatal mortality rate may be attributed to prematurity.[23]

The second meta-analysis pooled data from 11 cohort studies (8,209 twin gestations), of which 2,484 were intended for planned VD and 5,725 for planned CD. Twin TOLAC was associated with a higher risk of uterine rupture (OR 10.09, 95% CI 4.30–23.69; I2 = 68%) when compared to twin CD. Nonetheless, when compared with singleton TOLAC, twin TOLAC was not found to differ with regard to the rate of uterine rupture (OR 1.34, 95% CI 0.54–3.31). None of the other adverse outcomes were found to be different between twin TOLAC and CD, and the success rate of twin TOLAC was similar to that of singleton TOLAC (OR 0.85, 95% CI 0.61–1.18).[24] To conclude, it seems that twin TOLAC is a reasonable and safe option for women carrying twins who had a previous CD and that the risks and success rates are similar to those reported for TOLAC in singleton pregnancies.

Higher-Order Multiple Pregnancy

Several authors have attempted to assess the feasibility of VD in triplet pregnancies. All these studies are observational and are limited by small sample size. As for the guidelines, similar to MCMA twins, the NICE, ACOG and SOGC guidelines are uniform in their recommendation for CD in the case of triplets or higher-order multifetal gestations.[16,18,19]

Management Recommendations

- Twin delivery should be undertaken by an experienced practitioner competent in twin deliveries.
- Ultrasonographic examination is a useful adjunct prior to delivery (in order to assess fetal presentations, well-being and estimated fetal weights) and after delivery of the first twin in order to establish the fetal lie and presentation of the second twin. Depending on the gestational age, up to 20% of second twins will spontaneously change presentation once the first twin is delivered.[12]
- Intravenous access should be secured and blood sent for group and screen in anticipation of post-partum haemorrhage.

- The use of epidural, although not mandatory, is highly recommended. It is the authors' opinion that given the high likelihood for obstetrical intervention such as internal podalic version, breech extraction and/or operative delivery, adequate analgesia is essential.
- Continuous electronic monitoring is highly recommended. In order to increase maternal comfort by reducing the number of abdominal straps, and to better differentiate the two twins, the authors prefer a fetal scalp electrode on the leading twin once the membranes are ruptured.
- The use of oxytocin for augmentation may be advantageous, especially after the delivery of the first twin.
- We use double set-up (delivery in the operating room) for all twin gestations. The double set-up arrangement allows for a safe VD in the same setting of the delivery room, with extra care taken to provide for spousal chaperoning, skin-to-skin contact and so forth. On the other hand, if urgent obstetrical intervention is needed, all necessary personnel are in place and conversion to a CD is prompt.
- The third stage of labour should be managed actively to prevent blood loss, using oxytocin, uterine massage and other uterotonics as needed.

Key Points

- In women with uncomplicated DCDA or MCDA twin gestation, between 32 and 38 weeks of gestation, twin A in a cephalic presentation, and estimated fetal weights between 1,500 and 4,000 grams, a trial of VD should be offered.
- In women with twin and breech twin A, a caesarean section should be offered.
- Delivery of the second non-cephalic twin is probably safer using total breech extraction (with or without internal podalic version), rather than ECV.
- Although there is probably some association between the inter-twin delivery interval and deterioration of Apgar scores and umbilical cord pH, an exact threshold of the optimal time interval between the delivery of twins is not established.
- After delivery of the first twin, if there is concern about the well-being of the second twin, usually due to abnormal fetal heart rate tracing, delivery of the second twin should be expedited.
- There is scarce evidence regarding mode of delivery for MCMA twins, yet most guidelines recommend a caesarean section.
- The current data and recommendation regarding mode of delivery for MCDA twins suggest that it is no different than DCDA twins.
- Clear data concerning mode of delivery in preterm and low-birthweight twins is lacking, and individual management plans are recommended based on presentation, estimated fetal weight, gestational age, parity and so forth.
- Women with single previous low-segment caesarean section may be considered for a trial of VD in their subsequent twin gestation.
- There is scarce evidence regarding mode of delivery for higher-order multiple pregnancies, yet most guidelines recommend a caesarean section.

References

1. Barrett JFR, Hannah ME, Hutton EK et al. A randomized trial of planned cesarean or vaginal delivery for twin pregnancy. N Engl J Med 2013;**369**(14):1295–1305. https://doi .org/10.1056/NEJMoa1214939

2. Rabinovici J, Barkai G, Reichman B, Serr DM, Mashiach S. Randomized management of the second nonvertex twin: vaginal delivery or cesarean section. Am J Obstet Gynecol 1987;**156**(1):52–6. www .ncbi.nlm.nih.gov/pubmed/3799768

3. Rossi AC, Mullin PM, Chmait RH. Neonatal outcomes of twins according to birth order, presentation and mode of delivery: a systematic review and meta-analysis. BJOG 2011;**118**(5):523–32. https://doi.org/10.1111/ j.1471-0528.2010.02836.x

4. Zafarmand MH, Goossens SMTA, Tajik P et al. Planned cesarean or planned vaginal delivery for twins: a secondary analysis of a randomized controlled trial. *Ultrasound Obstet Gynecol* October 2019. https://doi .org/10.1002/uog.21907

5. Mei-Dan E, Dougan C, Melamed N et al. Planned cesarean or vaginal delivery for women in spontaneous labor with a twin pregnancy: a secondary analysis of the Twin Birth Study. Birth 2019;**46**(1):193–200. https://doi.org/10.1111/birt.12387

6. Mei-Dan E, Asztalos EV, Willan AR, Barrett JFR. The effect of induction method in twin pregnancies: a secondary analysis for the twin birth study. BMC Pregnancy Childbirth 2017;**17**(1). https://doi.org/10 .1186/s12884-016-1201-8

7. Asztalos E V, Hannah ME, Hutton EK et al. Twin Birth Study: 2-year neurodevelopmental follow-up of the randomized trial of planned cesarean or planned vaginal delivery for twin pregnancy presented at the annual pregnancy meeting of the Society for Maternal-Fetal Medicine, Atlanta, GA, Feb. 4, 2016.Am J Obstet Gynecol 2016;**214**(3):371.e1–371.e19. https://doi.org/10.1016/j.ajog.2015.12.051

8. Hutton EK, Hannah ME, Willan AR et al. Urinary stress incontinence and other maternal outcomes 2 years after caesarean or vaginal birth for twin pregnancy:

a multicentre randomised trial. BJOG 2018;**125**(13):1682–90. https://doi.org/10 .1111/1471-0528.15407

9. Schmitz T, Prunet C, Azria E et al. Association between planned cesarean delivery and neonatal mortality and morbidity in twin pregnancies. Obstet Gynecol 2017;**129**(6):986–95. https://doi .org/10.1097/AOG.0000000000002048

10. Hannah ME, Hannah WJ, Hewson SA, Hodnett ED, Saigal S, Willan AR. Planned caesarean section versus planned vaginal birth for breech presentation at term: a randomised multicentre trial. Term Breech Trial Collaborative Group. Lancet 2000;**356**(9239):1375–83. https://doi.org/10 .1016/s0140-6736(00)02840-3

11. Dotters-Katz SK, Gray B, Heine RP, Propst K. Resident education in complex obstetric procedures: are we adequately preparing tomorrow's obstetricians? *Am J Perinatol* 2020;**37**(11):1155–9. https://doi .org/10.1055/s-0039-1692714

12. Chervenak FA, Johnson RE, Berkowitz RL, Hobbins JC. Intrapartum external version of the second twin. *Obstet Gynecol* 1983;**62** (2):160–5. www.ncbi.nlm.nih.gov/pubmed/ 6866357

13. Aviram A, Lipworth H, Asztalos EV et al. The worst of both worlds – combined deliveries in twin gestations: a subanalysis of the Twin Birth Study, a randomized, controlled, prospective study. Am J Obstet Gynecol 2019;**221**(4):353.e1–353.e7. https://doi.org/10.1016/j.ajog.2019.06.047

14. Schneuber S, Magnet E, Haas J et al. Twin-to-twin delivery time: neonatal outcome of the second twin. Twin Res Hum Genet 2011;**14**(6):573–9. https://doi.org/10.1375/ twin.14.6.573

15. Cukierman R, Heland S, Palmer K, Neil P, da Silva Costa F, Rolnik DL. Inter-twin delivery interval, short-term perinatal outcomes and risk of caesarean for the second twin. Aust New Zeal J Obstet Gynaecol 2019;**59**(3):375–9. https://doi .org/10.1111/ajo.12867

16. National Institute for Health and Care Excellence. NICE guideline 137: twin and

triplet pregnancy. 2019;(March):1–69. www
.nice.org.uk/guidance/ng137

17. Bisschop CNS, Vogelvang TE, May AM,
Schuitemaker NWE. Mode of delivery in
non-cephalic presenting twins: a systematic
review. Arch Gynecol Obstet 2012;**286**
(1):237–47. https://doi.org/10.1007/s00404-
012-2294-6

18. Barrett J, Blocking A. Management of twin
pregnancies (part I). J SOGC 2000;**22**
(7):519–29. https://doi.org/10.1016/s0849-
5831(16)30135-5

19. Practice Bulletin No. 169: multifetal
gestations: twin, triplet, and higher-order
multifetal pregnancies. Obstet Gynecol
2016;128(4):e131–e146. https://doi.org/10
.1097/AOG.0000000000001709

20. Aviram A, Lipworth H, Asztalos EV et al.
Delivery of monochorionic twins: lessons
learned from the Twin Birth Study,
a randomized, controlled, prospective
study (unpublished data). Toronto, 2019.

21. Dagenais C, Lewis-Mikhael AM,
Grabovac M, Mukerji A, McDonald SD.
What is the safest mode of delivery for

extremely preterm cephalic/non-cephalic
twin pairs? A systematic review and
meta-analyses. BMC Pregnancy Childbirth
2017;**17**(1). Article number 397. https://doi
.org/10.1186/s12884-017-1554-7

22. Grabovac M, Karim JN, Isayama T,
Liyanage SK, McDonald SD. What is the
safest mode of birth for extremely
preterm breech singleton infants who are
actively resuscitated? A systematic review
and meta-analyses. BJOG 2018;**125**
(6):652–63. https://doi.org/10.1111/1471-
0528.14938

23. Shinar S, Agrawal S, Hasan H, Berger H.
Trial of labor versus elective repeat cesarean
delivery in twin pregnancies after
a previous cesarean delivery: a systematic
review and meta-analysis. *Birth* 2019;
(April):1–10. https://doi.org/10.1111/birt
.12434

24. Kabiri D, Masarwy R, Schachter-Safrai N
et al. Trial of labor after cesarean delivery in
twin gestations: systematic review and
meta-analysis. Am J Obstet Gynecol
2019;**220**(4):336–47. https://doi.org/10
.1016/j.ajog.2018.11.125

Chapter 25

Practical Management of Vaginal Delivery in Multiple Pregnancy

Julian N. Robinson

The Facts

Mode of Delivery of Twins

The choice of mode of delivery in twin gestations can be a complicated decision. Many mothers strongly desire a vaginal delivery. However, some may have a belief in the safety of caesarean delivery. Such a conviction can be heightened by advancing age and fertility treatment. The obstetrician may be more comfortable with elective caesarean delivery for twins, and it is certainly convenient for both mother and obstetrician. There may be limitations to a delivery suite's depth of experienced obstetric providers to provide a service for twin vaginal delivery at all times. The most undesired outcome for most twin mothers is a vaginal delivery for the first baby and a caesarean delivery for the second; some lean towards caesarean delivery just to avoid this outcome. The significant increase in caesarean delivery rates for twins over the past 30 years is documented in Chapter 24: this increase has likely led to a loss of clinical skills. The recovery from an abdominal surgery will make the first weeks of mothering much more challenging and may have longer-term sequelae (especially if the mother already has young children). In 2014 a joint consensus statement from the American College of Obstetrics and Gynecology (ACOG) and the Society of Maternal Fetal Medicine (SMFM) emphasised that perinatal outcome is not improved by caesarean section for twin deliveries where the presenting twin is in the cephalic presentation and recommended that women with cephalic-presenting twins should be counselled to attempt vaginal delivery.[1] The National Institute for Healthcare Excellence (NICE) published similar guidance on this topic in 2020. 'There is no reason to recommend one type of delivery over another in a twin pregnancy (irrespective of chronicity) when the presenting fetus is in cephalic presentation after 32 weeks, when there are no additional obstetric complications and no significant discordancy in the size of the twins.'[2] Pregnant twin mothers should be counselled about the safety of vaginal birth and obstetric departments should strive to allow women to comfortably make such a choice.

Preparation

Informed consent is complicated in twins and time should be taken in this process. The consent should include the possibility of all obstetric interventions that may occur in the course of a twin delivery. Obviously if a provider does not offer interventions such as internal podalic version and breech extraction or cephalic displacement there is no need for such consent. However, if a procedure may occur, consent should be obtained, regardless of the likelihood or intent to use it. The accoucheur may approach the delivery of a low-risk multiparous woman with cephalic/cephalic presentation with the very reasonable expectation of a simple, uncomplicated, vaginal delivery; however, if an unexpected breech extraction ends up being performed, it is optimal to have had appropriate consent.

Labour

Many aspects of obstetric labour and delivery care warrant particular attention in twin pregnancy: consent, analgesia, fetal monitoring, delivery planning and delivery methodology.

Analgesia

The woman should be informed of all of the choices available for analgesia in labour from natural childbirth to epidural. A practical approach is to go through all of the possible scenarios and how they might play out with differing methods of analgesia, integrating the approximate chance of occurrence of intervention so that the woman can make an informed choice. Twin patients at our institution have delivered with natural childbirth, pudendal block and epidural analgesia and patients are counselled in an open and non-directional fashion. However, it is fair to note that the possibility of a breech extraction or operative vaginal delivery appears to weight the choice of analgesia and the vast majority of our patients choose epidural analgesia.

Labour Patterns in Twins

Leftwich et al., using data from the Safe Labor Consortium, compared the labour curves of 891 twin gestations with 100,513 singleton controls and found labour progression was slower in nulliparous twin gestations, with a greater median time for cervical dilatation at every centimetre interval up to 7 centimetres compared with singleton nulliparous pregnancies.[3] The provider should keep in mind the potential for a slower labour and integrate this into clinical management before making a diagnosis of failed induction or failure to progress.

Fetal Monitoring

Our recommended practice for fetal monitoring in twin labour is for continuous electronic fetal monitoring with artificial rupture of membranes and placement of a fetal scalp clip on the presenting twin early in labour. The use of a scalp clip reduces the risk of inadvertently monitoring a single baby, or one baby and the mother ('coincidence' monitoring). It is reasonable to do external monitoring for both if the patient prefers, as long as clear, continuous, distinct fetal heart tracings are obtained for both babies. Simultaneous or coincidence monitoring may be precipitated by transducer, maternal or fetal movement, and very rarely fetal demise. Techniques to investigate and avoid coincidence include maternal pulse examination, pulse oximetry, three-lead maternal electrocardiogram and ultrasound examination. Software algorithms for coincidence detection include comparisons of the averaged heart rates over time with an alarm if only 2–3 beats per minute (bpm) difference over a period of greater than 30 seconds and detection of synchronised heartbeat patterns for greater than a minute. Another method to avoid coincidence monitoring is the use of a heart rate 'offset' or 'shift' mode that increases the baseline of the second heart rate by 20 bpm. If using this latter technology, care should be taken not to misinterpret tachy- or bradycardia. In the delivery process electronic fetal monitoring can be substituted with intermittent ultrasound monitoring.

Delivery

Planning

The delivering obstetrician should ideally know from recent ultrasound the presentation, lie, orientation of the limbs and the estimated amniotic fluid volume for both babies. It is possible for these things to change in the course of a delivery, but it makes sense to be aware of them at the time of contemplating the plan for delivery.

Twin deliveries should take place in the largest operating room (OR) available. The rationale for this is purely to have more space. The number of participants in team care in the academic setting is large. The protocol should ensure a paediatric team present for every twin birth under 37 weeks of gestational age. The timing of the transfer to the OR is at the end of the second stage, just before delivery, but with adequate time for transfer and optimal preparation of the final delivery destination.

Well before transfer, the obstetric team should plan the exact personnel roles and logistics for the delivery – down to the location of individuals and equipment. Delivery on a surgical bed is recommended for access, speed and simplification of procedure in the setting of complications.

It is our usual practice to have the surgical technician aware that a twin delivery is occurring; however, we do not necessarily have them present and do not have a caesarean section kit open in the room. It may be that the presence of an open, prepared surgical kit enables a self-fulfilling prophecy. If an epidural is *in situ* the anaesthetic team is present on transfer of the patient to ensure that analgesia is adequate on arrival in the OR; however, they may elect not to stay in the room for the entirety of the delivery but are always immediately available. Most providers prefer to have an ultrasound machine present for the delivery for confirmation of the presentation of the second twin after delivery of the first, and to help with guidance of a trainee if an internal podalic version and breech extraction is being performed. The presence of bedside intra-partum ultrasound is not essential. However, performance of a recent ultrasound is recommended. These ultrasound images can be transferred to a mental visual model that can be recreated in the delivering physician's mind if extra- or intrauterine manipulation is needed.

Delivery Methodology

It is important to note that the 'hands on' methodology of delivery has experienced an anecdotal rather than evidence-based evolution and there is considerable institutional and geographic variation in practice. The monologue that follows attempts to provide a comprehensive overview of current practices.

There can be a tendency in obstetric practice for an accoucheur to have a preferred method and to use that technique broadly. Twin delivery is a setting where such habitual practice may not be ideal: there are differing twin delivery scenarios and each can change dynamically as the delivery progresses, making adaptation of clinical approach appropriate. To have a single technique for all twin deliveries may be an over-simplistic approach.

Cephalic/Cephalic

There are three common current techniques for the delivery of cephalic/cephalic twins.

Passive Approach

This approach is non-interventional and is particularly appropriate for multiparous mothers. The first twin is delivered in the normal singleton fashion by the primary accoucheur. An assistant can confirm persistent cephalic presentation of the second twin by clinical or ultrasound examination. This assistant may manually attempt the cephalic presentation of the second twin, but this may be impractical due to the length of time from the delivery of the first twin to rupture of the membranes. Cephalic presentation of the second twin can also be confirmed by digital examination from below. Expectant management is then followed while the uterine contractions effect descent of the fetal head until it is engaged in the pelvis. Uterine activity can be encouraged if needed by institution or augmentation of oxytocin infusion. The heart rate of the second twin is monitored externally throughout. Once the head of the second twin is clearly engaged in the pelvis, artificial rupture of the membranes can be carried out (if it has not occurred spontaneously). The second twin is then delivered spontaneously as in a singleton. The advantage of this method is that allowing the head to properly engage in the pelvis before the membranes are ruptured minimises the chance of fetal heart rate abnormality and cord prolapse. The disadvantage is that the process can take an unexpectedly long time.

Active Approach

The active approach is similar to the passive approach, except immediately after the delivery of the first twin the cephalic presentation of the second twin is confirmed and stabilised by an assistant and artificial rupture of the membranes is carried out almost immediately (when the presenting part may still be high). The advantage of this approach is that it decreases the time between delivery of the second twin and delivery of the first and it reveals the nature of the second twin's amniotic fluid early in the process (the presence of meconium may lead to less tolerance of an abnormal fetal heart tracing). The disadvantages of the early rupture of membranes are the risk of cord prolapse if the presenting part is high and the common occurrence of a fetal bradycardia as the fetal head descends relatively quickly through the maternal pelvis. If a bradycardia does occur, the fetal heart rate usually returns to normal in a few minutes and care can proceed as planned. After rupture of the membranes and descent of the head of the second twin, the delivery can then be continued as for a singleton. A lack of recurrence of effective uterine contractions may need augmentation with an infusion of oxytocin.

Cephalic Version

After delivery of the first twin external cephalic version of the second twin combined with internal podalic version and breech extraction is an efficient method of delivery of a cephalic-presenting second twin. The rationale behind this approach is to minimise the time interval between first and second twin delivery and therefore to curtail the opportunity for complication and combined vaginal and caesarean delivery. This rationale is robust. However, there are a number of prerequisites, which include provider experience and confidence and appropriate case selection. A multiparous patient with an expected straightforward course with cephalic/cephalic twins may not seem the ideal candidate for such an intervention when a normal delivery is likely without intervention. The ideal patient for this technique is the nulliparous mother with a high presenting part, lack of descent and a generous amniotic fluid volume in the second twin, and with the second twin not being significantly larger than the first (see later in this chapter). The technique for carrying out the cephalic displacement is a firm hand on the fetal vertex with intact membranes and a firm, strong and directly vertical push. Once the baby is transverse with one or two feet available, internal podalic version and breech extraction can be performed (see later in this chapter).

Cephalic/Non-cephalic

We use a twin discordance range of 25%[4] to 40%,[5] where the second twin is larger than the presenting twin to determine suitability for vaginal delivery where the second twin is in a non-cephalic presentation. Twenty-five per cent is for the less favourable obstetric candidate of the nulliparous woman and towards 40% is for the more favourable case of the multiparous patient.

Cephalic/Breech

The preparation and delivery of the presenting cephalic twin is identical to that described earlier in this chapter. After delivery of the first twin, the options for the second, breech-presenting baby are internal podalic version and breech extraction or external cephalic version. The preferred option will depend on both the clinical scenario and the provider's choice. The default technique at our institution is internal podalic version and breech extraction. However, an external cephalic version can be very simple and easy to do in a multiparous thin patient with generous amniotic fluid volume and a fetal lie with a lateral location of the back: the simplest and easiest approach is usually the best choice.

The time for consideration of episiotomy in a cephalic/breech delivery is at the time of crowning of the first cephalic twin: if the perineum is providing significant soft tissue resistance at this time, the obstetrician should consider the breech delivery to follow. If the first baby is delivered without an episiotomy, there is less likely to be a need for one for the delivery of the second baby.

External Cephalic Version

Assessment for external cephalic version (ECV) can be carried out immediately after the delivery of the first twin. If that assessment is that such a version would be simple and uncomplicated, it is appropriate to attempt the intervention. External cephalic version is best carried out with a forward roll if the fetal back is lateral with firm, but gentle pressure on the occiput. Traditionally in ECV a hand elevates the breech: this is often not needed in a second twin as the breech is often already high. Once the cephalic presentation is achieved the fetus can be held stable while another practitioner artificially ruptures the membranes (or the same provider can immediately carry out the rupture).

Internal Podalic Version and Breech Extraction

For internal podalic version and breech delivery of the second twin, the accoucheur inserts their dominant hand into the uterus with intact membranes to identify and grasp a fetal foot or both feet. If a contraction is present, the membranes may be tense, and it is best to wait for the contraction to pass. When carrying out this manoeuver it is useful to have a mental picture of the lie of the breech presenting fetus in one's mind and where the foot or feet are expected to be. If the membranes rupture spontaneously and frequent or sustained uterine contractions are making manipulation challenging, uterine relaxation can be considered with a tocolytic such as nitroglycerin. The original description of breech extraction was by

Ambroise Paré (1510–90), who described a technique where both feet are grasped. Much later the London obstetrician John Braxton Hicks (1823–97) described the technique of using only one foot. The choice of technique is provider driven. In our practice we aim to get a single foot, ideally the uppermost foot (i.e. the one nearest the anterior abdominal wall) as when the upper leg is pulled the fetus will descend in a rotating fashion that will ensure that the fetal back is uppermost as the procedure progresses. The disadvantage of the 'two foot' technique is complexity: the need to locate and grasp both feet. The disadvantage of the 'single foot' technique is an occasional later need for some improvisation with the delivery of the second leg. The accoucheur should have a mental image from prior ultrasound examination or ultrasound guidance as to where the foot will be located: their dominant hand can explore and identify a free appendage. Once an appendage is identified, the operator grasps the distal limb and feels for a heel (Figure 25.1). If no heel is identified the limb should be released and pushed away. If the heel is identified the foot is then firmly grasped in a clenched fist with the fetal leg between the operator's first and second finger (Figure 25.2). Once the fetal foot is in the obstetrician's grip it is held firmly and not released until the majority of the limb has been delivered. Firm and steady traction of increasing tension is then applied to deliver the leg. Traction can be increased until the membranes spontaneously rupture, or the membranes can be artificially ruptured. Once rupture has occurred, the amount of traction required becomes much less. With the Paré technique both legs are delivered together. With the Braxton Hicks approach there sometimes has to be some manipulation for delivery of the second leg. Occasionally the second foot comes down

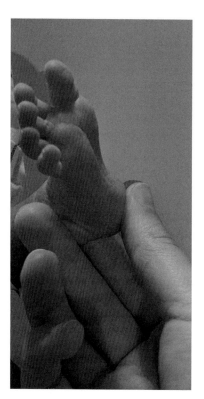

Figure 25.1 Locating the fetal heel

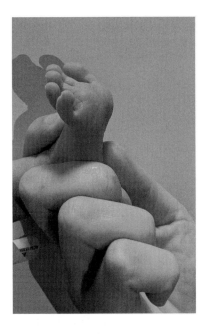

Figure 25.2 Grasping the foot prior to traction

with the first leg and can be grasped and both legs can then be delivered together. Sometimes the first leg delivers and the breech is visible, but the second leg is extended intra-utero: in this case, the breech is almost delivered and a hand can be passed into the vagina, the knee flexed, if needed, by popliteal fossa pressure and the leg delivered by a medial sweeping motion with the hand cupping the shin: the Pinard manoeuver (Aldolphe Pinard (1844–1934)). Once both legs and the breech are delivered the torso is gently grasped in a dry towel and steady traction is applied along the uterine axis: such traction should be slow and controlled. A nuchal arm is present in 0.5% of singleton breech deliveries and 9% of breech extractions – the higher incidence in breech extractions is likely due to the extraction process, present in one technique and not the other.[6] Fast extraction is more likely to elevate the arm and make a nuchal arm more likely. Once both scapulae are visible Lovset's manoeuver is performed (Jorgen Lovset (1896–1981)), rotating the torso and sweeping each arm down separately for delivery of the shoulders: the torso is rotated 90 degrees to one side and the arm is swept medially to deliver the arm and the shoulder and then the procedure is repeated for the other side with a 180 degree rotation, after which the baby is returned to the back-up lie. The head then often delivers spontaneously. The Bracht manoeuver for delivery of the aftercoming head (Erich Bracht (1882–1969)) is where, once the torso is delivered, the fetal hips are grasped between two hands and elevated and rotated towards the mother's abdomen. If the head does not deliver spontaneously and the Bracht manoeuver is not to be performed, the baby's body can be supported on the accoucheur's dominant forearm while the Mauriceau Smellie Veit manoeuver is carried out for delivery of the fetal head.[1] In this procedure the index and forefinger of the operator's dominant hand are used to place flexing

---

[1] Francois Mauriceau (1637–1709), William Smellie (1697–1703) and Gustave Veit (1824–1903) described the manoeuver independently and Mauriceau originally described it with the French physician André Levret (1703–80). The procedure may actually have originally been described by the French physician Jacques Guillemeau (1550–1613) – the son-in-law of Ambroise Paré.

pressure on the baby's maxilla while the other hand is used to apply gentle traction to one of the baby's shoulders and can also apply digital pressure with the forefinger to the occiput (increasing the flexion vector). Both the Bracht manoeuver and the Mauriceau Smellie Veit manoeuver can be assisted with supra-pubic pressure: Credé's manoeuver (Carl Credé (1819–92)). A twin second breech delivery is very different than a singleton breech delivery. The pelvis has just delivered one baby and most of another. The aftercoming head is not the same challenge as it can be in a singleton. Forceps almost never need to be applied for the delivery of the fetal head in a second twin.

A breech baby can be delivered in the occiput posterior position, although less orthodox: the Prague manoeuver is for this situation where a hand is inserted into the vagina posteriorly to deliver the shoulders with a lifting upward rotational movement while supra-pubic pressure is applied to facilitate delivery of the head. A planned occiput posterior breech delivery is not recommended.

As noted, a nuchal arm may occur in as many as 9% of breech extractions. This can be dealt with by identifying on which side the nuchal arm is, then rotating the torso to that side, almost to the point of complete rotation, until the shoulder can be identified and the arm reduced by hooking a finger gently over the crook of the elbow and sweeping the arm downward and medially. If unsuccessful the manoeuver can be repeated with ever-increasing rotation.

Cephalic/Oblique or Cephalic/Transverse

When the presenting twin is in the cephalic presentation and the second twin is oblique or transverse, careful consideration should be given to delivery planning. This constellation is where most problems or complications occur. An oblique lie can become a transverse lie after delivery of the first twin. If the back of the second fetus is towards the uterine fundus (back up) an internal podalic version and breech extraction can be relatively straightforward. If the fetal back is towards the accoucheur's hand (back down) delivery may be much more challenging (especially if the membranes rupture before a fetal foot is located). In this setting low amniotic fluid volume around the second twin will add to the degree of difficulty of manoeuvres. Such a fetus can be challenging to deliver even by caesarean section. In such cases many factors should be considered in the decision for planned mode of delivery (parity, estimated fetal weight discordance, amniotic fluid volume of the second twin, maternal BMI and provider experience). In these cases, where the fetal back is down, a planned caesarean delivery may not reflect a timid provider but rather demonstrate astute analysis and planning.

If an accoucheur does find themselves in the position of not being able to locate a fetal foot in a back-down transverse lie, the lie can sometimes be changed by cupping either pole of the fetus (head or foot) and attempting to change the lie with rotation. An external hand can aid the process by applying counter-rotational pressure to the opposite fetal pole.

Non-vertex Presenting Twin

The NICE guidelines recommend caesarean delivery for breech-presenting twins, and that is the practice at our hospital.[2] However, there is past[7] and recent literature[8] studying planned vaginal delivery in this setting. If planned or in an emergency presentation (delivering at presentation) the presenting breech is delivered as per a singleton: a passive non-interventionalist approach is recommended. No traction is applied, some manipulation may be needed for the delivery of the legs, Lovset's manoeuver is used for delivery of the shoulders, and the Mauriceau Smellie Veit, Bracht manoeuver or forceps may be needed for the aftercoming head. It is interesting that the primary reason for the caesarean delivery of breech-presenting twins is the rare incidence of locking of the heads, a phenomenon that cannot occur if the second baby is in the breech presentation.

Mode of Delivery in Triplets and Higher-Order Multiples

The evidence-based literature on triplet delivery is limited. A literature search on vaginal versus caesarean delivery of triplet pregnancy over the past 20 years where the data show the success rate of attempted vaginal delivery produces six studies. Four are very small case control or cohort studies and two are large studies. The four small studies amount to a total of 96 vaginal deliveries from 149 attempts (64%).[9,10,11,12] One of these studies had a higher rate of maternal transfusion and a trend towards higher composite neonatal morbidity and did not support vaginal delivery.[10] The remaining three were supportive of vaginal delivery. Of the two studies of larger numbers – a matched multiple birth database (1995–8) of 23,381[13] and a cohort study of 386[14] – the larger reported an increased risk of stillbirth (RR 5.7: 95% CI 3.63, 8.49), neonatal death (RR 2.83: 95% CI 1.91, 4.19) and infant death (RR 2.29 95% CI 1.61, 3.25) with planned vaginal delivery, and the smaller showed no advantage of Caesarean delivery. In short, in the past 20 years, one large, retrospective database study has shown planned caesarean delivery of triplets to be safer than planned vaginal delivery, one more modest-sized cohort study has shown no advantage, and three very small studies are supportive of vaginal delivery in this setting. A look into the more historic literature found five further controlled studies, the largest with a planned vaginal delivery group of 39. Both the numbers and ages of these studies have led to their not being included in this monologue. The remaining literature is cases series and reviews. There have been no randomised trials studying route of delivery in triplets to date. A synthesis of this data today makes it challenging to be a champion of planned vaginal delivery of triplet gestations.

A fundamental concern in modern obstetric practice for labouring triplet pregnancies is the issue of fetal monitoring in labour. If the standard of care in a unit is for twins to have continuous electronic fetal monitoring in labour, it should be the same for triplets. It is questionable whether continuous fetal heart traces of adequate quality can reliably be obtained for this population throughout labour. The shorter labours associated with multi-parity and higher chance of success with a previous vaginal delivery would make this a preferred population for those obstetricians wanting to provide this service. From current twin practice, it would seem intuitive to limit the practice to pregnancies with a presenting triplet in the cephalic presentation, and a constellation of the manoeuvres listed earlier in this chapter can be used after the delivery of the first baby. Proponents of the practice often state that after the first delivery it is the same as twins; however, external manipulation after delivery of the first twin, with two fetuses still present, will be more challenging. Regardless of case selection, in an age of evidence-based medicine it would seem both from the paucity of data and the historical context of the literature reviewed here that if vaginal delivery of triplet pregnancy is to be carried out it would perhaps be most appropriately carried out in a prospective research setting with appropriate ethics approval and with a randomised design. There appears to be no literature reporting or advocating vaginal delivery of quadruplets and higher-order multiple pregnancies in the US National Institutes of Health's National Library of Medicine. As such, the topic is not be explored further here.

Uterine Incision

There is very little in the literature, and nothing with robust numbers or design, regarding optimal uterine incision in multiple pregnancy. Our preference is lower-segment transverse incision in both twins and triplets unless the lower segment is diminutive (such as in significant prematurity).

The Issues

The issue with twin delivery over the past 30 years has been the increased use of caesarean section. Our leading professional organisations and many champions in the field are supportive of offering vaginal delivery for those who so choose. As such, departments of obstetrics should be advocating vaginal delivery of twins. A number of resources and interventions are available to institute in an attempt to increase the percentage of twin mothers having vaginal deliveries. Resources for patient information and education in addition to real-time counselling by their obstetric care provider include handouts and internet sources. Aids to help obstetricians include a questionnaire needs assessment (to identify areas of concern or weakness), expert clinical lectures, clinical protocols, webpages with videos, simulation sessions, establishing a dedicated twin clinic and availability of an experienced back-up team. The simulation approach has proven successful in at least a trainee population.[15] An experienced provider back-up programme may seem to be a challenging enterprise; however, our experience has been that expertise becomes swiftly adopted and multiplies quickly through the department. In our department such a programme changed the twin vaginal delivery rate from 32% to 44% over six years.

Key Points

- Current evidence shows no benefit of caesarean delivery if the presenting fetus is in the vertex presentation. A mother with twins with the first twin in the vertex presentation should be counselled on the safety of vaginal delivery.
- The data regarding safe delivery of triplet pregnancies are limited and the largest study supports planned caesarean delivery over planned vaginal delivery.
- Vaginal delivery of multiple pregnancies greater than triplets is not supported by scientific evidence.
- There are a number of different techniques for delivering twins and the accoucheur should be aware of all and use the most appropriate to the case and the moment.
- A programme of needs assessment, education, simulation and backup support can increase a hospital's vaginal delivery rate of twins.

References

1. Caughey AB, Cahill AG, Guise JM et al. Safe prevention of the primary cesarean delivery. Am J Obstet Gynecol 2014;**210**:179–93.

2. Gibson JL, Castleman JS, Meher S, Kilby MD. Updated guidance for the management of twin and triplet pregnancies from the National Institute for Health and Care Excellence guidance, UK: what's new that may improve perinatal outcomes? Acta Obstet Gynecol Scand 2020;**99**:147–52.

3. Leftwich HK, Zaki MN, Wilkins I, Hibbard JU. Labor patterns in twin gestations. Am J Obstet Gynecol 2013 Sep;**209**(3):254.e1–5.

4. Peaceman AL, Kuo L, Feinglass J. Infant morbidity and mortality associated with

vaginal delivery in twin gestations. Am J Obstet Gynecol 2009;**200**:462 e1–6.

5. Houlihan C, Knuppel RA. Intrapartum management of multiple gestations. Clin Perinatol 1996;**23**:91–116.

6. Cheng M, Hannah M. Breech delivery at term: a critical review of the literature. Obstet Gynecol 1993 Oct;**82**(4 Pt 1):605–18.

7. Blickstein I, Goldman RD, Kuofermic M. Delivery of breech first twins: a multicenter retrospective study. Obstet Gynecol 2000;**95**:37–42.

8. Korb D, Goffinet F, Bretelle F et al. First twin in breech presentation and neonatal mortality and morbidity according to planned mode of delivery. Obstet Gynecol 2020 May;**135**(5):1015–23. https://doi.org/10.1097/AOG.0000000000003785

9. Alran S, Sibony O, Lutun D et al. Maternal and neonatal outcome of 93 consecutive triplet deliveries with 71% vaginal delivery. Acta Obstet Gynecol Scand 2004;**83**:554–9.

10. Lappen JR, Hackney DN, Bailit JL. Maternal and neonatal outcomes of attempted vaginal compared with planned cesarean delivery in triplet gestations. Am J Obstet Gynecol 2016;**215**:493e 1–6.

11. Peress D, Dude A, Peaceman A, Yee LM. Maternal and neonatal outcomes in triplet gestations by trial of labor versus planned cesarean delivery. J Matern Fet Neonatal Med 2019;**32**:1874–9.

12. Machtinger R, Sivan E, Maayan-Metzger A, Moran O, Kuint J, Schiff E. Perinatal, postnatal, and maternal outcome parameters of triplet pregnancy according to the planned mode of delivery: results of a single tertiary center. J Matern Fetal Neonatal Med 2011;**24**:91–5.

13. Vintzileos AM, Ananth CV, Kontopoulos E, Smulian JC. Mode of delivery and risk of stillbirth and infant mortality in triplet gestations: United States, 1995 through 1998. Am J Obstet Gynecol 2005;**192**:464–9.

14. Mol BW, Bergenhenegouwen L, Velzel J et al. Perinatal outcomes according to the mode of delivery in women with a triplet pregnancy in the Netherlands. J Matern Fetal Neonatal Med 2019;**32**:3771–7.

15. Easter SR, Gardner R, Barrett J, Robinson JN, Carusi D. Simulation to improve trainee knowledge and comfort with twin vaginal birth. Obstet Gynecol 2016;**128**:34s–39s.

Neonatal Care Aspects of Multiple Pregnancy

Alejandra Barrero-Castillero and DeWayne M. Pursley

The Issues

Few clinical events are more challenging than the resuscitation and stabilisation of a critically ill patient. In paediatrics, the management of multiple-gestation newborns can present an even more formidable task. While the majority of these infants will only require routine nursery care, because of their greater prevalence of high-risk conditions, the likelihood of emergent care is higher in multiple births. This is owing to higher rates of complications during pregnancy, delivery and the neonatal period. Sound preparation is essential, as is the need for the nursery staff to quickly identify these conditions and provide effective neonatal management. Multiple-pregnancy newborns make up only 3.5% of all live births but account for up to 15% of neonatal intensive care unit (NICU) admissions.[1,2]

Adverse Outcomes (Compared to Singletons)

Multiple pregnancies have an increased risk of adverse outcomes, including intrauterine growth restriction, preterm delivery (PTD), preterm and premature rupture of membranes (PPROM) and congenital anomalies, compared to singleton pregnancies. All have potential clinical implications for the multiple infant.

Perinatal Morbidity and Mortality

Morbidity

A study evaluating a comprehensive financial and health services evaluation of multiple-pregnancy and higher-order multiples in 2014 found that multiple-pregnancy infants consume significantly more health resources during the newborn period and the first year of life.[3] Even though multiple-gestation newborns are statistically at a higher risk for morbidity, this association is highly confounded by the associated adverse factors.

In general, multiple-pregnancy newborns, especially twins, do well, experience little morbidity and develop normally. Because of the association between morbidity and long-term development, this relationship is important to examine. Newborns born from multiple pregnancy may experience serious complications associated with prematurity, including respiratory distress syndrome, that may progress to chronic lung disease, apnoea, hypoglycaemia, intraventricular and intra-parenchymal haemorrhage, periventricular leukomalacia, asphyxia and other complications that can result in long-term developmental problems. These are described in more detail later in this chapter.

Mortality

Most complications and adverse outcomes of multiple-pregnancy newborns are associated with gestational age and birthweight, the most important predictors of infant mortality. Overall mortality in premature infants has declined due to developments in neonatal and obstetric care, including the use of antenatal glucocorticoids, exogenous surfactant and improved ventilatory care.

In 2017 almost three-quarters of all infant deaths in the United States occurred in preterm infants, with the highest rates experienced by extremely premature infants born at 28 weeks or less (183 times the rate for term infants).[4] Among higher-order multiple births, the increased risk of infant mortality appears to be largely due to the lower birthweight distribution and shorter gestation among these infants. When matched for gestational age, race, gender and mode of delivery, preterm twins appear to have similar outcomes to singleton infants. On the other hand, monochorionic and monoamniotic twins have higher risk for both morbidity and mortality compared to dichorionic twins. Death of both twins is higher with gestation associated with monochorionic placentation.[5]

Prematurity

Prematurity (birth before 37 weeks of gestation) is one of the leading causes of morbidity and mortality in children younger than five years worldwide. It is well known that multiple pregnancies are associated with a higher risk of preterm delivery compared to singleton pregnancies. The pathogenesis of premature delivery remains unclear, and it is difficult to predict which multiple pregnancies will result in preterm birth.[6] Some suggest that uterine over-distension, mechanical stretching of the cervix and decreased uterine blood flow – consistent with the observation that the number of fetuses present is inversely proportional to the gestational age at birth – may explain the increased risk of prematurity in multiples.

In the United States in 2018, when preterm births accounted for 10% of all live births, twins were almost eight times more likely to be born preterm than singletons: 60.3% compared with 8.2%. The incidence of preterm birth increases with plurality. Of all live births in the United States in 2018, 96.6% were singletons and 3.4% were multiple births. In 2005 the mean gestational age for twin delivery was 35.2 weeks, and for triplet delivery it was 31.9 weeks, for quadruplet delivery it was 29.8, and for quintuplet delivery and higher it was 27.4 weeks compared to 38.7 weeks for singletons.[7]

Complications in premature infants after birth are mainly due to difficulties in extra-uterine life adaptation as well as to a spectrum of multiple organ immaturity that is inversely proportional to gestational age at birth. Thanks to advanced intensive care, even infants who are born very prematurely are more likely to survive today than some years ago. Figure 26.1 describes the classification of prematurity by gestational age and birthweight and the most common and expected complications after birth. It is important to note that incidence and severity of complications decrease as gestational age increases.

Abnormal Fetal Growth (Intrauterine Growth Restriction and Discordant Growth)

We use several terms that describe the overall weight at birth independent of gestational age (*low birthweight*, *very low birthweight* and *extremely low birthweight*), and we use others to describe weight by gestational age, which include *small for gestational age* (SGA) (weight at < 10th

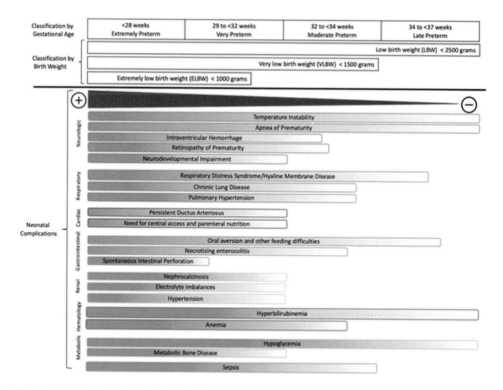

Figure 26.1 Neonatal complications broadly associated with gestational age and birthweight ranges

percentile for gestational age), *large for gestational age* (LGA) (weight at > 90th percentile for gestational age) and *appropriate for gestational age* (AGA). Additionally, we use either *fetal growth restriction* (FGR) or *intrauterine growth restriction* (IUGR) to describe delayed growth in utero. While many SGA infants have evidence of IUGR and many IUGR infants are SGA, they are not exclusive.

The weight at birth of multiple-pregnancy infants is less than the weight of singletons, in part due to shorter gestational age at birth. The birthweight of multiples is comparable to singletons up to 30–34 weeks of gestation, at which point multiples begin to have delayed growth. This growth restriction in twins and higher-order multiples may be explained by limited placental growth due to overcrowding, relative utero-placental insufficiency with inadequate nutrition consumption and insufficient blood flow to support the rate of growth seen in singletons.

Discordant growth in multiples is generally indicative of growth restriction in one of the fetuses and is defined as a difference in weight of more than 15%, 20% or 25% between fetuses, depending on the classification used. Individual IUGR is when one of the fetuses' weight falls below the 10th percentile of weight for gestational age. Growth restriction in both twins may reflect utero-placental dysfunction while discordant growth may be due to several factors like selective placental dysfunction (only in one placenta), genetics or an unequal vasculature share in a monochorionic placenta.[8] A growth discordance of more than 30% has been associated with higher mortality in the smaller twin and higher morbidity in both twins.[9]

Congenital Anomalies and Early Malformations

Congenital anomalies are more likely to occur in multiple-pregnancy infants than in singletons. This increased rate is largely associated with monozygotic twins. These defects can develop early in gestation due to abnormal placental vascular anastomoses (discussed later in this chapter), or late in gestation due to constraints in the physical environment. The anomalies developed early in gestation may be incompatible with life and account for the overrepresentation of monozygotic twins among spontaneous abortions. Severe structural defects in monozygotic twins include acardia or hemicardia, anencephaly, holoprosencephaly malformation sequence, sacrococcygeal teratoma, exstrophy of the cloaca malformation sequence, VACTERL association, caudal regression syndrome (including sirenomelia) and conjoined twins. Most of these cases are present in one twin but occur in both in 5–20% of cases. Even in cases where both infants have the defect, one may be less affected than the other. Finally, due to environmental constraints and uterine crowding, some twins may present with deformations like positional plagiocephaly, bowing of the limbs or clubfeet, developing later in gestation.[6,10]

Conjoined Twins

Conjoined twins (see Chapter 10) are a rare event and represent an infrequent complication of monozygotic twinning. Two theories explain conjoined twins. The first one is 'fission theory', where it occurs around day 13 to 15 after fertilisation when the embryonic discs (monozygotic twins) fail to separate. A second theory, called 'fusion theory', describes two separated embryonic discs that fuse in areas where ectoderm is absent.[11] Most commonly these twins are joined at the thorax, but they can be joined at the head, buttocks and other sites. Partial or complete duplication of only the upper or lower body parts may also take place. There is a 10–20% occurrence of major defects in addition to the defect related to the site of juncture, and this condition is more common in females than in males (3:1).[11,12]

Adverse Events due to Placental Vascular Anastomoses

Placentation is a major determinant of mortality in twins, with monochorionic twins experiencing greater morbidity and mortality than dichorionic-monozygotic or dizygotic twins. Vascular interconnections occur in almost all monochorionic twins and rarely in dichorionic multiples.[6] Vascular connections between the two fetal circulations can be artery-to-vein shunts (twin–twin transfusion syndrome and twin anaemia-polycythaemia sequence), which are more common, and artery-to-artery shunts, which can range from no clinical significance to very severe disorders such as twin-reversed arterial perfusion (TRAP) sequence.

Twin–Twin Transfusion Syndrome and Twin Anaemia-Polycythaemia Sequence: Artery-to-Vein Anastomoses

Occurring in monochorionic twinning, artery-to-vein anastomoses are the basis of twin–twin transfusion syndrome (TTTS) in which blood vessels connect within the placenta and divert blood from one fetus to the other. During pregnancy, anastomoses are common and usually go through a placental cotyledon. Their size, number and direction, as well as the period of time over which the transfusion occurs, determine their consequences. Twin–twin transfusion syndrome has a spectrum of possible clinical outcomes and happens in about 15% of twins with a shared placenta. Clinically, the vascular shunt with many or large anastomoses will appear as hypovolemia, anaemia and paleness at birth in the 'donor' twin and hypervolemia, polycythaemia and plethora in the 'recipient' twin. An inter-pair difference in haemoglobin may be more than 5 grams/100 ml, and there may be discordant amniotic fluid volumes (polyhydramnios and oligo- or anhydramnios) and birthweight differences of more than 1,000 grams.[6]

Over time, the cardiovascular system of the recipient fetus may become overloaded from chronic transfusion, and increased urine output may result in polyhydramnios. These infants are usually larger and they may develop polycythaemia (which may lead to jaundice or thrombosis postnatally), hypervolemia and cardiac hypertrophy. The volume overload may result in cardiac dysfunction that may progress to anasarca and hydrops. In the meantime, the donor fetus may develop a severely low blood volume, decreased urine output and oligo- or anhydramnios. These infants tend to be smaller (severe growth restriction) and may develop anaemia, hypovolemia that may progress to renal insufficiency, decreased organ mass and amnion nodosum (impacted vernix). While there are therapies to treat TTTS during pregnancy (discussed in previous chapters), these twins often must be delivered early to avoid stillbirth.

Management in the delivery room and after birth depends on the clinical presentation. The recipient twin with polycythaemia may have severe hyperviscosity syndrome that may require partial exchange transfusion. The donor twin may present with hypotension or poor perfusion due to chronic hypovolemia that may require immediate volume expansion and, at times, red blood cell transfusion. Both infants may present with severe respiratory distress, cyanosis, poor feeding, hypoglycaemia, jitteriness, lethargy, hypotonia and seizures. Later they are at risk for hyperbilirubinemia.

In some cases there is a recently described atypical chronic and milder form of TTTS, called twin anaemia-polycythaemia sequence (TAPS) that may be spontaneous, or a result of laser therapy for TTTS, where the arterio-venous placental shunt is through very narrow-calibre vessels causing a very slow transfusion that only causes anaemia and polycythaemia in the donor and recipient, respectively. Management in the NICU may include transfusion for the donor twin and partial exchange transfusion for the recipient twin.[13] Additionally, the donor twin may present with growth restriction and hypoglycaemia.

Vascular Disruption Sequence (Artery-to-Artery Shunts)

Artery-to-artery anastomoses between two fetal circulations are common and often have no major clinical significance. However, on some rare occasions these connections may cause acute problems during labour and delivery, causing exsanguination of the donor twin. If this shunt develops early in gestation, it may lead to severe hemodynamic shifts, chronically perfusing the lower part of the recipient twin's body, resulting in deterioration of tissues and severe malformations. This vascular disruption is variable, but in extreme cases it may result in an acephalic, acardiac or amorphous twin. This disorder is called twin-reversed arterial perfusion (TRAP) sequence. While the recipient twin may present with acardia, the donor twin (called the pump twin) may present with a structurally normal heart but with an excessive cardiovascular load that may result in cardiac dysfunction and progress to hydrops with very high mortality.[6] Given the risk for cardiac overload, if surviving, donor (pump) twins in TRAP sequence should be evaluated for congestive heart failure.

Cord Complications in Monoamniotic Twins

In addition to the baseline risk factors and potential complications of multiple-pregnancy newborns, monoamniotic twins have unique risk for severe complications that contribute to a higher risk of perinatal morbidity and mortality among all multiple-pregnancy newborns, including cord complications. Cord complications and accidents include rupture of a vasa previa, cord entanglement and cord prolapse.

Respiratory Distress and Perinatal Depression to the Non-presenting Twin

Non-presenting newborns are generally considered at higher risk for morbidity and mortality. In infants born via vaginal delivery respiratory distress syndrome and perinatal depression tend to occur less frequently in the first or presenting twin, who may receive the full benefits from labour (the presenting twin has a higher lecithin–sphingomyelin ratio in amniotic fluid and higher cord-blood cortisol compared to the non-presenting twin after labour). This effect is particularly seen in premature infants who are at higher risk of respiratory distress syndrome and perinatal depression at baseline.[14] The effects of perinatal depression can be ameliorated with readily available team(s) present at delivery and neonatal intensive care.

Increased Risk for the Surviving Twin in the Presence of Fetal Demise

As noted previously, monochorionic twins are at increased risk of mortality. In some cases one of the fetuses will die, placing the surviving twin at higher risk of mortality and adverse outcomes after birth. Co-twin demise may result in a capacitance effect or disseminated intravascular coagulation from emboli of the demised twin entering the surviving twin's circulation. This may increase the risk of serious defects like porencephalic cyst, hydranencephaly, limb amputation, aplasia cutis, gastroschisis or intestinal atresia. This presentation has been associated with an increased risk of cerebral palsy.

Long-Term Outcomes

In addition to the increased risks of morbidity and mortality during the neonatal period, multiple-pregnancy newborns are at increased risk for long-term neurodevelopmental deficits and poor growth. These deficits, however, may be largely explained by the multitude of genetic, perinatal and neonatal morbidity and the associated medical and social risk factors that can affect multiples, not associated with plurality. For example, preterm delivery is associated with increased risk for short-term outcomes such as high-grade intraventricular haemorrhage and periventricular leukomalacia[15] and long-term neurodevelopmental deficits. Further, congenital anomalies are more common in twins and some anomalies like congenital heart disease are independently associated with increased risk of neurodevelopmental delays.

Long-term outcomes are difficult to evaluate, much less apply to a single infant or group of infants. Systematic reviews of long-term neurodevelopmental outcomes of multiples compared with singleton newborns have not reported conclusive findings. Most studies control for birthweight and gestational age, have poor or borderline power to detect differences, and fail to include additional variables that may contribute to neurodevelopmental delays.[16] While overall the prevalence of cerebral palsy is low, some population-based studies have shown an increased risk of developing cerebral palsy in twins compared to singletons. Prospective cohort studies, however, have not found a higher incidence of cerebral palsy or seizure disorders in twins.[17]

One exception has been seen in fetal demise of a twin and history of TTTS (with or without fetal demise) where there is a risk of long-term neurodevelopmental outcomes like cerebral palsy (cognitive and neuromotor disabilities) reported in the surviving twin. Intrauterine therapies (e.g. amnioreduction) are not consistently associated with improvements in long-term neurodevelopment.[17] As with other outcomes, no studies have reported increased risk in autism among multiples when adjusted for prematurity and older parental age.

Though not specific for twins, in addition to the increased risk for neurodevelopmental delay, premature and very low birthweight babies have an increased risk of rehospitalisation in the first year of life compared to newborns with normal weight.[18] These infants may also be at a greater risk for child abuse and neglect.

Recent studies have shown that the majority of adults who were born preterm are healthy and well with a slight but significant increased risk of developing chronic and metabolic disorders, as well as neuropsychological and behavioural problems earlier in life compared to adults who were born at term, but there is little evidence that this is an independent risk factor for former multiple-pregnancy infants.[19]

Management of Multiple-Pregnancy Newborns

Multiple-pregnancy deliveries should occur in hospitals with appropriate staff to provide the appropriate level of care and ensure optimal outcomes. Although potential complications can never be fully anticipated for any delivery, given the range of risks for multiples, it is essential that the staff are fully aware of and prepared to respond to potential concurrent clinical challenges. The delivery site must be capable of providing risk-appropriate care for known fetal or anticipated delivery complications, and this may require transfer to a higher level of perinatal care.

Antenatal Consultation

The anticipated birth of multiple-pregnancy newborns may result in questions and uncertainly about possible outcomes, type of delivery and complications that may develop during pregnancy, at the time of birth or in the neonatal period. Referral to a paediatric provider or neonatal intensive care team should be considered, depending on the potential need for specialised care. Antenatal consultation provides an opportunity to create a relationship between the parents and the neonatal clinicians, setting the groundwork for a therapeutic relationship and a shared decision-making approach to care before and after the delivery, as well as an opportunity to educate and support decisions like breastfeeding. The maternal medical record should be carefully reviewed by the neonatal care team prior to the consultation to provide appropriate care recommendations and initiate planning for delivery room management and immediate neonatal care. Additionally, if there are significant conditions or congenital anomalies that will require early paediatric medical subspecialty or surgical specialty care consultation, referral should be directed to those specific disciplines for counselling, planning and follow-up care.

Delivery Room Management

Delivery room management is especially important for multiple-gestation newborns given their higher likelihood of preterm delivery and greater risk for perinatal depression. Appropriately trained personnel must be in attendance, and in complex cases preparation may benefit from a pre-delivery huddle of the multidisciplinary team. Problems must be anticipated and prevented if possible, not simply treated. In infants for whom NICU admission is likely, a NICU delivery room team is required for each newborn.

The immediate postnatal goals are the same for multiples as for singletons, including resuscitation and stabilisation. Interventions in the delivery room will depend on gestational age at birth and clinical presentations. Resuscitation principles, as outlined in the Neonatal Resuscitation Program, include establishing an airway to support adequate oxygenation and ventilation, ensuring an effective cardiac output and maintaining appropriate temperature through drying and providing radiant heat. When respiratory support is necessary, a pulse oximeter and, at times, a cardiac monitor should be used for continuous respiratory and cardiac monitoring.

A physical assessment should be undertaken in the delivery room to identify malformations that were not prenatally diagnosed. A detailed newborn examination and careful observation may reveal subtle or delayed findings associated with a variety of anomalies and conditions.

Neonatal Intensive Care Unit Admission

Because multiple-pregnancy newborns are at greater risk of preterm birth, low birthweight, anomalies and other pathologic conditions, NICU admission is common. Preterm multiples of course require the same attention and care as preterm singletons, but the concurrent admission of high-risk multiplies may tax the personnel and resources of some units.

During the first hours of life in the NICU, multiple-pregnancy infants may require an array of diagnostic studies and procedures – including x-rays, central line insertion, endotracheal intubation, surfactant therapy and respiratory support – which may happen simultaneously and demand the specialised efforts of a limited group of individuals. Even after clinical acuity subsides, nurses at the bedside must constantly strive to ensure every opportunity for substantive family involvement by synchronising feeding schedules and coordinating bed placement so that siblings are proximately located in the unit.

After the initial hours and days of stabilisation, close monitoring for common setbacks must occur:

- Preterm, SGA and growth-restricted infants will require a thermal neutral environment with either a radiant warmer or a closed incubator that additionally will offer the advantage of decreased insensible water loss and provide a barrier to infection.
- Oxygen therapy, exogenous surfactant and assisted ventilation may be required to maintain adequate oxygenation. Continuous positive airway pressure or surfactant therapy may be indicated for infants with respiratory immaturity.

- A patent ductus arteriosus will often develop in the second to third hospital day. Some will require a prostaglandin antagonist such as indomethacin or ibuprofen, and surgical ligation may rarely be indicated should medical treatment fail.
- Whether enteral or parenteral, early nutrition is recommended. This may be limited by the inability of the preterm infant to suck and swallow effectively or to tolerate enteral feedings and may require parental nutrition and/or gavage feeding. Feedings should be initiated early and advanced cautiously, especially in growth-restricted newborns.
- Hyperbilirubinemia is inevitable in the smallest preterm infants and is generally managed effectively through careful monitoring of bilirubin concentrations and thoughtful use of phototherapy.
- Infection should always be considered in the preterm infant and many infants may receive short courses of antibiotics until blood cultures return negative.
- Immunisations should be administered in a full dose based on chronologic, not post-conceptional age.
- Infants at risk for retinopathy of prematurity, intraventricular haemorrhage and hearing deficit should be screened.

Admission of multiple-pregnancy newborns may present additional logistical challenges, particularly when the infants are at varying stages of illness and may require bed locations in the acute and convalescent sections of the unit. Some of these infants may qualify for transfers closer to the family's home or back to the birth hospital. Siblings seldom meet discharge criteria simultaneously and one infant is ready to be discharged or transferred before the other or others, separating multiples for days or even weeks. The NICU staff must make efforts to support parents through these difficult and vulnerable times in a caring and compassionate way.

Discharge Home and Follow-Up

Multiple-pregnancy infants born prematurely may be vulnerable and have an increased risk for long-term neurodevelopmental deficits.[20] These infants are not only at increased risk for post-neonatal illness and rehospitalisation, particularly in the first year of life, but they may also be at greater risk for child abuse and neglect.[18] Close follow-up by a primary care provider specialised in paediatrics or a medical provider with experience in complex care when appropriate, early intervention services and multidisciplinary infant follow-up may improve the infants' potential for normal development. Focused discharge planning is essential to ensure the family is ready and well supported for the transition to home.

Breastfeeding

Human milk and breastfeeding is the recommended standard infant nutrition by the World Health Organization (WHO) and the American Academy of Pediatrics (AAP). Evidence has demonstrated short- and long-term benefits of breast milk, particularly in preterm infants, including gut and lung anti-inflammatory properties, better cognitive outcomes, breast cancer protection for mothers and even lower risk for long-term adverse health outcomes like diabetes and obesity in adulthood. While there is strong evidence to support breastfeeding among all infants, women may have unique challenges associated with multiple birth, including frequent suckling, coordinating multiple needs and prematurity, where acute illness, NICU admission and mother–infant separation may delay and restrict breastfeeding. There are multiple options to support mothers with breast milk expression, lactation, use of pasteurised donor breast milk and different methods of supplementary feedings that may be considered.

A recent Cochrane review on breastfeeding education and support for women with twins or higher-order multiples found little consistent evidence about effective education and support practice, with evidence particularly lacking for effective interventions to support multiples.[21] On the other hand, support and education have been found to improve the duration of breastfeeding in healthy term infants.

Parental Support

Having a child admitted to the NICU can be very stressful and isolating, due not only to the very technical environment, but also to the uncertainty and disrupted parental bond. Parents of multiple infants may have additional stressors compounded by having more than one infant, possibly at varying stages of illness. Many families in the NICU may have social and cultural backgrounds that may add additional barriers. Barriers like communication with families with limited local language proficiency can be bridged with translated materials and trained interpreters.

Occasionally infants may be placed in different areas of the unit and very frequently one of the infants meets discharge criteria before the sibling. The NICU staff must make efforts to support families through the stresses inherent in 'leaving a baby (or babies) behind' and managing time between the baby(ies) at home and the one(s) still in the NICU. In worse circumstances, some families experience the emotional trauma resulting from the loss of one or more of the infants.

The mental health impact on parents, particularly of mothers, has been studied as the rate of multiple pregnancies has increased. Most studies that have compared mental health outcomes in parents of multiples versus parents of singletons found that parents of multiples experience heightened symptoms of stress, anxiety and depression. In the outpatient setting after discharge the paediatric provider should be attentive to identifying and addressing maternal depression in multiple-birth families.[22]

Financially, compared with singletons, multiple-birth infants consume significantly more hospital resources (e.g. increased length of stay and readmissions), particularly during the neonatal period and the first year of life. This might represent to the families a burden not only from healthcare costs, but also from lost days of earning.[4]

Key Points

- Multiple pregnancy is relatively common and most infants do well.
- The most common neonatal complication of multiple births is prematurity, which is the primary factor for elevated morbidity and mortality risk.
- Overall, morbidity and mortality in premature infants, including multiple-pregnancy infants, has improved due to advances in obstetric and neonatal care.
- Problems more likely to be seen in multiples compared to singletons include congenital anomalies, intrauterine growth restriction, placental complications, hypoxia and prematurity-related conditions.
- Because of the prevalence of high-risk conditions of multiple-gestation newborns, nursery staff must be prepared to identify and effectively manage the complications seen in these infants.

- Delivery room management of multiples requires individual teams to attend to the needs of the individual newborns.
- Parents of multiples may require specialised teaching, counselling and additional psychosocial support.

References

1. Martin JA, Osterman MJK. Is twin childbearing on the decline? Twin births in the United States, 2014–2018. NCHS Data Brief. 2019.

2. Murray SR, Stock SJ, Cowan S, Cooper ES, Norman JE. Spontaneous preterm birth prevention in multiple pregnancy. Obstet Gynaecol J Contin Prof Dev from R Coll Obstet Gynaecol 2018;20(1):57–63. https://doi.org/10.1111/tog.12460

3. Adashi EY, Gutman R. Delayed childbearing as a growing, previously unrecognized contributor to the national plural birth excess. Obstet Gynecol 2018;132(4):999–1006. https://doi.org/10.1097/AOG.0000000000002853

4. Chambers GM, Hoang VP, Lee E et al. Hospital costs of multiple-birth and singleton-birth children during the first 5 years of life and the role of assisted reproductive technology. JAMA Pediatr 2014;168(11):1045–53. https://doi.org/10.1001/jamapediatrics.2014.1357

5. Ely DM, Driscoll AK. Infant mortality in the United States, 2017: data from the period linked birth/infant death file. Natl Vital Stat Reports 2019;68(10):1–20.

6. Benirschke K, Kim CK. Multiple pregnancy. 1. N Engl J Med 1973;288(24):1276–84. https://doi.org/10.1056/NEJM197306142882406

7. Fuchs F, Senat M-V. Multiple gestations and preterm birth. Semin Fetal Neonatal Med 2016;21(2):113–20. https://doi.org/10.1016/j.siny.2015.12.010

8. Martin JA, Hamilton BE, Osterman MJK, Driscoll AK. Births: Final data for 2019. Natl Vital Stat Reports 2021 Apr;70(2):1–51.

9. Hubinont C, Lewi L, Bernard P, Marbaix E, Debiève F, Jauniaux E. Anomalies of the placenta and umbilical cord in twin gestations. Am J Obstet Gynecol 2015;213(4 Suppl):S91–S102. https://doi.org/10.1016/j.ajog.2015.06.054

10. Boghossian NS, Saha S, Bell EF, et al. Birth weight discordance in very low birth weight twins: mortality, morbidity, and neurodevelopment. J Perinatol 2019;39(9):1229–40. https://doi.org/10.1038/s41372-019-0427-5

11. Benirschke K, Kim CK. Multiple pregnancy. 2. N Engl J Med 1973;288(25):1329–36. https://doi.org/10.1056/NEJM197306212882505

12. Spitz L, Kiely EM. Conjoined twins. JAMA 2003;289(10):1307–10. https://doi.org/10.1001/jama.289.10.1307

13. Tollenaar LSA, Slaghekke F, Middeldorp JM et al. Twin anemia polycythemia sequence: current views on pathogenesis, diagnostic criteria, perinatal management, and outcome. Twin Res Hum Genet Off J Int Soc Twin Stud 2016;19(3):222–33. https://doi.org/10.1017/thg.2016.18

14. Arnold C, McLean FH, Kramer MS, Usher RH. Respiratory distress syndrome in second-born versus first-born twins: a matched case-control analysis. N Engl J Med 1987;317(18):1121–5. https://doi.org/10.1056/NEJM198710293171805

15. Leonard CH, Piecuch RE, Ballard RA, Cooper BA. Outcome of very low birth weight infants: multiple gestation versus singletons. Pediatrics 1994;93(4):611–15.

16. Babatunde OA, Adebamowo SN, Ajayi IO, Adebamowo CA. Neurodevelopmental outcomes of twins compared with singleton children: a systematic review. Twin Res Hum Genet Off J Int Soc Twin Stud 2018;21(2):136–45. https://doi.org/10.1017/thg.2018.3

17. Lorenz JM. Neurodevelopmental outcomes of twins. Semin Perinatol 2012;36(3):201–12. https://doi.org/10.1053/j.semperi.2012.02.005

18. McCormick MC, Shapiro S, Starfield BH. Rehospitalization in the first year of life for high-risk survivors. Pediatrics 1980;**66**(6):991–9.

19. Raju TNK, Buist AS, Blaisdell CJ, Moxey-Mims M, Saigal S. Adults born preterm: a review of general health and system-specific outcomes. Acta Paediatr 2017;**106**(9):1409–37. https://doi.org/10.1111/apa.13880

20. Litt JS, McCormick MC. Preterm infants are less likely to have a family-centered medical home than term-born peers. J Perinatol 2018;**38**(10):1391–7. https://doi.org/10.1038/s41372-018-0180-1

21. Whitford HM, Wallis SK, Dowswell T, West HM, Renfrew MJ. Breastfeeding education and support for women with twins or higher order multiples. *Cochrane Database Syst Rev* 2017 Feb 28;**2**(2): CD012003. https://doi.org/10.1002/14651858.CD012003.pub2

22. Wenze SJ, Battle CL, Tezanos KM. Raising multiples: mental health of mothers and fathers in early parenthood. Arch Womens Ment Health 2015;**18**(2):163–76. https://doi.org/10.1007/s00737-014-0484-x

Lifestyle Considerations for Multiple Pregnancy

Nathan S. Fox

Introduction

Currently, twin pregnancies represent approximately 3% of all births in the United States. Women with multiple pregnancies are at increased of nearly every pregnancy complication, most notably preterm birth and fetal growth restriction, but also hypertensive disorders of pregnancy, gestational diabetes, congenital anomalies and stillbirth. Twins are at increased risk of neonatal morbidity and mortality, mostly due to preterm birth, growth restriction and congenital anomalies. Despite the knowledge that multiple pregnancies are at higher risk of these complications, efforts aimed at reducing these risks have mostly not been effective. In unselected twins, the use of cerclage, pessary, bed rest and tocolysis have not been shown to reduce the risk of preterm birth or neonatal morbidity or mortality.

This chapter focuses on twin pregnancy given the paucity of evidence-based literature for triplets and higher-order pregnancies. To some degree, the advice given can be extrapolated to higher-order pregnancies on a common-sense basis, with perhaps more limited expectations for exercise and travel. Regarding lifestyle modifications for women with twin pregnancies, there are unfortunately few evidence-based recommendations even for singleton pregnancies. Therefore, aside from recommending folic acid to reduce the risk of neural tube defects, avoidance of alcohol and other potentially teratogenic exposures, avoiding injury and infections and staying current with vaccination recommendations, it is difficult to make lifestyle recommendations based on high-quality evidence to any pregnant woman, let alone one with a twin pregnancy.

Yet pregnant women do seek this information and increasingly they will turn to other sources online, in the lay press or from friends and family. While this is not problematic per se, it is important for obstetricians, midwives and other prenatal providers to let pregnant women with twins know what we do know and what we do not know, and at least what our best advice is under the circumstances.

Nutrition and Weight Gain

The Facts (What We Know)

The National Academy of Medicine published gestational weight gain recommendations for women with twin pregnancies, based on the pre-pregnancy body mass index (BMI):

- BMI < 18.5 kg/m2 (underweight): No recommendation made due to insufficient data.
- BMI 18.6–24.9 kg/m2 (normal weight): 37–54 lb (16.8–24.5 kg).
- BMI 25.0–29.9 kg/m2 (overweight): 31–50 lb (14.1–22.7 kg).
- BMI 30.0 kg/m2 or higher (obese): 25–42 lb (11.4–19.1 kg).

A few things should be noted regarding these recommendations. First, these recommendations were not based on high-quality studies demonstrating improved outcomes with these weight gain parameters, but rather on how much weight most women with twin pregnancies gain. In fact, the specific recommendations simply represent the 25th to 75th percentile for women with twin pregnancies. Second, these recommendations assume a pregnancy of 37–42 weeks. Therefore, for women with a normal pre-pregnancy BMI, the recommendation of 37–54 lb weight gain over pregnancy comes out to *at least* a pound per week. Since many women have difficulty gaining much weight in the beginning of pregnancy, this could be difficult to achieve without significant effort. Third, the recommendations do not address *when* it is best to gain weight in pregnancy. Are there times in pregnancy when weight gain is more important, or is it best to have a steady weight gain, or does it not matter? Finally, it is also possible that weight gain is a sign of a healthy pregnancy and not a cause of a healthy pregnancy. Even if a certain amount of weight gain might be *associated* with good outcomes, it does not necessarily follow that manipulating a woman's weight gain (increasing it or decreasing it) to fall within these windows will actually *cause* improved outcomes. This is a shortcoming of all observational studies.

Despite the lack of high-quality evidence used to derive these recommendations, several studies have examined these recommendations retrospectively and have shown that in women with twin pregnancies, achieving these weight gain recommendations is in fact associated with many improved outcomes. Achieving the minimum amount of weight gain is associated with a decreased risk of fetal growth restriction and a decreased risk of preterm birth. For example, we have published several retrospective studies of our own twin pregnancy experience and have consistently found a positive association between average weekly weight gain and improved outcomes in twin pregnancies. In our first study in 2010, we examined weight gain in 297 twin pregnancies and found that women with normal pre-pregnancy BMI who met the minimum weight gain guidelines were at significantly decreased risk of preterm birth < 32 weeks and fetal growth restriction and delivered babies with larger birthweights.[1] On the opposite end of the weight gain spectrum, in 2011, we published a study of 170 women with twin pregnancies who delivered at 37 weeks or greater and found no adverse outcomes associated with excessive weight gain as defined by the guidelines.[2]

For women with pre-pregnancy overweight or obese BMI, we also found that achieving the recommended weight gain was associated with improved outcomes. In a study of 252 overweight or obese women with twin pregnancies, women who achieved the minimum recommended weight gain had lower rates of spontaneous preterm birth, preterm premature rupture of membranes and fetal growth restriction.[3] Adequate or excessive weight gain was not associated with an increased risk of pre-eclampsia or gestational diabetes.

In our first attempt to study the timing of weight gain in twin pregnancies in 2014, we published a study of 382 women with twin pregnancies and a normal pre-pregnancy BMI and found that weight gain from before pregnancy to 16 weeks had a significant association with preterm birth.[4] In this study, the risk of spontaneous preterm birth < 32 weeks increased significantly with poor weight gain from before pregnancy to 16 weeks (Table 27.1).

Table 27.1 Weight gain from before pregnancy to 16 weeks

	≤ 2.0 lb N = 68	2.1–5.5 lb N = 65	5.6–10.0 lb N = 70	≥ 10.1 lb. N=73
Spontaneous preterm birth < 32 weeks	14.7%	9.2%	4.3%	2.7%

Risk of spontaneous preterm birth < 32 weeks in twin pregnancies, based on the weight gain from before pregnancy to 16 weeks of gestation

The results of this study were unexpected as we did not expect to find such a strong correlation between *early* weight gain and spontaneous preterm birth and we could not identify a confounding factor to explain these findings. However, since this was a retrospective study, it is uncertain if efforts to increase weight gain early in a twin pregnancy would be successful in reducing preterm birth, or even if they would be successful in actually achieving more weight gain.

In a larger follow-up study on gestational weight gain patterns, we examined weight gain in 609 women with twin pregnancies and a normal pre-pregnancy BMI.[5] We found that maternal weight gain from 0 to 16 weeks and from 16 to 24 weeks was most associated with improved fetal growth, whereas maternal weight gain from 24 weeks to delivery was most associated with a reduced risk or preterm birth.

In 2003, Barbara Luke and colleagues published outcomes for twin pregnancies managed in the Michigan Multiples Clinic, a specialised prenatal clinic for women with twin pregnancies that included the following:[6]

- Twice-monthly visits that included meeting with a registered dietician and a physician.
- Additional maternal education.
- Modification of maternal activity (work leave by 24 weeks, decreased strenuous activities).
- Individualised dietary advice.
- Multi-mineral supplementation.
- Serial monitoring of nutritional status.

The dietary and weight gain advice was comprehensive. For example, for women with a normal pre-pregnancy BMI, the recommendations included an intake of 3,500 calories a day and weight gain of 1.0–1.75 lb/week based on the gestational age. They published outcomes for 190 women with twin pregnancies enrolled in this programme compared to 339 women with twin pregnancies who were not enrolled in this programme and instead received usual care (study participants were not randomised). They found that women enrolled in this programme had lower rates of preterm birth, pre-eclampsia, growth restriction, NICU admission and neonatal morbidity. Programme participants delivered on average eight days later with birthweights on average 220 g (8 oz) larger.

Similar results were seen in the Higgins Nutritional Intervention Program in Montreal, which had similar recommendations as the Michigan Multiples Clinic.[7] In their study, which was also not randomised, they found that participants had a significantly reduced risk of preterm birth and low birthweights.

The Issues (What We Do Not Know and Problems)

Even if we accept that for women with twin pregnancies, improved weight gain is associated with improved outcomes, several important questions remain:

- Do attempts to achieve these weight gain goals lead to improved outcomes? This is really two different questions. First, do these attempts even lead to the desired weight gain? Second, would the desired weight gain lead to the improved outcomes? At this time, neither is certain, but most experts (including this author) believe both are true. It is possible to improve nutrition and weight gain in most women with twins, and it likely would lead to improved outcomes.
- What is the ideal diet for women with twin pregnancies? Although many scholars have put forth recommendations, there are no high-quality studies to guide recommendations for caloric intake, nutrient composition and micronutrient requirements.
- Are there times in pregnancy when nutrition or weight gain has the greatest impact, and might those times differ for different outcomes such as preterm birth and fetal growth?
- What is the impact of 'excessive' weight gain in twin pregnancies? Is there a point when weight gain becomes detrimental?

Management Options

In our practice, for women with twin pregnancies, we recommend the following:

1. We review the current weight gain guidelines for twin pregnancies. It is usually easier to present them in average weight gain per week rather than over the entire pregnancy.

   - BMI 18.6–24.9 kg/m2 (normal weight): 1.0 lb per week.
   - BMI 25.0–29.9 kg/m2 (overweight): 0.75–1.0 lb per week.
   - BMI 30.0 kg/m2 or higher (obese): 0.5–0.75 lb per week.

   For women with an underweight pre-pregnancy BMI (< 18.6 kg/m2), we recommend the same weight gain as for women with a normal pre-pregnancy BMI. We base this on the results of a study we published examining outcomes in underweight women with twin pregnancies.[8] In this study, we found that underweight women with twin pregnancies who achieve similar weight gain to normal-weight women with twin pregnancies had similar outcomes. Therefore, we do not recommend a higher weight gain for underweight women with twin pregnancies.

2. We recommend formal nutritional counselling for all women with twin pregnancies. We do this for several reasons. First, nutritional counselling takes time, and if it had to be covered thoroughly in a prenatal visit, it likely would either not be given enough attention or it would reduce the time needed for other important counselling. Second, it imparts on the patient the significance of this aspect of prenatal care. Third, the studies that showed improved outcomes with formal twin programmes all included dedicated nutritional counselling sessions.[6,7] Finally, not all prenatal providers have the expertise to help women with their nutritional concerns, especially those with specialised diets (plant-based, gluten-free, certain allergies etc.) or difficulty consuming food due to nausea or early satiety, both of which are common in twin pregnancies.

3. For women with twin pregnancies whose weight gain *exceeds* the recommended weight gain, as long as they are maintaining a healthy diet and remaining active, we do not attempt to modify their diet to reduce weight gain.

4. Regarding micronutrient consumption, if a woman is taking a prenatal vitamin and has a well-balanced diet, we only recommend supplementation with calcium (to achieve 1,000–2,000 mg daily). We only recommend supplemental iron if she is anaemic. Since our patients all have formal nutritional counselling, we try to have women receive their other micronutrients by eating a well-balanced diet. If they are unable to do so, we recommend supplementation as needed. We do not routinely measure serum vitamin levels in women with twin pregnancies.

Activity and Exercise

The Facts (What We Know)

Recommendations regarding activity in women with twin pregnancies are often restrictive and not based on high-quality studies. A Cochrane review found no benefit to routine hospitalisation or bed rest in women with twin pregnancies.[9] In routine pregnancies, women should try to achieve on average 20–30 minutes of moderate-intensity exercise four or five times a week.[10]

The Issues (What We Do Not Know and Problems)

Since women with twin pregnancies are at increased risk of preterm birth, it is unclear if regular exercise is beneficial, harmful or neither. It is also unclear if activity recommendations for women with twin pregnancies can and should be individualised based on history, symptoms, cervical length or other variables.

Management Options

In our practice, for women with twin pregnancies, we recommend the following regarding activity in pregnancy.

1. We do not routinely recommend bedrest.

2. We do not routinely recommend stopping working. However, we discuss the high likelihood that working full time will become more difficult as pregnancy progresses. Each woman will have to individualise her work schedule based on her specific job requirements, commute, and symptoms.

3. We do not place restrictions or limitations on sexual activity, aside from the typical restrictions for women with a singleton pregnancy, such as placenta praevia after 20 weeks, vaginal bleeding, preterm labor or ruptured membranes.

4. We recommend exercise similar to women with singleton pregnancies: an average of 20–30 minutes of moderate-intensity exercise 4–5 times a week. As with singleton pregnancies, the exact exercise, intensity, and amount of time will vary based on her prepregnancy exercise habits, her overall health status, and how far along she is in pregnancy. Women with twin pregnancies often have to modify their routines due to increasing uterine size and increasing fatigue.

5. For women with twin pregnancies and other factors concerning for preterm birth, such as contractions or a short cervical length, we do recommend modifying activities. There is no exact definition for 'modify' and it will likely differ for each woman. A good working definition would be a level of activity greater than complete bedrest, but less than whatever level brings about symptoms such as pressure or contractions. For some women that is very light activity, for other women it might allow for somewhat increased activity.

Travel

The Facts (What We Know)

Airline travel is considered safe in pregnancy, but since all pregnant women are at increased risk of thrombosis, and twin pregnancies especially so, it is probably prudent for women with twin pregnancies to take precautions to lower their risk of thrombosis, including compression stockings or periodic walking. Cosmic radiation is below the threshold level for fetal concerns. Women with twin pregnancies may go through security metal detectors as well. The radiation exposure from the newer backscatter units is 5 microrem, which is 1/600 the amount of cosmic radiation from the flight itself (3 milirem).

In regard to the travel destination, pregnant women should be aware of the potential infection exposures as well as the available medical care at each individual destination. Also, as pregnancy progresses, the risk of several pregnancy complications increases. Therefore, while there is no exact gestational age after which women cannot travel, each pregnant woman must balance the benefit of the trip with the potential risk of a complication at her destination.

The Issues (What We Do Not Know and Problems)

Since women with twin pregnancies are at increased risk of complications such as preterm birth and hypertension, it is unknown when exactly they should stop travelling, and whether this should be individualised based on history, symptoms, cervical length or other factors.

Management Options

In our practice, for women with twin pregnancies, we recommend the following in regards to travel:

1. In general, airline travel is safe in pregnancy.
2. Women with twin pregnancies should take extra precautions to prevent thrombosis, including frequent ambulation during awake hours on the plane. Since we recommend low-dose aspirin (81 mg) to all women with twin pregnancies, this might be preventative as well.
3. There is no exact gestational age below which women with twin pregnancies can be guaranteed that travel will be uncomplicated. Therefore, we advise women with twin pregnancies never to travel to areas without access to good medical care. When travelling to areas with access to good medical care, each woman must decide for herself the benefit of the travel versus the potential for a complication at that destination and how stressful or inconvenient that would be for her. In general, in an uncomplicated twin pregnancy, most women will travel within the United States and to developed countries until 28–32

weeks. After this time, usually they will not travel or will only go for short trips of great importance to them. Women with bleeding, a short cervix, preterm labour or other significant risk factors for preterm birth usually do not travel at all.

Key Points

- Women with twin pregnancies are at increased risk of pregnancy complications.
- There are very few high-quality studies to direct recommendations for lifestyle modifications in women with twin pregnancies.
- Improved nutrition and proper weight gain might be beneficial to women with twin pregnancies.
- In the absence of complications, most women with twin pregnancies can exercise regularly, continue working and have no restrictions in sexual activity.
- Most women with twin pregnancies can travel up to 28–32 weeks, provided they have access to medical care, do not have other significant complications and accept the small possibility of a complication at their destination.

References

1. Fox NS, Rebarber A, Roman AS, Klauser CK, Peress D, Saltzman DS. Weight gain in twin pregnancies and adverse outcomes: examining the 2009 Institute of Medicine guidelines. Obstet Gynecol 2010;**116**:100–6.

2. Fox NS, Saltzman DH, Kurtz H, Rebarber A. Excessive weight gain in term twin pregnancies: examining the 2009 Institute of Medicine definitions. Obstet Gynecol 2011 Nov;**118**(5):1000–4.

3. Liu LY, Zafman KB, Fox NS. Weight gain and pregnancy outcomes in overweight or obese women with twin gestations. J Matern Neonat Fetal Med 2019 [in press].

4. Fox NS, Stern E, Saltzman DH, Klauser CK, Gupta S, Rebarber A. The association between maternal weight gain and spontaneous preterm birth in twin pregnancies. J Matern Fetal Neonatal Med 2014;**27**(16):1652–5.

5. Liu LY, Zafman KB, Fox NS. The association between gestational weight gain in each trimester and pregnancy outcomes in twin pregnancies. Am J Perinatol 2019 [in press]

6. Luke B, Brown MB, Misiunas R et al. Specialized prenatal care and maternal and infant outcomes in twin pregnancy. Am J Obstet Gynecol 2003 Oct;**189**(4):934–8.

7. Dubois S, Dougherty C, Duquette MP, Hanley JA, Moutquin JM. Twin pregnancy: the impact of the Higgins Nutritional Intervention Program on maternal and neonatal outcomes. Am J Clin Nutr 1991 Jun;**53**(6):1397–1403.

8. Liu L, Zafman KB, Fox NS. Weight gain and pregnancy outcomes in underweight women with twin pregnancies. J Matern Neonat Fetal Med 2018 [in press].

9. Crowther CA, Han S. Hospitalisation and bedrest for multiple pregnancy. Cochrane Database Syst Rev. 2010 Jul 7;(7): CD000110. https://doi.org/10.1002/146518 58.CD000110.pub2

10. American College of Obstetricians and Gynecologists. Physical activity and exercise during pregnancy and the postpartum period. Committee Opinion No. 650. Obstet Gynecol 2015;**126**:e135–e142.

Emotional and Mental Well-Being in Multiple Pregnancy

Chapter 28

Lala Langtry White

Introduction

Pregnancy and parenting in any form continuously challenge and influence parents' mental and emotional well-being – as a collective family unit and as individuals – in a way few other life events do. The benefits of a parent-centred, holistic approach to healthcare in supporting the mind–body duality are no longer in question. Integrated care is crucial to support both aspects of an individual's well-being.

The additional mental and emotional considerations for families pregnant with or parenting multiples may be as unique as the person themselves, but, in my experience as a parent of twins and a parent of multiples (PoMs) support specialist, there are considerable commonalities that are rarely fully understood outside the multiple birth community. Families face significant and specific challenges during pregnancy and the first years of their babies' lives. A lack of quantitative research and feedback within this context contributes to a continued lack of sufficient appreciation, empathy and support. Using primarily an empirical and anecdotal approach, this chapter aims to highlight common concerns, observations and perspectives and provides considerations for healthcare professionals to better support the mental and emotional well-being of the mother and family – from pregnancy to parenting – following these fundamental steps: recognise, empathise, signpost and reflect.

Antenatal Considerations

Recognise and Empathise

As a healthcare provider, your first interaction with PoMs is likely to be discovery of multiples during a scan. Whether you are supporting a family with a genetic predisposition towards multiples, a pregnancy resulting from assisted reproductive techniques (ART) or a spontaneous planned or unplanned pregnancy, it is very likely discovering twins, triplets or more elicits a range of emotions that battle to be recognised simultaneously. If the information is first imparted within an empathic space allowing parents to process and validate new and possibly unexpected feelings and reactions, this paves a positive pathway for future emotional well-being, shaping the mental health support offered by healthcare professionals. Whoever gives this news sets the tone of all subsequent interactions.

Historically, societal reactions have varied greatly, from seeing multiples as symbols of luck to a fascination that has seen them subjected to anything from questionable exposure to a type of reverence. More common in modern, Western society is the culture of negatively clichéd statements such as 'double trouble'. Rarely amusing or helpful, these statements reiterate the 'rather you than me' ostracism parents of multiples (PoMs) often feel. Equally, if parents struggle with accepting the news, overly enthusiastic statements may also be inappropriate. Instead, allowing parents to form their own reactions, addressing their concerns and providing unbiased support and links to peers who may better understand or have shared a similar reaction, sets up a supportive approach from the outset.

Signpost

Being proactive in referring families to local, national and international organisations and support groups is essential (see Chapter 30). In addition, linking PoMs to well-established online social media groups provides an instant connection to other PoMs. This becomes more pertinent the rarer the subset: higher-order multiples, loss within a multiple pregnancy, twin–twin transfusion syndrome (TTTS), twin anaemia-polycythaemia sequence (TAPS) or parenting children with special needs. The possibilities are multiple. Finding others who share a similar experience can be an essential part of coping with the psychological component. While PoMs undoubtedly face a surfeit of challenges, there is also an unquestionable joy in parenting multiples. While this chapter may focus on mitigating the more challenging physical and psychological tolls of parenting two or more babies simultaneously, it is important to connect parents to the joys too. As a mother of two singletons as well as twins, I have observed a unique kinship between PoMs that simultaneously normalises, sometimes bemoans, but revels in the privilege of parenting multiples.

> I could reach out online, day or night, and without fail find someone, somewhere, instantly combatting my feelings of isolation who shared similar feelings of being overwhelmed. That non-judgemental understanding was (and continues to be) a lifeline for my mental health at some really challenging times. Though I never met the majority of parents in person, some were even on opposite sides of the world, we have bonded and followed one another through the challenges and the mini triumphs that may seem insignificant to other parents. We have supported and celebrated each other in a way I don't share with my friends who don't have multiples.

Many questions are likely to arise, for multiple pregnancy brings multiple scenarios of placentation, gender and fetal and maternal health alongside varied financial and familial dynamics. Many parents may be unaware of these differences and the implications for their healthcare requirements during pregnancy. The disproved theory that all monozygotic twins share a placenta still prevails, even within the obstetric and medical communities. Zygosity is important to know in terms of the medical and genetic implications, but also as part of the psychology of being or parenting multiples. Yet zygosity testing is not routinely offered to parents or comes at considerable cost, illustrating a lack of awareness of the effects on both child and parent. It is a belief of the International Council of Multiple Birth Organisations (ICOMBO) that same-sex multiples with undetermined zygosity have a human right to establish zygosity.[1]

While the potential obstetric risks of a multiple pregnancy are well documented and care plans are in place, the risks to parental well-being in relation to isolation, perinatal anxiety and depression are often overlooked. Although specific studies are lacking, the majority of evidence gathered to date suggests parents of twins or more are at increased risk.

A published study showed a large, unmet need for mental health treatment in parents of multiples during the perinatal period, especially the early post-partum months.[2] Two hundred and forty-one parents of multiples completed survey questionnaires: 197 were the mother and 44 were spouses/partners. The survey identified the first three months as the hardest, with few participants receiving any form of mental health support. The most common barrier to care was a lack of time. Forty-eight per cent would have been interested in some type of mental health treatment during pregnancy or the first year after birth. Participants reported a wide range of concerns, including elevated symptoms of depression/anxiety and stress levels, relationship issues and 'managing having multiples'. The lead author, a mother of twins, identified that 'eHealth strategies seem particularly feasible and acceptable in this population and may help circumvent common barriers to care'. A further small qualitative study in 2020 by the same lead author reiterated these findings, identifying 'experiences that were unexpected and unique to parenting multiples and indicated numerous desired aspects of mental health treatment. Interest in internet-delivered care was especially high.'[3]

Patient Psychosocial Considerations

From the outset, the path to parenting multiples may come with an increased incidence of emotionally challenging factors that may complicate parental well-being. The parental unit may not be limited to the mother. Establishing a psychosocial history whereby parents can choose the disclosures they wish to share with their medical care team would benefit all concerned. This would be achieved through a form with options to provide information such as:

- Language barriers, disability or learning support needs.
- Any influencing or additional factors the mother and supporting family dynamic would prefer healthcare providers were aware of. These may include ART, surrogacy, previous loss, trauma or abuse, female genital mutilation, financial disadvantage, familial and/or housing and living circumstances, insurance issues, cultural beliefs or practices relating to pregnancy and birth or LGBTQI+ parenting.
- How they would like to be referred to, encouraging inclusivity.
- Who will be part of the decision-making process relating to pregnancy, birth and care of the babies.
- Any areas in which they would like further support or signposting to additional services such as mental health support, breastfeeding education, antenatal classes for multiples, peer support groups and so forth.

This is simple, cost-effective and unanimously applicable. It provides an opportunity for healthcare professionals to take proactive, sensitive steps towards individualised emotional support in tandem with physiological care. Failure to recognise and address these areas can mar pregnancy and the parenting experience from the start with long-reaching and potentially devastating consequences continuing throughout the post-partum period.

This measure could be further evolved into identifiable visual prompts on paper or electronic health records so that parents need to provide this information only once. This can be applied to many of the aforementioned scenarios such as parenting after infertility, loss and surrogacy.

For example, in the case of families who wish their care team to be aware they are parenting after loss, UK-based organisations such as Dear Orla and SANDS offer identifiable, downloadable stickers to place on or within patient records to notify professionals that the parents in their care may require additional understanding and sensitivity. This is especially pertinent for parents who have lost one or more babies during multiple pregnancy, either spontaneously or through fetal reduction, and who may have to continue the pregnancy and give birth to both living and deceased babies. A unique potential dynamic in multiple parents is managing grieving for one or more babies while caring for one or more surviving babies. Giving emotional space to parents who experience loss at any stage and validating their experience and feelings along with offering signposting to specialised professional and peer support is essential.

The same sensitive acknowledgement could easily be applied to any influencing scenarios. Another area of awareness within multiple pregnancy is the lasting emotional impacts of infertility (see Vignette 1).

Vignette 1

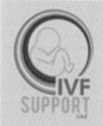

After undergoing a prolonged infertility journey there may be continued mental health issues to be considered, especially in the case of a multiple pregnancy. Issues of anxiety will tend to be amplified in these cases. Often there are medical issues which have prevented spontaneous conception resulting in the birthing person feeling like they have already failed as a parent. When pregnancy is finally achieved these feelings of inadequacy do not simply disappear. The person may well be more concerned than someone who has not had ART for the health of herself and her pregnancy. She may have over informed herself on potential risks of a multiple pregnancy and have many concerns and questions. Thoughtful, attentive listening, giving parents a sense that all their questions and concerns are valid and welcomed, being empathic and reassuring whenever possible is key in enabling the birthing person to relax into their pregnancy experience. IVF and other methods of assisted reproduction can be an incredibly stressful experience. The pregnancies that result from them are often beginning from a place of anxiety and stress which may continue through pregnancy and into parenthood. An understanding of that situation is important to families who are navigating their multiple pregnancy. This may be particularly challenging to identify within parents who have travelled overseas for fertility treatment due to restrictions within their own country and may feel unable to freely express how they're feeling.

Cassie Destino, mother of twins and founder of IVF Support UAE

Psychological Impact of the High-Risk Label: When Does Awareness Become Anxiety?

Though not specific to families of multiples, Wright et al examined the effects of high-risk pregnancy on the parental adaptation process.[4] The families included all had full-term, healthy infants, yet the appearance of high obstetrical risks appeared to negatively influence the perception of parental competence beyond pregnancy and into parenting. Further studies, articles and observations support this theory.

Most multiple pregnancies are automatically categorised as high risk. Attached from the outset, this label can provoke a range of reactions. Not all parents expressed a negative connotation: some embraced the feeling of uniqueness and heightened medical vigilance while others were ambivalent. Others reported feelings of increased vulnerability, hypervigilance, anxiety, resentment or disempowerment due to the change in expectations of pregnancy and birth. We know increased anxiety can result in detrimental physiological responses such as increased blood pressure, shortness of breath, increased cortisol levels and generally lower levels of physical comfort and mental clarity. This association extends to feelings of guilt, responsibility, helplessness and anxiety reported from birth partners.

An article by the Association for Improvements in the Maternity Services (AIMS) reflected that 'with the "high risk" label comes an additional reliance on care providers for information and guidance. The content and emotional tenor of this advice will be heavily influenced by the clinicians' background and experience. 'I saw two consultant obstetricians at two different Trusts and they were each concerned about entirely different aspects of my twin pregnancy! Nevertheless, the experience of talking to them was positive and I felt that they respected my right to make "unusual choices". I know this is not the experience many women have of maternity services.'[5]

Supporting parents psychologically so they can make an informed choice is especially important when considering the profound long-term consequences of fetal reduction. It is essential that healthcare professionals are knowledgeable about the potential for complications and it is equally important that they can inform and offer non-directive counsel to parents clearly, sensitively and without exerting personal bias (see Vignette 2).

The potential implications of this were raised in an article by Zager:[6]

Vignette 2

We were under the care of a respected fertility doctor when we became pregnant with our triplets following IUI. Our doctor strongly recommended fetal reduction to improve our chance of a pregnancy without complications. After considering our own circumstances [and] feelings and speaking to other triplets mothers, we declined fetal reduction and made this clear to our doctor. However, I was continually reminded of the hypothetical risks at each appointment, and felt stressed by the pressure exerted to reconsider; I was made to feel I was making a poor choice in continuing with expectant management in place of reduction. Although I am eternally grateful to our doctor for our treatment and resulting pregnancy, I would like to see a more individual, unbiased and respectful approach to counselling families on their options and supporting their subsequent choices.

Suman Manning, mother of triplets and founder of Twins Plus Arabia

For the woman pregnant with two or more fetuses, issues of termination for one or more of them produce anxiety, guilt, and the need to cope with decisions well beyond those of a usual pregnancy, particularly when they have resulted from infertility or similar treatments. The decision to terminate selectively certain of the fetus(es) so that one (or more) can be carried more viably to term represents a significant stress. The woman may continue the pregnancy with the remaining fetus(es), but she probably will be assailed with feelings of responsibility for the death(s) of the other fetus(es); feelings of sadness, guilt, grief, and mourning for them must co-exist with the more expected and positive anticipatory ones in the usual, wanted pregnancy. She will also be beset with increasing anxiety over the fate of the remaining fetus(es).

Studies within pregnancies deemed high risk (not specific to multiples) consistently report increased maternal depression and anxiety. It is therefore reasonable to assume that the high-risk label may influence perinatal psychological well-being and contribute to a lack of confidence emotionally and physically to trust in the body's ability to grow two or more babies without complication or intervention. In turn, this and the need for specialised medical support may cultivate a passivity in decision-making surrounding care choices for pregnancy and birth and unintentionally undermine parental instincts from the outset, potentially leading to a negative or disconnected birth or parenting experience.

If we take a family who has had a fertility-assisted path to conception, a high-risk, medically intense pregnancy who potentially began parenting within the neonatal intensive care unit (NICU), we can see that parental instinct and involvement can be unintentionally undermined by the necessary processes of medical care and a belief that the medical care teams at each stage know best. As a result, often women and parents perceive their role in the pregnancy according to the inverted pyramid model (see Figure 28.1). In this traditional paradigm, parents' personal knowledge, choices and instinct regarding their own and their babies' well-being are perceived as of lower value than those of the experts caring for them (see Vignette 3).

The question to ask as part of this team is: how can we lessen the culture of fear, anxiety and anticipation around the high-risk label in multiple pregnancy, increase the normalcy of

---

Vignette 3

From the very beginning of my egg-donation twin pregnancy, I felt I lost my ability to make sound decisions. I refused to invest – financially or emotionally – in my impending mother-hood and was consumed with fear. I feared pregnancy failure because I believed that my pregnancy was 'against nature'. As a 45-year-old woman in possession of one partial ovary, I had no usable eggs of my own. I believed that I was flaunting nature in being pregnant and that this would have a price. I feared the price might be pregnancy failure; what I see now looking back is that the price was my own ability to accept and enjoy my pregnancy and early motherhood. I felt that I could not have any natural motherly instincts as nothing about my pregnancy was natural. In pregnancy this meant I did not engage in the decision-making process. In early motherhood this meant I felt afraid and barely capable of parenting. In both phases I preferred to wholly trust and leave choices to medical experts believing they knew better than me. I regret not playing more of an active role in my pregnancy and allowing others to do so much of the mother role for me instead of in support alongside me. I am certain that my negative experience of pregnancy and the first year of motherhood was because I did not feel like a mother because I was not able to be a 'real' mother. Five years later, I am still not wholly rid of this belief.

E, mother of twins

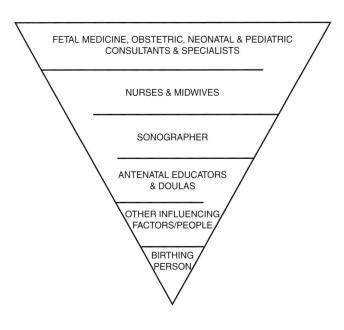

Figure 28.1 Provider Involvement in patient wellbeing

multiple pregnancy and create a more engaged and empowering experience for parents while maintaining a watchful awareness of potential issues?

Encouraging multiple pregnancy to be viewed as a variation within the norm rather than simply 'high risk' and ensuring parents understand the potential risks/complications in relation to their individual pregnancy plays an important role in framing parental confidence. We can help families understand that an increased *chance* of something happening does not mean it *will* happen and that awareness of potential complications does not equate to a self-fulfilling prophecy. Giving parents confidence to ask questions and feel fully informed rather than fearful creates a culture of trust. This may require providing longer appointment times for PoMs so that their questions and concerns can be addressed without feeling rushed as well as contact details for families to utilise outside of appointments if needed.

Reassurance that every element of the surrounding team is there to support them and their babies' well-being through pregnancy, birth and into parenthood as opposed to waiting to diagnose potential complications is desirable. Encouraging co-decision-making without dissolving the doctor–patient relationship builds confidence and trust in both the medical team and themselves as parents (see Figure 28.2).

Emotional Impact of Contested Interventions

This area continues to raise much debate within both the medical and PoMs communities. The recommendations of contested interventions such as bed rest, cerclage, progesterone treatment, high-protein diets and so forth are routine within certain care environments. While evidence for the physical benefits may be debateable, the emotional implications are varied and complex. Some parents report these interventions gave them a feeling of

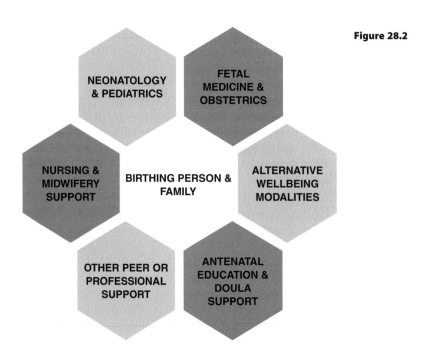

Figure 28.2

regaining control over their well-being. Conversely, others felt undue pressure and responsibility that their immediate actions could harm their babies in some way.

> My doctor recommended cerclage, progesterone and strict bed rest from 12 weeks of my IVF triplet pregnancy and I trusted she had our best interests in mind. I felt certain that this, coupled with a high-protein diet, were what got me through to my planned birth at 34 weeks. I felt I was taking every necessary and possible precaution to give my babies the best chance of being born at a good gestation and good birthweight.

Bed rest is notoriously challenging to mental health and often misunderstood by those who haven't experienced it as an 'opportunity to put your feet up and do nothing'. Individual circumstances may require consideration, but the disparity in blanket recommendations, particularly for triplets and higher-order multiples, from region to region or doctor to doctor raises concerns within the PoMs support networks. Some parents are adamant that it has/will lead to a healthy pregnancy/babies, while others who have not had such recommendations fear they may be jeopardising their babies' well-being by not doing so. For others, it may have ramifications on family life with older siblings, potential loss of earnings or early forced maternity leave diminishing the time allowance once the babies are born.

> My doctor recommended a cerclage would be prudent during my spontaneous triplet pregnancy. I did my own research and felt there was not enough evidence to support its use within my individual pregnancy. I presented my research and my doctor was supportive of my decision. I ended up carrying my triplets to week 36 without bed rest, interventions or a deliberate course of action other than listening to my body and not overdoing it.

Further clarity about such interventions would be beneficial for all parties, particularly in relation to the emotional impacts it has both on those to whom they are recommended and on those who worry about the lack of such recommendations.

Emotional Consequences of Physical Challenges

While it is important to recognise that many enjoy a comfortable and uncomplicated pregnancy, multiple pregnancy often increases the incidence and the severity of 'normal' physical pregnancy symptoms such as nausea, vomiting, muscle cramps, fatigue, haemorrhoids, pelvic and back pain, constipation, heartburn and varicose veins. Without generalising the distress these can cause, we must acknowledge that these physical tolls can enormously impact emotional well-being. Feedback from mothers showed many felt their challenges in this area were dismissed or downplayed; there was a 'just get on with it' attitude which significantly marred their enjoyment of and emotional well-being within pregnancy. It was especially highlighted by those who had experienced a singleton pregnancy and were taken aback by the difference in carrying twins or more. Listening with empathy, normalising without being dismissive and discussing ways to alleviate symptoms is desirable. Equally, be aware of perinatal specialists in alternative modalities such as chiropractic, osteopathy, acupuncture, reflexology and so forth that may help physically and provide an additional layer of emotional support.

Here too peer support can be of enormous, cost-free value and offer a perspective from others who have shared similar struggles. As mentioned previously, being informed of online and in-person support groups and, where possible, offering a space for regular meet-ups within your facilities is a responsible and proactive move towards ensuring greater social support for PoMs. Various evidence, as summarised by a Cochrane review, confirms that for 'women at low risk of complications and some at increased risk, but not currently experiencing problems', the midwifery-led model of care increased positive parent experiences.[7] It also led to fewer preterm births and fetal and NICU deaths. In multiple pregnancy, while specialist obstetric care may be essential, where possible, a multidisciplinary care model involving a midwife may offer additional support and serve to normalise pregnancy and postnatal experiences. Parents can raise questions they may feel more comfortable addressing with a midwife, meet other PoMs and benefit from group discussions and signposting to further mental health support services.

Antenatal Education

Antenatal education classes, whether in person or through eLearning, can be important for parents to develop well-being strategies. They can also provide information about local parenting networks and events which, for some families, are the beginning of their parent peer support community. Parents of multiples often report that while generalised antenatal classes are helpful to a point, segregation from singleton parents can exist and multiple parenting was an insufficiently covered addendum or an exception to 'the norm'.

During pregnancy is when PoMs generally have greater ability to take classes that are applicable to all modalities of parenting and classes that are more pertinent within the context of parenting multiples. For example, while statistically one in nine babies are born prematurely, NICU parenting is unlikely to be covered in depth within routine antenatal classes whereas around 40% of multiples require NICU or special care support after birth. Understanding factors regarding timing and mode of birth can encourage PoMs to find confidence in their decision-making. Likewise, mothers of multiples need breastfeeding education specific to multiples.

Multiple-specific antenatal education may manage parental expectations, emphasise mental well-being, raise awareness of symptoms for parents to be aware of and provide pre-emptive signposting to mental health support, as well as encourage self-confidence, self-reliance and inclusion. Incorporating classes within your practice or knowing where to refer to externally or online would be a proactive and positive approach.

Not Just One Day in Your Life: Making Birth More Parent Centred

Mode of Birth

Birth is unique and transformational for all parents, no matter whether they are parents to a single baby or to multiples. How a mother is engaged with, supported and cared for will have a lasting impact long beyond the day of birth. Within the context of twin births, we know there are many influencing factors when it comes to deciding the optimal timing and mode of birth. Ensuring these factors are fully understood by a family and framing the conversation so that they can take an active role in the decision-making process is important. An informed, competent parent should be the appropriate decision maker about what is best for their birth, with the support, expertise and guidance of their care team. Empowering parents in the decision-making process is essential in starting the parenting journey engaged and with confidence.

It is important that as guidelines are updated they are represented in the options given to families. Evidence shows caesarean birth is not the safest mode of birth as a blanket rule, but it remains the preferred mode of birth in many healthcare settings. As we continue to see high rates of caesarean birth for twin births, where all influencing factors are optimal, we need to question whether further professional development is required to improve confidence levels in changing practice. No parent wants to ask their care team to support them in a choice they don't feel competent or confident in, or to knowingly jeopardise the well-being of their babies, but we routinely see bias exerted and parents pressured to make decisions based on outdated practice, scaremongering or convenience. Parents who have gone through an ART journey often hear the phrase 'precious babies' used to influence a decision. While it stands to reason that no one would be any more cavalier with care for babies conceived spontaneously, once that hint of doubt or fear creeps in it is hard to make a choice based upon evidence and parental preference. This is another scenario where care shared between a multidisciplinary team of fetal medicine and obstetric consultants, together with midwives, may be beneficial not only psychologically but also physically (see Vignette 4).

Vignette 4

During the course of my MCDA twin pregnancy, I moved between two countries, experiencing a multidisciplinary midwifery/obstetric care model and then a purely obstetric-led system. Although a language of risk and a strong bias towards caesarean birth prevailed under both systems, my maternal wishes for vaginal birth felt more understood by midwives, who recognised and prioritised my informed birth choices as integral to my birth experience and birth outcome. I was fortunate that my pregnancy was uncomplicated and my first baby presented head down so that circumstance and perseverance together led me to a vaginal birth by induction, with an intervention- and trauma-free second-stage labour at 35 weeks. This enabled me to immediately follow my babies into the NICU, initiate breastfeeding without disruption and recover in good time to meet the physical, mental and emotional demands of caring for two premature newborns. My gratitude for my labour extends far beyond the birth experience; it served me and my babies in the immediate aftermath of my birth and set a foundation for the strongest possible start from which two lives could flourish. Having benefitted from the best of both, I would confidently advocate for an integrated care system which balances the obstetric expertise of intricate twin pregnancies with the parent-centred approach for which midwives are deservedly recognised. For, alongside medical aptitude, women-centred care that recognises each woman's social, emotional, physical, spiritual and cultural needs is vital for mothers faced with the unique risks, challenges and promise of birthing and raising multiples.

Brit Williams, perinatal fitness author and mother of twins

To be accompanied by Figure 28.3

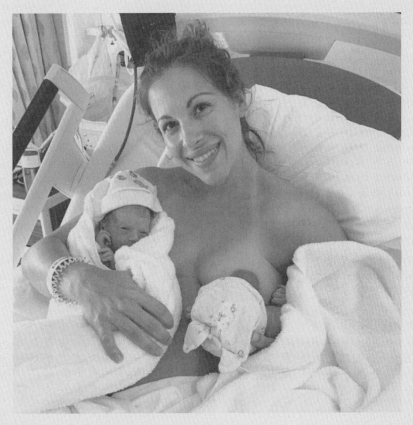

Figure 28.3

Changing the Language around Birth

Babies are not pizzas; they are born not delivered.

Rebecca Dekker, PhD, RN, founder of Evidence Based Birth

Small differences in language can have a big impact on how engaged and empowered a parent feels in the birth experience. Parents need to be supported with appropriate expertise rather than 'managed'. You may support a person's birth, but no matter how that baby is born, framing it as their birth rather than your delivery changes the onus enormously back to it being the parents' active experience than something in which they played a passive, secondary role.

Birth Support

Within the context of birth of multiples, other small differences can have a great impact on creating a parent-centred experience. An additional support person, whether family, friend or doula, in a multiple birth scenario may result in more positive birth experiences for PoMs.

> Due to circumstances in my pregnancy, my partner and I understood it was likely our babies would be born prematurely and would need to go to [the] NICU. It was my partner's preference that I went with the babies straight after birth and remained with them initially. My concern at that point was primarily for my partner's well-being and I felt hesitant at the thought of leaving her side. We chose to employ the support of a doula who was experienced in supporting multiples, who would remain beside my partner in theatre and into recovery, while I stayed with the babies. This was invaluable in making the day of our children's birth a fully supported experience of excellent medical and emotional care. I found great comfort and confidence knowing there was someone there to support us both, who understood what that day might look like for us from an emotional perspective and whose focus was solely on our emotional well-being. She was able to help my wife establish early expressing of colostrum and act as a liaison between me in [the] NICU and my wife in recovery.
>
> Father of twins

Allowing parents to create their own support framework, within logistical reason, enables them to continue to have choices, even when they may have felt restricted by the circumstances of their multiple pregnancy. For parents from the LGBTQI+ community, parents of colour, parents from indigenous or minority ethnic groups, parents with particular religious or cultural influences or parents birthing via surrogacy or from other minority demographics, allowing greater choice in framing the support system may be an important step in recognising individuality and fostering early parenting confidence without compromising the work and expertise of the medical team.

Birth Environment

Encouraging parental input and choice wherever possible can have a significant impact on how engaged parents feel, especially where parents may not have been able to choose the mode of birth they would have liked due to maternal or fetal factors. For example, they can choose who is there to support them, opt to make the environment and lighting more sympathetic and less clinical, make informed choices about pain relief and, crucially, provide informed consent at every stage of labour and/or birth.

> Being able to choose the song that each of our babies was born to was a small detail that made a big impact on reclaiming some individuality and choice in an otherwise, highly medicalised, caesarean birth experience for us as parents. Cutting the umbilical cord was something I'd always imagined doing as a father. Our doctor respected our wish for delayed cord clamping of two minutes and then cut the cords to be long so that I could cut them shorter up on the warmer which meant a lot to me and helped normalise and personalise our birth experience.

Navigating the Emotional Roller Coaster of the NICU and Special Care

Mental Health Support

A 2018 survey by UK-based charity BLISS revealed that 80% of parents whose babies were admitted into neonatal care think that their mental health suffered after their experience.[8] Some were formally diagnosed with PTSD and postnatal depression while many felt they had developed a mental health condition but were not formally diagnosed. The vast majority of families did not have access to formal psychological support during their time in the unit or once discharged home. With twins 10 times and triplets 30 times more likely to be born preterm, it is logical to take a pre-emptive approach towards addressing the psychological strain of parenting in the NICU. This preparative approach could be incorporated in the aforementioned antenatal classes specifically for PoMs, healthcare-facilitated group support meetings and peer support systems. Further research is needed to understand the unique dynamic that parenting multiples in the NICU presents.

Issues repeatedly raised by families of multiples with one or more babies in the NICU include but are not limited to:

- Feeling disempowered and helpless as parents.
- The emotional implications of having babies separated, be it to different beds, rooms or units within a hospital, or to a different hospital entirely.
- The additional financial strain and time constraints for both parents.
- The challenges of balancing older siblings alongside one or more babies in the NICU.
- Staggered discharge and the effects on parental ability to spend adequate time with either baby once one or more of a set of multiples is home when one or more remains within special care.
- The challenge of expressing for two or more babies.
- Establishing breastfeeding, especially when rooming in or parent accommodation is not available.

Starting any parenting journey within the NICU or special care is emotionally challenging. It may mean parents are separated from their baby having barely seen them, and this may continue for some hours or days depending on the health of the mother. Even parents who felt they had prepared for a NICU journey report being overwhelmed by the actual experience.

Even though we had older children and we had met the neonatology team and discussed what those first few days might look like, I was emotionally floored by the difference in experience from my previous births. Recovering from a caesarean birth, being separated from my babies, being placed in a busy ward with other mothers who had their babies with them, trying to express precious colostrum … the whole experience was incredibly traumatic and, I felt, the catalyst for my poor mental health in those early months.

It is essential that psychological support for the whole family be made a priority alongside the physical care of the babies in NICU. Where professional support within a unit is not possible, partnering with local or national psychological support centres and systems should be investigated and encouraged (see the list of support organisations at the end of this chapter). In addition to multiple-specific support communities, NICU support organisations provide another avenue for peer-to-peer support.

Family-Integrated Care

We know the evidence to support kangaroo care as a means of therapeutic and bonding practice for both parents and neonates is overwhelming (see Figure 28.4). However, parents consistently report feelings of anxiety or a lack of support in carrying out this practice. One reason seems to be the lack of clarity surrounding the stability criteria for babies before carrying out kangaroo care. Further research and clearer guidelines would benefit both staff and parents. It is also an area that parents who experience the death of one or more of their multiples during or after birth, particularly in relation to infection, may struggle with when caring for surviving multiples, and awareness of this and specialised support within units is essential. Understanding the benefits and risks of tandem or more kangaroo care with multiples needs to be similarly explored.

Involving parents in other aspects of their babies' routine care is also shown to have benefits both within NICU and longer term, post discharge. Most parents are not aware of

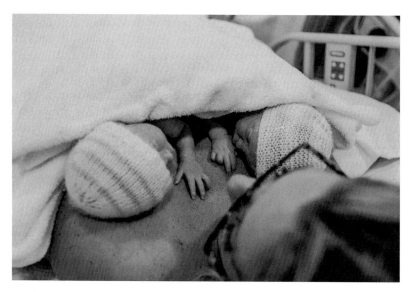

Figure 28.4 Skin to skin

how they can care for their baby when they first enter the ward; typically they express feelings of helplessness and being overwhelmed. Having supportive and encouraging staff to guide their involvement as early as possible is an essential way to care for both parents' and babies' emotional well-being. Taking time to show parents how to care for, feed, clean and hold their baby fosters parental confidence. It is also important to recognise that parents may feel they have surrendered much of their hopes of parenting and that important firsts such as first feed, first bath or first cuddle are momentous and must be respected and celebrated appropriately.

> Although I was rooming in at the hospital, I was shocked to come up to the NICU one night to feed my babies only to have a nurse share with delight that my babies had just enjoyed their first bath. To say I was devastated is an understatement, and I was so angry that my consent had not been sought, nor my desire to be involved even considered! I don't doubt she had my babies' best interests in mind, but I felt it was at the expense or ignorance of my well-being and [I was] robbed of another 'first' for my babies that should have been with me.

Parents who are encouraged to spend time observing their baby are more intuitive and often the first to notice if their baby is 'out of sorts', potentially enabling earlier medical intervention where needed. Offering signposting/access to specialised mental health support and allied healthcare professionals would be beneficial. Early lactation support for expressing and guidance in initiating non-nutritive sucking and then breastfeeding is especially valuable at this early stage. Acknowledging the mother's wish to work towards exclusive breastfeeding is imperative to ensure that her goals are aligned with those of the babies' weight gain and well-being. Many mothers report feeling that the goal within the NICU was to grow the babies to a healthy discharge weight and that this sometimes came at the expense of establishing breastfeeding. Creating a plan with the mother and care team to support both goals benefits babies' and mothers' well-being. Helping parents to understand the roles of allied professionals such as physiotherapists, dieticians and occupational and speech therapists creates a clear support structure for parents with babies who may have longer-term support needs from birth. It also offers a chance for parents to avail of additional emotional support within one place and before the time constraints of full-time care of multiples makes this more challenging.

Acknowledging Twinship While Cultivating Individuality

Parents of multiples describe feeling that their babies draw comfort from one another after birth and often find it distressing to see their babies separated, especially when this may mean hours of distance between them. While this may be unavoidable, reuniting parents and babies within a single unit must be a priority. The evidence to support co-bedding of twins or more in relation to co-regulation or therapeutic benefits is conflicting and in short supply. A Cochrane review raises the issues of infection, medication errors and caregiver satisfaction.[9] On the basis of the available evidence, the authors could not make recommendations for or against co-bedding and recommended further research. Parental feelings should be considered as the majority of parents embrace the concept of their babies co-bedding in the NICU, as long as it poses no risk to the babies' well-being. Where parents cannot be with their babies full-time, comfort may be drawn from the fact the babies have physical contact with one another, a unique advantage to parenting multiples.

While PoMs may be keen to keep their babies together, having them recognised as individuals within the NICU and during their follow-up healthcare is often felt to be in stark contrast to single babies. It would be surprising for a single baby to be referred to generically as 'baby' for an extended duration after birth rather than by name; however, multiples are often referred to as twin 1 or 2 for days, weeks or months after birth. While identifying multiples can be challenging and a clear difference in identification is undoubtedly needed for clinical care purposes, individualised care has a big emotional impact for parents. Having a simple white board or sticker system for each incubator or cot that identifies the baby's name, parents' names and multiple siblings' names where appropriate is a simple way to make an alien environment feel more personal and a way for parents to communicate with healthcare professionals when not with their baby.

Bereavement

Small differences in personalising care make a big emotional impact on parents. This is never more crucial than when supporting parents through the loss of one or more of their babies. The Purple Butterfly Project in the UK is one organisation concentrating on increasing bereavement support for families who lose one or more of their twins, and their awareness videos are an essential watch for anyone caring for multiples in an NICU setting.

One of their simple suggestions is offering a card or sticker with, for example, a purple butterfly to be placed on or within the cot of a surviving twin to acknowledge their bereavement and the twinship of the surviving baby/ies. Specialised bereavement support services that recognise the unique dynamic of caring for one or more babies when one or more babies has died are essential. Many hospitals offer memory boxes or memory making for bereavement and it is important where possible to take photos alongside their twin as this holds enormous value not just for parents, but also for surviving multiples. Parents often struggle to comprehend memory making at the time but almost always later report that it brings enormous comfort. Explaining this in a sensitive, unhurried manner and repeating, if necessary, so that parents understand all options available to them, is essential.

It is also a crucial role of the medical team caring for the surviving baby that they feel confident to engage with the parents who may want to talk about the baby they have lost, helping them to care for their grief within their unique context as PoMs. Where possible, providing privacy for families within the ward environment is beneficial. Be mindful that parents may have to return to the ward where they have lost a baby, or to see another baby in the cot or space where their baby had been while visiting their surviving twin, and this may be extremely traumatic. Empathy, validation and continued support are critical, especially when many families report having to 'keep it together' for the sake of their surviving baby and may seem to be coping on the surface. An instantly identifiable visual reminder such as the aforementioned purple butterfly helps staff to identify where additional sensitivity is required.

Acknowledging External Strains and Stressors

Additional time and financial pressures exaggerated by having two or more babies in the NICU are significant contributing risk factors to parental well-being. Alleviating stressors on parents at a basic level such as reduced parking costs and longer or more flexible appointment times should be considered wherever possible. Advocacy or lobbying for

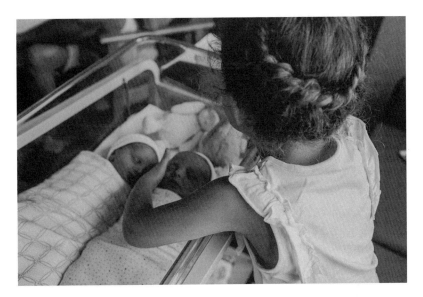

Figure 28.5 Sibling with twins in cot

better parental leave – both within individual scenarios through proof of medical care letters for employers and on a governmental policy level for parents of preterm babies and multiples – as well as for more comprehensive insurance coverage, where applicable, may shift the landscape of early parental support and well-being within the context of parenting multiples in the NICU. Family dynamics such as older siblings should be equally taken into consideration and helpful childcare strategies established, as well as ways to include them, focusing on the well-being of the family as a whole as they navigate the NICU together (see Figure 28.5).

> Our time spent in the NICU was a really emotional journey for our whole family. Our older children had limited access to us as parents and they were not allowed into the NICU to meet their siblings due to infection control policies. They had to be content with photos of the babies and a team effort of extended family and friends to keep their day-to-day routines running while we drove back and forth from hospital. Taking small steps to include them such as having them draw pictures and print photos of themselves that we could laminate and stick on the incubators, and in turn taking photos back to them, telling them how much their baby siblings loved them, went some small way to helping them feel included in caring for babies they had never even met.

This challenge only continues when one baby is discharged ahead of its multiple sibling(s); hospital policies vary enormously on the protocol for visiting the NICU with a discharged baby. Where there is no provision for support or care for the discharged twin, it creates additional emotional pressures and stress on parents, particularly in the context of older siblings and/or single parenting or where one parent has had to return to work. Offering options for rooming in or parent accommodation may not be feasible or practical in all scenarios, but it would be an important consideration for supporting physical and emotional recovery and the transition to parenting should parents desire this option.

Post-partum Well-Being

Post-partum Recovery and Adjusting to Parenting

A published study concluded that PoMs had 43% greater odds of moderate to severe post-partum depressive symptoms at nine months compared with mothers of singletons and that greater attention is needed in paediatric settings to address maternal mental and emotional well-being in families with multiples.[10]

Parenting rarely has a gentle introductory period, and this is never more so than with multiples. For a significant majority of mothers, it may also include the discomfort, restrictions and physical recovery period associated with caesarean or assisted birth. It is important that when discussing mode of birth prenatally, families understand these considerations as far as possible and the implications they can have for caring for two or more newborn babies as well as for their own sleep, physical comfort and emotional well-being. Though research regarding mode of birth as a risk factor for post-partum depression is varied, some empirical studies report that mothers who give birth by caesarean section are more likely to experience a negative self-image and anxiety. No matter the mode of birth, it is important that every mother be made aware of what the short- and longer-term birth recovery period may look like from both a physical and an emotional standpoint. Parents need to understand the role adjusting hormones play in emotional well-being – particularly over the first fortnight – how to recognise the 'baby blues' and how to differentiate between them and post-partum depression or anxiety. Although it is important not to generalise distress or expectations of the post-partum period, parents need to understand what those early weeks may look like, what is 'normal', how to cope with the extremes of exhaustion associated with caring for multiple newborns and when and how to seek professional support. Involving birth partners and those who will be closely involved in supporting the parents in the early days in this awareness is important for whole family's well-being and encourages active involvement and self-confidence in co-parenting.

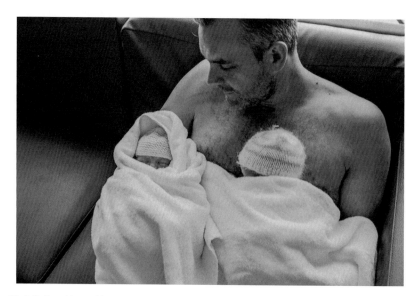

Figure 28.6 Father skin to skin

Demographics vary greatly from family to family and region to region, and the expectation of involvement and support from the wider family and surrounding community can have a big impact on the availability of support in the early days. It would be beneficial to encourage parents to consider in advance where they may be able to afford to hire help or draw support from willing helpers, whether that's practical support with the babies, meals for parents, housework and laundry or care of pets or older children.

Whether or not parents have invested time and money in gathering knowledge, researching and preparing for parenthood, once their babies are born and discharged from hospital the abstract and theoretical very quickly become reality. While all parents may feel overwhelmed as they adjust to life at home with a new baby, PoMs have an even greater adjustment to life as a family. While most parents will undoubtedly be happy and relieved to be at home with healthy babies, they may carry trauma from the experience of their path to conception, pregnancy and birth. Parents may have experienced the neonatal loss of one or more babies or be parenting a baby with special or high-dependency needs.

> I found it really hard to say out loud that I was finding caring for my baby challenging as it immediately raised feelings of guilt. I should have been caring for two babies and would have given anything for my other twin to have survived and things to feel even more overwhelming. I felt by voicing my struggles it might mean or be perceived that I didn't wish every second that he was there too. It was extremely confusing and I found very few people I felt brave enough to confide my feelings in. It accounted for a very difficult time for me emotionally.

The intense early weeks of caring for a newborn, or for two or more, may allow little time to process those emotions or in the case of loss, may serve as a constant reminder of what parents are missing. Parents of multiples are more likely to report low confidence and feeling overwhelmed.

Breastfeeding Two or More Babies

One of the most intense and emotive areas postnatally surrounds breastfeeding. Women need proper information about the value of breastfeeding twins or more, for both mother and babies, and about the risks of choosing not to breastfeed, in order to make an informed choice. Too often the perception or the societal bias is that breastfeeding multiples is not possible or is unrealistic, which undermines maternal confidence. In reality, breastfeeding multiples can be enormously challenging. A mother of newborn twins is likely to offer 16–24 feeds every 24 hours, and that number increases with each additional baby. Success is often let down by unrealistic expectations coupled with a lack of effective education and support.

Access to prenatal and early postnatal specialised support from a lactation consultant or breastfeeding counsellor (clinical background or peer based) confident in supporting mothers of multiples is a crucial provision for all families wishing to breastfeed their multiples. Parents of multiples are more likely to have preterm and/or low-birthweight babies, which can have significant impact on feeding efficacy and the early success of exclusive breastfeeding. Effective education and support in hand expressing, providing access to and explaining how and when to use a breast pump, giving practical help in tandem or individually positioning babies at the breast, explaining how to safely store milk and how to offer supplementary feeds where necessary, without potentially compromising breastfeeding goals, and mixed feeding all play an enormous role in success rates and maternal confidence. This in turn has enormous influence on emotional well-being in mothers wishing to breastfeed their babies. Lack of confidence, concern around adequate infant weight gain, worrying about milk supply and the challenge of transitioning from bottle to breast are standout challenges to maternal mental health for breastfeeding mothers of multiples in the early postnatal period. Acknowledging maternal feelings and goals and offering unbiased support, reassurance and encouragement are highly valued by mothers.

A published study[11] reported that women commented more positively on support from breastfeeding counsellors than on support from healthcare professionals, and they showed an appreciation of the counsellors' knowledge, experience, reassurance, non-judgemental approach and preparation to listen; another study found higher levels of breastfeeding knowledge and positive attitudes in peer supporters compared to student midwives.[12] This may be attributed to the fact that many peer counselling training programmes have a requirement that counsellors have personal experience of breastfeeding. Expanding peer counselling training within multiple birth support initiatives and improving accessibility to peer counsellors both in and out of clinical settings would benefit parents and alleviate pressures on healthcare services. We also know that breastfeeding success is greater when co-parents are supportive, so including them within the education and support framework is important (see Vignette 5).

Parents who choose not to breastfeed their babies also require support and clarity around safely preparing and offering feeds. Since the introduction of formula preparation machines and hands-free feeding pillows and aids a lack remains of clear knowledge and guidance on safe preparation and feeding practices. Parents are naturally inclined towards streamlining and efficiency when parenting multiples given the additional demands on their time. Understanding parental choices without exerting judgement while supporting safe practice is important in not undermining parental confidence while ensuring the well-being of their babies.

Vignette 5

This is more than a beautiful photo capturing a precious moment with my babies. It embodies everything I wanted motherhood to be and everything I worked hard to achieve as a single parent: the ability to give life to new humans, to feed them with my own body and to watch them grow and thrive. But this moment would never have happened without the help of an amazing breastfeeding counsellor and doula. She knew I didn't get the support I needed post partum from the hospital, their lactation team or our paediatrician. She understood that I was heartbroken, frustrated and lost. She helped me to latch and position my twins for the first time and then captured the moment in an image that will be a part of my heart forever. The care and attention I received when pregnant with my twins was intense. The number of doctors' visits and scans makes you feel deeply cared for and paid attention to. But the instant I gave birth I felt this virtually vanished. Post-partum care is very little about you anymore, other than the physical basics, and all about the babies, but as a new mother you still need care too. I felt tired, often lost, overwhelmed and sleep deprived. I felt I, like many multiples mothers I have spoken to, was left to slip through the cracks by the professionals and discouraged from breastfeeding as 'too hard'. This peer supporter and this moment shows that with time, patience and the right support everything is possible

To be accompanied by Figure 28.7.

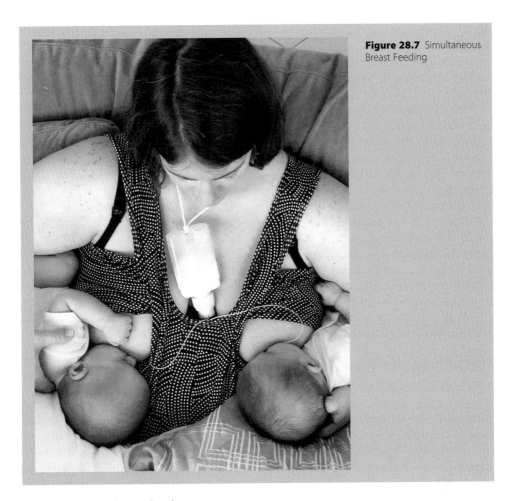

Figure 28.7 Simultaneous Breast Feeding

Safe Sleep with Multiples

Not many families have the luxury of space to easily accommodate two, three or more cots within their bedroom for the recommended six months of rooming in. The Lullaby Trust has one of the most comprehensive guides for parents of multiples and acknowledges the challenges associated with adhering strictly to all recommended guidelines; however, the guidelines are still very much directed towards singletons.[13] The realities of parenting newborn multiples mean co-sleeping is often key to precious additional sleep. However, the majority of multiples fall into the low birthweight and/or preterm category, for whom it is contraindicated, and there is a demographic of parents more likely to have anxiety relating to their babies' well-being or vulnerable child syndrome. Research into safe sleeping practices that accommodate the realities of multiple parenting is important both from a safety aspect and to better support parent post-partum adjustment, confidence and well-being.

Encouraging Postnatal Support Frameworks and Fostering Self-Confidence

It is not always an easy adjustment to go from the intensity and frequency of antenatal healthcare appointments, possibly preceded by a fertility journey and then followed with a

NICU journey, and then transition to life at home without the same routine level of contact and reassurance from healthcare experts. Helping parents to understand that it may be a period of adjustment and guiding them on where they can reach out for help is important in mitigating feelings of abandonment, uncertainty, self-doubt and isolation in their new, parent-led dynamic.

Given the significantly increased time and financial constraints of multiple parenting it is not uncommon to see parents place less emphasis on their own well-being and they are unlikely to be motivated or feel able to seek help, particularly during the early months, outside of routine or necessary appointments for their babies. In these settings it would be prudent for healthcare providers who are likely to be in contact with parents during pregnancy, through birth, the NICU and into parenthood to consider additional measures they can put in place to offer tangible support or signposting where necessary.

Where it is not possible to offer individual support sessions to families postnatally, alternative methods of support should be considered such as finding collective group support facilitated by a healthcare professional, encouraging parents to be proactive in getting together and exploring further the efficacy of e-consultations, e-counselling, tele-therapy or cyber-counselling for mental well-being, lactation and general parenting support. This is particularly pertinent for families recognised as suffering from or vulnerable to PTSD, anxiety and postnatal mood disorder/depression, especially if those families have self-identified and requested support.

Life with Two or More Babies

Within this same context it is important to normalise with empathy the exhaustion of parents caring for two or more babies who may likely have independent sleep and feeding routines, certainly initially. This is where peer support is of undeniable value as it really is hard to comprehend quite how much more challenging multiple parenting can be in terms of sleep deprivation unless you've experienced it first-hand. Understanding subtle differentiations that have a big emotional difference is important. For example, since the majority of multiples are likely to be born before 37 weeks and are at increased risk of developmental delays, it may be months of keeping up with the physical and emotional demands of parenting before you get those heart-warming smiles that punctuate the natural take-take character of a newborn. Families who have parented one or more children previously frequently report being surprised by the big differences in parenting twins or more, but also tend to show a greater resolve to 'just get on with it', knowing it will eventually get easier.

> I underestimated how much more challenging it would be co-parenting twins. With our first child I willingly helped out ad hoc at nights when my partner needed support but with our twins it was clear we needed to work as a team day and night. The unrelenting exhaustion for both of us put a strain on our relationship, our family and work, but I'm proud that we all got through it and I believe it ultimately made us all a stronger, more bonded family for it.

Effective co-parenting may look different for every family and may not be an option for everyone, but it is prudent to discuss and encourage it wherever possible. In turn, the greater toll on *both* parents' mental and emotional well-being is important to recognise. Though parenting multiples often comes with challenges, raising multiples brings many joys. Most parents feel incredibly privileged to parent multiples and to observe the growing interaction between their babies as they discover one another and become playmates. Some parents report assuaged negative emotions at leaving their babies or returning to work because the babies have one another for comfort and company, a point that also raises the understandable resentment PoMs may have at having no different parental leave than parents of a singleton. As with all parenting, the challenges of the early months may lessen as others evolve. Parents of multiples have an increased chance of parenting children with moderate or severe developmental delays or dependency needs. Simple family outings can often result in being treated as or perceiving themselves as a nuisance with larger strollers, greater noise volume, extra pairs of hands to fiddle or children to keep an eye on.

Conclusion

There is no better demographic than PoMs themselves from which to gain first-hand knowledge about the mental and emotional considerations that come with parenting multiples. I would encourage you to take the steps outlined at the beginning of this chapter and adopt them into your care: recognise, empathise, signpost and reflect.

References

1. http://icombo.org/wp-content/uploads/2010/11/Declaration-of-Rights.pdf

2. Wenze SJ, Battle CL. Perinatal mental health treatment needs, preferences, and barriers in parents of multiples. J Psychiatr Pract 2018 May;24(3):158–68. https://doi.org/10.1097/PRA.0000000000000299. PMID: 30015786

3. Wenze SJ, Miers QA, Battle CL. Postpartum mental health care for mothers of multiples: a qualitative study of new mothers' treatment preferences. J Psychiatr Pract. 2020 May;26(3):201–14. https://doi.org/10.1097/PRA.0000000000000469. PMID: 32421291

4. Wright J, Belanger C, Delude D. The effects of pregnancy complications on the parental adaptation process. J Reprod Infant Psychol 2000;18(1):5–20. https://doi.org/10.1080/02646830050001645

5. Whistler J. Are twins always high risk? AIMS J 2011;23(4).

6. Zager R. Glob. libr. women's med. (ISSN: 1756-2228) 2009. https://doi.org/10.3843/GLOWM.10155

7. Sandall J, Soltani H, Gates S, Shennan A, Devane D. Midwife-led continuity models versus other models of care for childbearing women. Cochrane Database Syst Rev 2016;(4). Art. No.: CD004667. https://doi.org/10.1002/14651858.CD004667.pub5

8. www.bliss.org.uk/news/bliss-releases-new-research-on-mental-health

9. Lai N, Foong S, Foong W, Tan K. Co-bedding in neonatal nursery for promoting growth and neurodevelopment in stable preterm twins. Cochrane Database Syst Rev 2016;(4). Art. No.: CD008313. https://doi.org/10.1002/14651858.CD008313.pub3

10. Choi Y, Bishai D, Minkovitz CS. Multiple births are a risk factor for postpartum maternal depressive symptoms. Pediatrics 2009;123(4):1147–54. https://doi.org/10.1542/peds.2008-1619

11. Graffy J, Taylor J. What information, advice and support do women want with breastfeeding? Birth 2005;32(3):179–86. https://doi.org/10.1111/j.0730-7659.2005.00367.x

12. Darwent KL, Kempenaar LE. A comparison of breastfeeding women's, peer supporters' and student midwives' breastfeeding knowledge and attitudes. Nurse Educ Pract 2014;14(3):319–25. https://doi.org/10.1016/j.nepr.2014.02.004. Epub 2014 Feb 19.

13. www.lullabytrust.org.uk/safer-sleep-advice/twins

GLOBAL SUPPORT RESOURCES FOR FAMILIES WITH PREMATURE/ SICK BABIES

Argentina
http://psicologialp.blogspot.com

Australia
www.lifeslittletreasure.org.au
www.miraclebabies.org.au/index.php
www.pipa.org.au
www.prembaby.org.au

Austria
www.frueh-r-leben.at
www.kleine-helden.at

Belarus
www.facebook.com/rano.by
http://premature.by/en/1183-2

Belgium
www.vvoc.be

Brazil
www.prematuridade.com

Bulgaria
www.premature-bg.com

Canada
www.cpbf-fbpc.org
www.lifewithababy.com

Chile
www.facebook.com/asprem.chile.2
www.neovidas.cl

Colombia
www.milagrosdevida.org

Costa Rica
https://m.facebook.com/fundaprema

Croatia
https://palcici.hr

Cyprus
www.facebook.com/morathavmata

Czech Republic
www.nedoklubko.cz

Denmark
https://praematur.dk

Dominican Republic
http://pequenasvidas.weebly.com

Estonia
www.facebook.com/EnneaegsedLapsed

Finland
www.kevyt.net

France
www.sosprema.com/page/173781-accueil

Germany
www.fruehgeborene.de

Ghana
www.afpncvoice.org
http://littlebigsoulsghana.com

Greece
http://ilitominon.org

Hungary
https://koraszulott.com
www.mellettedahelyem.hu

Iceland
www.fyrirburar.is

Ireland
www.inha.ie

Israel
https://pagim.net

Italy
www.fruehgeborene-suedtirol.com
www.nostrofiglio.it/neonato/prematuro/bambini-prematuri
www.piccinopiccio.it/home.html
www.progettopulcino.org
www.vivereonlus.com

Kazakhstan

www.vivereonlus.com

Latvia

www.esmu-klat.lv

Lithuania

www.neisnesiotukas.lt

Mexico

http://conamorvenceras.org

https://sites.google.com/site/proyectonacertemprano/mision

Netherlands

https://beta.prematurendag.nl

www.care4neo.nl

www.kleinekanjers.nl

https://nee-eten.nl

New Zealand

www.neonataltrust.org.nz

Nigeria

www.littlebigsouls.org

North Macedonia

www.lulka.org/index.php/mk

Norway

www.prematurforeningen.no

Poland

www.fundacjaswiadomirodzice.pl

https://wczesniak.pl

Portugal

www.nascer-prematuro.pt

www.xxs-prematuros.com

Romania

https://asociatiaprematurilor.ro

http://babycaresibiu.ro/en/home

https://unusiunu.com

Russia

https://fond-providenie.ru

http://pravonachudo.ru

www.sunlightfond.ru

Slovakia
www.malicek.sk

South Africa
www.facebook.com/preemieconnect

Spain
http://aprem-e.org

https://prematura.info

www.seneo.es

Sweden
http://prematurforbundet.se

www.prematurmirakel.se

Taiwan
www.pbf.org.tw

Turkey
https://elbebekgulbebek.org

Ukraine
www.facebook.com/ranniptashky

United Kingdom
www.bliss.org.uk

www.leosneonatal.org

www.smallandmightybabies.com

www.tinylife.org.uk

www.tommys.org

United States
https://grahamsfoundation.org

www.handtohold.org

www.marchofdimes.org

https://nicuparentnetwork.org

Uruguay
www.facebook.com/aupaprem

Vietnam
www.newbornsvietnam.org

SUPPORT AND RESOURCES FOR SPECIFIC CONDITIONS

Gestational Diabetes
www.diabetes.org/diabetes/gestational-diabetes

www.gestationaldiabetes.co.uk/gestational-diabetes-support

Necrotising Enterocolitis

www.necuk.org.uk

Pre-eclampsia

https://action-on-pre-eclampsia.org.uk/public-area

www.preeclampsia.org

Primary Immunodeficiencies

https://ipopi.org

Spina Bifida and Hydrocephalus

www.ifglobal.org

Twin Anaemia-Polycythaemia Sequence (TAPS) Support

www.tapssupport.com

Twin–Twin Transfusion Syndrome (TTTS)

See Facebook for closed parent support communities worldwide.

www.facebook.com/groups/tttsfoundation

www.facebook.com/Twin-to-Twin-Transfusion-Syndrome-TTTS-Parents-Arabia

www.facebook.com/Twin-to-Twin-Transfusion-Syndrome-Support-Page

www.tttsfoundation.org/index.php

Support Resources for Loss/Bereavement
International

www.stillbirthalliance.org

Australia

www.bearsofhope.org.au

www.theperinatallosscentre.com.au

www.pregnancylossaustralia.org.au

www.sands.org.au

Italy

www.ciaolapo.it

Kenya

https://stillamum.com

United Kingdom

https://babyloss-awareness.org

www.childbereavementuk.org

http://childdeathhelpline.org.uk

www.miscarriageassociation.org.uk

www.neonatalbutterflyproject.org/about-us

https://petalscharity.org

www.sands.org.uk

United States

www.the2degrees.org/nj-support-groups.html

http://nationalshare.org

https://pregnancyafterlosssupport.org

https://starlegacyfoundation.org/for-families-and-friends

www.walkinsunshinecharity.org

Singapore

www.cbss.sg

www.facebook.com/AngelHearts.SG

www.facebook.com/groups/240500147193415/?source_id=53462200688

Spain

www.umamanita.es

New Zealand

www.babyloss.co.nz

www.miscarriagesupport.org.nz

Pregnancy, Birth and Parenting Equity

https://birthequity.org

https://blackmamasmatter.org

http://blackmothersbreastfeeding.org

www.sistamidwife.com

LGBTQI+

www.facebook.com/148739775166504/videos/1465806753615504

www.familyequality.org/family-building/path2parenthood

www.hrc.org/resources/professional-organizations-on-lgbt-parenting

www.proud2bparents.co.uk/home.html

www.psychology.org.au/getmedia/9ea8dd55-7c2b-4653-8371-b1f732b70b58/LGBT_pregnancy_loss.pdf

Termination of Pregnancy Support

www.aheartbreakingchoice.com

www.arc-uk.org/for-parents/ending-a-pregnancy

www.safeabortionwomensright.org

Twinless Twins

www.twinlesstwins.org

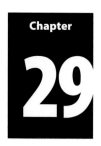

Chapter 29

New Frontiers in Multiple Pregnancy Management

Caroline J. Shaw and Christoph C. Lees

The Facts

Multiple pregnancy is widely understood to carry higher risks – that increase with the number of fetuses – of adverse perinatal outcome when compared to singleton pregnancy. While this is due to higher rates of premature delivery, fetal growth restriction and congenital malformations, it is also important not to underestimate the impact of complications uniquely associated with monochorionic placentation irrespective of fetal number. Even in the context of current assisted reproductive technology, about one-fifth of twins are monochorionic. The fall in overall twin pregnancy perinatal mortality in the UK following the introduction of evidence-based, chorionicity-specific national standards for antenatal care is an important achievement. However, it clearly demonstrates the burden of monochorionicity, and this may explain why research in multiple pregnancy appears disproportionally focused on the development of diagnostic and treatment modalities for monochorionic twins or dichorionic triplets when compared to dichorionic twins or even trichorionic triplets. Although the 'hidden mortality of monochorionic twins' was a phrase coined more than two decades ago, its message holds true.

The excess mortality of monochorionic multiple pregnancy is attributable to complications of a shared placental circulation; anastomoses between the vessels of what ideally should be separate circulations are found in up to 90% of monochorionic placentae. They may form artery to artery (AAA), artery to vein (AVA) or vein to vein (VVA), and have been found both superficially and deep within the placental cotyledon.[1] The consequences of a shared placentation and the presence of placental vascular anastomoses include twin–twin transfusion syndrome (TTTS), twin anaemia-polycythaemia sequence (TAPS), twin-reversed arterial perfusion (TRAP) sequence, selective intrauterine growth restriction (sIGUR) and a risk of co-twin death or ischaemic-hypoxic brain or organ injury in the event of a single intrauterine fetal death (sIUFD). Of these, TTTS is the leading cause of perinatal mortality in all twins.

The Issues

The disparity in second-trimester fetal loss between monochorionic and dichorionic twins – or mono/dichorionic and trichorionic triplets – is acknowledged to be primarily due to TTTS, a disease which currently cannot be screened for, nor can patient risk stratification be performed. Management strategies are based on regular review to detect early disease stages by ultrasound examination and timely intervention where indicated. Fetoscopic laser has emerged as the leading intervention, rather than amnioreduction or selective termination of one fetus with radiofrequency ablation (RFA) or bipolar cord occlusion. This is despite a 2013 Cochrane review demonstrating neither a survival advantage nor a reduction in major neurological abnormality at the age of six years when treatment with fetoscopic laser is compared to amnioreduction.[2] Fetoscopic laser treatment of TTTS continues to be recommended as it reduces the rate of minor neurological abnormalities at the age of six years.

A current Cochrane review identifies that further research is needed in the appropriate treatment for less severe disease (stages I–II); this is an advance from the previous version, which concluded that further research was needed only for the appropriate treatment of stage I disease. These conclusions infer a more basic lack of medical and scientific knowledge: the natural history of TTTS remains unclear. While the Quintero stage at diagnosis is prognostic of perinatal outcome, a nearly equal chance remains that stage I disease will remain stable, regress or progress once diagnosed. Hence, for any particular family, specific – or customised – outcomes remain difficult to approximate, making the burden of choosing between the risks of expectant management and intervention a heavy one. Similarly, in pregnancies diagnosed with TRAP sequence, a one-third chance remains of spontaneous resolution with invasive treatment, but determinants on which families can choose to safely pursue expectant management remain uncharacterised. So too, in the management of selective growth restriction, where termination of the growth-restricted fetus can be considered to prevent the potential consequences of sIUFD to the appropriately grown surviving twin, there is little understanding of why some co-twins suffer hypoxic-ischaemic injury, but the majority do not.

These questions shine a light on perhaps the least understood area of monochorionic pregnancies: the function of the placental vasculature within the shared placental portion. Histological and dye injection studies have demonstrated the anatomical structure of the monochorionic placenta with its multiple anastomotic connections; however, there is very limited functional assessment of the placenta in vivo. How a vessel that is histologically a vein functions when connected to another vein may, for example, be different to how it functions when it is anastomosed to an artery. Veins used as conduits for arterial flow have been shown to have greater incidence of endothelial injury due to haemodynamic stresses when compared to arteries, as well as poor elastic recoil, increased stiffness and turbulent flow beyond the point of anastomosis with a reduction in the mean blood flow velocity, yet none of these features have been described in placental AVAs to date.

Here, then, is our first frontier: a better understanding of the pathophysiology of disease in monochorionic placentae is needed. For this, a better understanding of normal and abnormal function of the shared circulation in the monochorionic placenta is a prerequisite. The lack of a preclinical model for the monochorionic placenta which mimics the gross shape, the haemochorial nature of the materno-fetal interface and the anatomy of shared placental portion has limited the amount of basic scientific research in this field.[3] However, the National Institute of Child Health and Human Development (NICHD) Human Placenta Project, which aspires in part to develop new technologies for real-time assessment of placental development across normal and abnormal pregnancies, has regenerated a timely interest in technologies for both ex vivo models and in vivo assessment of the human placenta, which may be applicable to the monochorionic placenta.[4] Only with better understanding of the pathophysiology of monochorionic placental disease can we move from observational, population-based statistics to individualised assessment of likely outcomes.

Closely related is our second frontier: how to ease the burden of decision-making on families with multiple pregnancies. Even if supplied with customised prognostications of disease outcome, many of the available interventions intended to further inform or reduce the risks associated with multiple pregnancy involve invasion into the intrauterine space, requiring the acceptance of the risk of associated iatrogenic miscarriage or pregnancy loss if they are chosen over expectant management. As the research revealing high levels of support among women for non-invasive prenatal testing for chromosomal anomaly compared to chorionic villous sampling (CVS) or amniocentesis has shown, concerns related to miscarriage are a key motivator in rejecting invasive procedures. Given that CVS, amniocentesis, fetoscopic laser, radio-frequency ablation and in utero transfusion are already minimally invasive procedures and remain associated with iatrogenic pregnancy loss, this suggests the focus should be on non-invasive therapies or techniques to mitigate the damage caused by intrauterine invasion. While decisions regarding individual fetuses within a multiple pregnancy have additional complexities of bereavement reactions despite ongoing pregnancy, reducing the risk of procedure-related pregnancy loss can only be a benefit.

Research Avenues

Assessment of Multiple-Pregnancy Placental Vasculature and Function Using Diagnostic Imaging

In a research setting the structure and, to a lesser degree, the function of placental anastomoses within the shared region of the monochorionic placenta have been investigated using both Doppler ultrasound and MR angiography. Additionally, the function of the materno-fetal interface in both monochorionic and dichorionic twin pregnancy has been assessed using MRI.

Standard 2D colour and pulse-wave Doppler techniques can be used to identify both AAAs and AVAs.[5-7] The AAAs appear easier to locate with a sensitivity of 85% and specificity of 97% compared to placental injection studies,[5] while AVAs have a lower sensitivity of 50% but retain a reported specificity of 93–97%.[6,7] Recently the use of 3D high-definition flow between the cord insertions of the twins co-registered with tomographic ultrasound imaging (TUI) has improved the sensitivity for AVAs to 88% while maintaining a high sensitivity.[8] Tomographic ultrasound imaging combines spatial tracking of the ultrasound probe (typically using spatial sensors attached to the probe) with the diagnostic imaging obtained during the probe movements. This offers the possibility of ultrasound post-processing, as in this application, to display multiple parallel sections of the placenta, allowing identification of both superficial and deep anastomoses.

Innovation in colour Doppler imaging may also have a role to play in this field. Conventional colour Doppler imaging within obstetrics employs a wall filter to reduce motion artefacts and remove low-flow 'noise' that could contaminate the ultrasound signals so as to optimise identification of high-flow vessels within the fetal circulation and umbilical cord. However, the loss of the low-flow signal compromises the imaging capabilities for microvascular circulations such as placental vessels and anastomoses. Colour Doppler applications such as superb microvascular imaging (SMI) or advanced dynamic flow (ADF) focus on flow distribution in the region of interest using a high-density ultrasound system architecture.[9,10] This enables the processed ultrasound image to identify and remove global motion signals while preserving very low-flow (SMI < 1 cm.s^{-1}) and low-flow components (ADF < 10 cm.s^{-1}), hence enabling visualisation of placental microvasculature with a much greater degree of clarity than simply reducing the scale of conventional colour Doppler (Figure 29.1).[11]

In all these studies, sensitivity and specificity values were determined by comparison of the number and type of anastomoses detected on postnatal dye injection studies – which

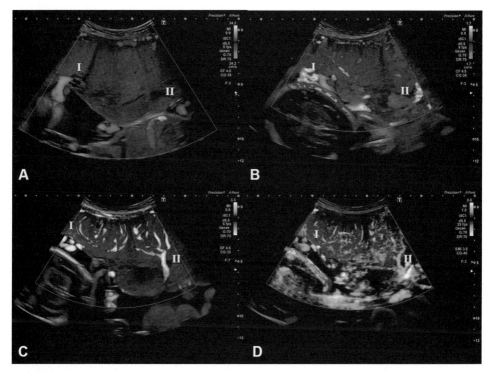

Figure 29.1 Comparison of colour Doppler imaging modalities to identify placental vasculature (A black and white version of this figure will appear in some formats. For the colour version, please refer to the plate section.)

The ultrasound images were taken from a monochorionic twin pregnancy with no features of twin–twin transfusion syndrome at 25+6 weeks' gestational age using:

(A) conventional colour Doppler with default obstetric mode settings (scale −34.2–34.2 cm.s^{-1}). Here the umbilical cord insertions (denoted as I and II) can be seen at the placental-amniotic interface; however, little colour signal is visible within the placental tissue.

(B) conventional colour Doppler with scale reduced to capture low flow (scale −1.7–1.7 cm.s^{-1}). In this image there is aliasing at the sites of the umbilical cord insertion into the placenta (denoted as I and II) and more vessels are seen within the placental tissue. However, the quality of the image is greatly reduced by motion artefact and signal noise and detail of the placental angio-architecture cannot be ascertained.

(C) Advanced dynamic flow with default settings (scale −3.3–3.3 cm.s^{-1}). Here the umbilical cord insertions are again seen at the placental-amniotic interface (denoted as I and II). However, in this image the branching vessels within the placenta can be seen in continuity from the cord insertions towards the materno-fetal interface, with minimal motion artefact or signal noise.

(D) Superb microvascular imaging with default settings (scale −0.8–0.8 cm.s^{-1}). Here the umbilical cord insertions can again be defined by colour signal intensity (denoted I and II) and there is an appearance of branching vessels from the cord insertions towards the materno-fetal interface, with many more and smaller vessels seen compared to ADF. In this instance there is significant motion artefact despite the relatively high frame rate.

Ultrasound images were obtained using a 1.8–6.2 MHz convex probe (i8C1, Aplio i900, Canon Medical Systems) and are reproduced here with written consent from the patient.

showed only superficial anastomoses – to the number and type predicted based on previous ultrasound assessments, which should have identified both superficial and deep anastomoses. These studies also did not provide any functional assessment of the in vivo direction or nature of flow through the anastomoses, nor their contribution to the disease processes (sIUGR, TTTS, TAPS) within the population studied. None of these studies have determined whether the structure of a placental vessels – be it arterial or venous – within the monochorionic placenta corresponds absolutely to either the direction or pattern of the blood flow within it in utero. This is a major and frequently overlooked fact. Hence we are able to conclude from these important studies that it is possible to see opposing arterial-arterial and arterial-venous flow as vessels of the two fetal circulations meet. They do not, however, elucidate why the proportion of monochorionic placentae with AVAs far exceeds those that will develop TTTS. Nor do they explain why hypoxic-ischaemic injury following sIUFD is fivefold more likely in pregnancies affected by TTTS than sIUGR.

While rarely challenged, it should be recalled that the role of AAAs, AVAs and VVAs in the development of disease in monochorionic twins has not been demonstrated in vivo and remains speculative to an extent. For example, a study in which intra-amniotic Doppler was performed in a series of three patients affected by TTTS showed that the net direction of blood flow in TTTS was from the recipient to the donor, contrary to received wisdom.[12] Why, for example, could a 'recipient' twin not maintain the blood supply of a donor with a poor share of the placenta – the latter explaining its inability to grow or produce urine?

While this novel application of Doppler remains unvalidated, and the findings may be affected by fluctuations in flow or skewed by AVAs not identified on fetoscopy, it remains an intriguing counterpoint to received wisdom regarding the pathogenesis of TTTS. In fact, while reasonable correlations based on that same received wisdom have been drawn between the findings of Doppler ultrasound antenatally and superficial dye injection studies postnatally, the ability to ascribe a specific Doppler waveform recorded antenatally to a particular vessel within a post-delivery placenta is limited unless that vessel is described relative to a landmark such as the cord insertion. This truly would be an important next step in understanding the function of placental anastomoses.

Such a technology remains elusive, but the advances in co-registration techniques suggest it may be possible. A novel simulator showing a fetoscopic view of the placental surface has been described using MRI-derived imaging of the placenta co-registered with 3D ultrasound imaging overlaid (Figure 29.2).[13] While this system, by design, focuses on showing the position of surface placental vessels within the body of the uterus for the purpose of treatment planning and training of fetoscopic laser techniques, there is potential for it to be adapted. It is a significant advance on the 3D representations of the monochorionic placenta previously produced, using software modelling of overlapping image layers. This 'virtual fetoscopy' technique was reported to allow identification of the umbilical cord insertions and placental equator, but was unable to characterise the nature of the anastomoses seen, as blood flow within the vessels could not be assessed to be arterial or venous.[14]

Such co-registration techniques, between Doppler ultrasound, which assesses the direction and characteristics of anastomotic blood flow, and B-mode or MRI to show the structure of placental tissues and the uterus raise the possibility of a meaningful study of the in vivo assessment of placental anastomotic function, although quantification of blood flow remains problematic. A study quantified blood flow through AVAs and both shared and non-shared cotyledons in MCDA placentas, and then correlated the ultrasound findings with histological examination of the placenta.[7] However, both vessel size (a circular

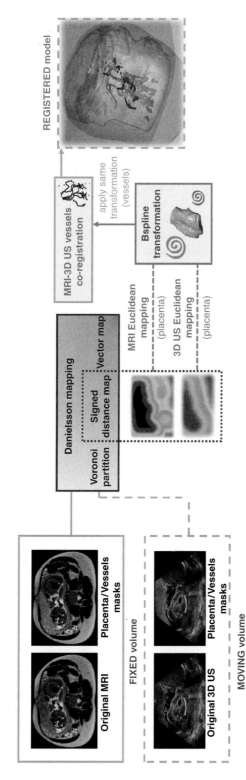

Figure 29.2 Schematic overview of the proposed MRI – 3D US registration methodology (A black and white version of this figure will appear in some formats. For the colour version, please refer to the plate section.)

Source: Torrents-Barrena et al. 2019 (13). TTTS-GPS: Patient-specific preoperative planning and simulation platform for twin-to-twin transfusion syndrome fetal surgery. Computer Methods and Programs in Biomedicine, 179, 104993 (Reuse licence 4784840550036)

vessel was assumed and calculated from the radius) and velocity (not angle corrected, measured with Doppler optimised for higher flows than observed) calculations involved assumptions. These were appropriate methodologies employed to overcome the technical limitations of Doppler at the time, but potentially explain why the flow velocities recorded were inconsistent with previous studies where cotyledonary flows are typically reported around 3 ml/min, compared to the authors' findings of around 31 ml/min in this study, which appear supra-physiological. To date, there remains no accepted quantification of the flow through placental anastomoses or between monochorionic twins in complicated or uncomplicated pregnancies.

As a body of evidence, therefore, these studies remain a proof of principle that anastomoses can be identified but do not suggest a standard procedure to identify, type and record the presence of placental anastomoses – the basis of making an ultrasound 'map' of the placenta for use as a reproducible screening tool. Without this the value of such studies as prognostic indicators of pregnancy outcomes cannot be inferred.

While MRI has not been the leading technology in assessment of placental anastomoses, both diffusion-weighted (DWI-MRI) and blood-oxygenation-level-dependant (BOLD-MRI) imaging have been used to investigate the function of the materno-fetal interface in multiple as well as singleton pregnancies.

The DWI-MRI is a measure of tissue integrity; this can be assessed quantitatively as the apparent diffusion coefficient (ADC), where the impedance of water molecules due to tissue cellularity and the presence of intact cell membranes is calculated. The ADC is not thought to change during placental maturation despite progressive structural changes, increase in parenchyma and angiogenesis during gestation in singleton pregnancies. Neither is ADC affected by uncomplicated twin pregnancy, in either monochorionic or dichorionic twin pregnancy.[16] However, ADC is different between the recipient and donor portions of a monochorionic placenta affected by TTTS, a disparity not seen in uncomplicated monochorionic pregnancy. The ADC is also different in the donor portion of the placenta, but not the recipient portion, when compared to uncomplicated MCDA placentae, which suggests an accumulation of tissue damage within the donor portion of the placenta.[17]

Independent assessment of placental damage may be a useful adjunct in understanding whether TTTS is likely to progress, remain stable or spontaneously improve, although there is currently no evidence to support this. Multiple groups investigating the cardio-vascular function of twins affected by TTTS have reported that placental impedance has a role to play in cardiac remodelling, acquired right ventricular outflow tract abnormalities and the risk of fetal demise following intrauterine procedures or the death of a co-twin. Placental damage such as that suggested by ADC could feasibly account for such acquired placental impedance; however, this remains speculative in the absence of further evidence.

The BOLD-MRI is a tool for visualising tissue and placental oxygenation, exploiting the differences in T2* weighted signal of deoxy- and oxyhaemoglobin in blood. As such, it provides an alternative to gadolinium-enhanced MRI, given the associated risk of adverse pregnancy and neonatal outcomes associated with gadolinium usage. In both monochorionic and dichorionic twins, inter-twin differences in placental oxygen time-to-plateau maps were independent predictors of sIUGR and enhanced the sensitivity and specificity of ultrasound-based estimation of discrepancy in estimated fetal weight alone.[18,19] The use of BOLD-MRI has not been reported in TTTS at the time of writing.

Non-invasive Diagnosis of Chromosomal Abnormality and Genetic Disease

Non-invasive prenatal testing for chromosomal abnormalities and non-invasive prenatal diagnosis (NIPD) are the most obvious non-invasive fields in which multiple pregnancy management lags behind that of singleton pregnancy. Non-invasive prenatal testing is currently recommended with caution in twin pregnancies as it has poorer sensitivity and specificity than in singleton pregnancy, but it is still superior to other available screening modalities.

Existing NIPT providers use a variety of platforms to perform screening: next-generation targeted SNP-based, targeted and massively parallel shotgun sequencing methods have all been reported by companies, each used with its own proprietary algorithms to interpret the results. Research groups have reported that SNP-based NIPT techniques appear to have high specificity for trisomies 21, 18 and 13 in addition to zygosity and fetal sex in both monochorionic and dichorionic twins.[20] There is potentially a limited role for assessment of zygosity using NIPD. As previously discussed chorionicity is the most important predictor of outcome in multiple pregnancy and therefore dictates the intensity of antenatal screening. In situations where it is not possible to assign chorionicity with ultrasound such a technique could provide additional information.

A key issue when understanding NIPT usage in multiple pregnancy is that while maternal serum has an overall higher fetal fraction when compared to singleton pregnancy, there is a smaller contribution per fetus, making failure more likely. It may be possible to overcome this limitation using low-coverage, paired-end, whole-genome sequencing of maternal plasma: in one study a sufficient fetal fraction was obtained for screening of triplet, quadruplets, sextuplets and octuplets in addition to twins as a proof of principle. It is therefore possible to envisage a situation in which NIPT could play a larger role in diagnosis of aneuploidy and genetic conditions in multiple pregnancies.

Non-invasive Intrauterine Treatments

In the past decade high-intensity focused ultrasound (HIFU) has been proposed as a non-invasive treatment which may be suited for use in fetal and placental therapies. It is an established non-invasive method of ablating soft tissue and occluding blood vessels which has been in clinical usage since the 1990s. It uses ultrasound waves generated by an externally placed ultrasound transducer to produce localised tissue necrosis at depth due to a combination of thermal and/or mechanical effects. The ultrasound energy ideally passes through overlying tissue without causing damage to converge in a small region (the focus) where the increase in temperature or changes in pressure is sufficient to ablate tissue or occlude vessels. As such, HIFU technology is reliant on diagnostic imaging modalities such as ultrasound or MRI to direct the HIFU focus to the target tissue.

In obstetrics and gynaecology HIFU has been used for the treatment of uterine fibroids, endometriosis, adenomyosis and caesarean scar pregnancy, using MRI guidance, with a low rate of complications.[21] In a research setting ultrasound-guided HIFU has been reported as the treatment for monochorionic twins with TRAP sequence: in about half of these cases blood flow to the acardiac twin was successfully occluded and no significant maternal or fetal adverse outcomes were reported.[22] In this application researchers used HIFU to target the soft tissues surrounding the cord insertion of the acardiac twin to effect cord occlusion.

This ultrasound-guided HIFU technique could be adapted to perform selective fetal reduction when indicated.

High-intensity focused ultrasound has also been suggested as a non-invasive method of treating fetal conditions such as TTTS, where access to blood vessels is restricted or associated with the risks of iatrogenic pregnancy loss.[23,24] Recently preclinical studies have been used to demonstrate the feasibility, high efficacy and materno-fetal safety of using ultrasound-guided HIFU to selectively occlude placental blood vessels in an animal model.[25,26,27] In these studies colour Doppler was used to identify placental vessels and direct the HIFU focus in order to occlude them through intact maternal abdominal skin. High rates of successful selective occlusion (93–100%) of targeted placental vessels were reported without excessive destruction of placental tissue. In later studies persistent vascular occlusion of placental vessels for up to 21 days was also demonstrated histologically. A combination of invasive and non-invasive techniques was employed to monitor maternal and fetal cardiovascular, metabolic, acid-base, stress responses and fetal growth and development patterns both during and following HIFU medicated placental vascular occlusion. The overall conclusion of this work was that HIFU mediated selective placental vascular occlusion appeared to be well tolerated in the mother and fetus in both the short and long term with no discernible adverse effects. However, as in the treatments for TRAP sequence, maternal abdominal skin erythema did result in a proportion of exposed subjects.[22]

Based on this research the clinical applications are clear and could in addition to HIFU include non-invasive treatment for TRAP and selective reduction in monochorionic pregnancy. A phase 1a clinical trial is currently being designed for the non-invasive treatment of TTTS using HIFU in human pregnancy.[28] The intention is to target the HIFU focus using colour Doppler modalities optimised to the low-flow placental vessels. If non-invasive ablation of blood vessels using ultrasound-guided HIFU was successful, this would represent a paradigm shift in the treatment of the condition. As previously discussed, fetoscopic laser has not been shown to confer a survival advantage when compared to amniodrainage, in part due to the associated risk of procedure-related pregnancy loss.[2] Hence a treatment which is able to occlude placental anastomoses without breaching the intrauterine space would have the potential to deliver the therapeutic benefit of anastomotic occlusion without the associated risks of invasive fetoscopy itself. Such a treatment also lends itself better to retreatment of recurrent disease. Furthermore, following fetoscopic laser, 5–35% of monochorionic placental retain residual anastomoses deep within the placenta,[29] and up to 16% of cases have recurrent disease due to this, which has been shown to have a worse prognosis.[30] Given that laser as a technology has a limited depth to which it can ablate tissue, there is again a case for a technology such as HIFU which can occlude vessels at any depth within the placental tissue.

References

1. Bajoria R, Wigglesworth J, Fisk NM. Angioarchitecture of monochorionic placentas in relation to the twin–twin transfusion syndrome. Am J Obstet Gynecol 1995;172(3):856–63.

2. Roberts D, Neilson JP, Kilby MD, Gates S. Interventions for the treatment of twin–twin transfusion syndrome. Cochrane Database Syst Rev 2014;1:CD002073.

3. Grigsby PL. Animal models to study placental development and function throughout normal and dysfunctional human pregnancy. Semin Reprod Med 2016;34(1):11–16.

4. Kaiser J. Reproductive biology. Gearing up for a closer look at the human placenta. Science 2014;**344**(6188):1073.

5. Taylor MJ, Denbow ML, Tanawattanacharoen S, Gannon C, Cox PM, Fisk NM. Doppler detection of arterio-arterial anastomoses in monochorionic twins: feasibility and clinical application. Hum Reprod 2000;**15**(7):1632–6.

6. Machin GA, Feldstein VA, Van Gemert MJ, Keith LG, Hecher K. Doppler sonographic demonstration of arterio-venous anastomosis in monochorionic twin gestation. Ultrasound Obstet Gynecol 2000;**16**(3):214–17.

7. Wee LY, Sullivan M, Humphries K, Fisk NM. Longitudinal blood flow in shared (arteriovenous anastomoses) and non-shared cotyledons in monochorionic placentae. Placenta 2007;**28**(5–6):516–22.

8. Sun W, Cai A. OP12.03: 3D high-definition flow combined with tomographic ultrasound imaging in observation of placental vascular anastomoses in monochorionic twins. Ultrasound *Obstet Gynecol* 2019;**54**(S1):124-.

9. Sato T. Technological description of advanced dynamic flow in the aplio diagnostic ultrasound system. eMedical Review, Toshiba Corporation, 2003.

10. Mack LM, Mastrobattista JM, Gandhi R, Castro EC, Burgess APH, Lee W. Characterization of placental microvasculature using superb microvascular imaging. J Ultrasound Med 2019;**38**(9):2485–91.

11. Girardelli S, Shaw C, Lees C. OP12.02: Mapping of the placental angioarchitecture in monochorionic twin pregnancies using different colour Doppler filters. Ultrasound *Obstet Gynecol* 2019;**54**(S1):123.

12. Nakata M, Martínez JM, Díaz C, Chmait R, Quintero RA. Intra-amniotic Doppler measurement of blood flow in placental vascular anastomoses in twin–twin transfusion syndrome. Ultrasound Obstet Gynecol 2004;**24**(1):102–3.

13. Torrents-Barrena J, Lopez-Velazco R, Piella G et al. TTTS-GPS: patient-specific preoperative planning and simulation platform for twin-to-twin transfusion syndrome fetal surgery. Comput Methods Programs Biomed 2019;**179**:104993.

14. Werner H, Dos Santos JL, Sa RA et al. Visualisation of the vascular equator in twin-to-twin transfusion syndrome by virtual fetoscopy. Arch Gynecol Obstet 2015;**292**(6):1183–4.

15. Denbow ML, Taylor M, Cox P, Fisk NM. Derivation of rate of arterio-arterial anastomotic transfusion between monochorionic twin fetuses by Doppler waveform analysis. Placenta 2004;**25**(7):664–70.

16. Shapira-Zaltsberg G, Grynspan D, Reddy D, Miller E. Apparent diffusion coefficient of the placenta in twin versus singleton pregnancies. Fetal Diagn Ther 2018;**44**(2):129–34.

17. Fu L, Zhang J, Xiong S, Sun M. Decreased apparent diffusion coefficient in the placentas of monochorionic twins with selective intrauterine growth restriction. Placenta 2018;**69**:26–31.

18. Poulsen SS, Sinding M, Hansen DN, Peters DA, Frokjaer JB, Sorensen A. Placental T2* estimated by magnetic resonance imaging and fetal weight estimated by ultrasound in the prediction of birthweight differences in dichorionic twin pairs. Placenta 2019;**78**:18–22.

19. Luo J, Abaci Turk E, Bibbo C et al. In vivo quantification of placental insufficiency by BOLD MRI: a human study. Sci Rep 2017;**7**(1):3713.

20. Norwitz ER, McNeill G, Kalyan A et al. Validation of a single-nucleotide polymorphism-based non-invasive prenatal test in twin gestations: determination of zygosity, individual fetal sex, and fetal aneuploidy. J Clin Med 2019;**8**(7).

21. Chen J, Chen W, Zhang L et al. Safety of ultrasound-guided ultrasound ablation for uterine fibroids and adenomyosis: a review of 9988 cases. Ultrason Sonochem 2015;**27**:671–6.

22. Seo K, Ichizuka K, Okai T et al. Treatment of twin-reversed arterial perfusion

sequence using high-intensity focused ultrasound. Ultrasound Obstet Gynecol 2019 Jul;**54**(1):128–34.

23. Shaw CJ, Ter Haar GR, Rivens IH, Giussani DA, Lees CC. Pathophysiological mechanisms of high-intensity focused ultrasound-mediated vascular occlusion and relevance to non-invasive fetal surgery. J R Soc Interface 2014;**11** (95):20140029.

24. Caloone J, Huissoud C, Vincenot J et al. High-intensity focused ultrasound applied to the placenta using a toroidal transducer: a preliminary ex-vivo study. Ultrasound Obstet Gynecol 2015;**45** (3):313–19.

25. Shaw CJ, Civale J, Botting KJ et al. Noninvasive high-intensity focused ultrasound treatment of twin–twin transfusion syndrome: A preliminary in vivo study. Sci Transl Med 2016;**8** (347):347ra95.

26. Shaw CJ, Rivens I, Civale J et al. Trans-abdominal in vivo placental vessel occlusion using high intensity focused ultrasound. Sci Rep 2018;**8**(1):13631.

27. Shaw CJ, Rivens I, Civale J et al. Maternal and fetal cardiometabolic recovery following ultrasound-guided high-intensity focused ultrasound placental vascular occlusion. J R Soc Interface 2019;**16**(154):20190013.

28. ISTCRN registry. Developing a non-invasive treatment for twin–twin transfusion syndrome. https://doi.org/10 .1186/ISRCTN33458649

29. Chmait RH, Assaf SA, Benirschke K. Residual vascular communications in twin–twin transfusion syndrome treated with sequential laser surgery: frequency and clinical implications. Placenta 2010;**31** (7):611–14.

30. Walsh CA, McAuliffe FM. Recurrent twin–twin transfusion syndrome after selective fetoscopic laser photocoagulation: a systematic review of the literature. Ultrasound Obstet Gynecol 2012;**40** (5):506–12.

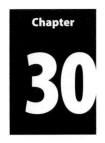

Multiple Pregnancy Resources for Professionals and the Public

Natasha Fenwick and Jane Gorringe

Multiple Pregnancy Care

Outcomes, Guidelines and Policies for Multiple Pregnancies

Twin and higher-order multiple pregnancies constitute a high-risk group, with stillbirth and neonatal death rates much higher than a singleton pregnancy. Although stillbirth rates fell by almost 50% and neonatal death rates fell by more than 30% between 2014 and 2016,[1] both rose slightly in 2017 and remain much higher than singleton rates.[2] Key guidelines, policies and programmes seek to address this inequality in order to make multiple pregnancy safer and to improve the chance of mothers having a positive birth experience and healthy babies. Guidelines for multiple pregnancies in the UK include the National Institute for Health and Care Excellence (NICE) Guideline 137 for Twin and Triplet Pregnancy,[6] the NICE Quality Standard 46 for Twin and Triplet Pregnancy (see Figure 30.1),[5] Green-Top guideline number 51 on the management of monochorionic pregnancy[4] and the International Society of Ultrasound in Obstetrics and Gynecology (ISUOG) practice guidelines on the role of ultrasound in twin pregnancy.[3] Meanwhile, elements of the NICE guidance such as personalised care, continuity of care and multi-professional working are known to reflect in improved maternity care.[7] Implementation of the NICE guidance is also recommended by the Saving Babies' Lives Care Bundle as an important step towards achieving best practice in antenatal care and meeting the aim of halving stillbirths by 2025.[8]

Multiple-Specific Care in Practice

In 2019 Twins Trust[10] conducted the BeCOME survey of more than 1,000 parents' and 76 health professionals' experiences of antenatal and neonatal care between January 2015 and April 2019, based on NICE quality standard 46. The survey found that approximately a third of multiple pregnancies were seen by a multidisciplinary specialist core team, with a decrease in the number seeing a specialist obstetrician since the previous survey in 2015. Discussions about the risks and signs of preterm labour only took place before 24 weeks in 28% of pregnancies. These rates are worryingly low given that Twins Trust's Maternity Engagement Quality Improvement project produced clear evidence that following the NICE guidelines for the antenatal care of multiple pregnancies will improve the outcomes of those pregnancies.[9] The survey also showed that health professionals are likely to overestimate the level of NICE adherence in their hospital.

Qualitative feedback from parents demonstrated that they truly value NICE implementation and feel reassured that specialist care is available to help them through their high-risk pregnancy. Continuity of care allows them to maximise time to address concerns during

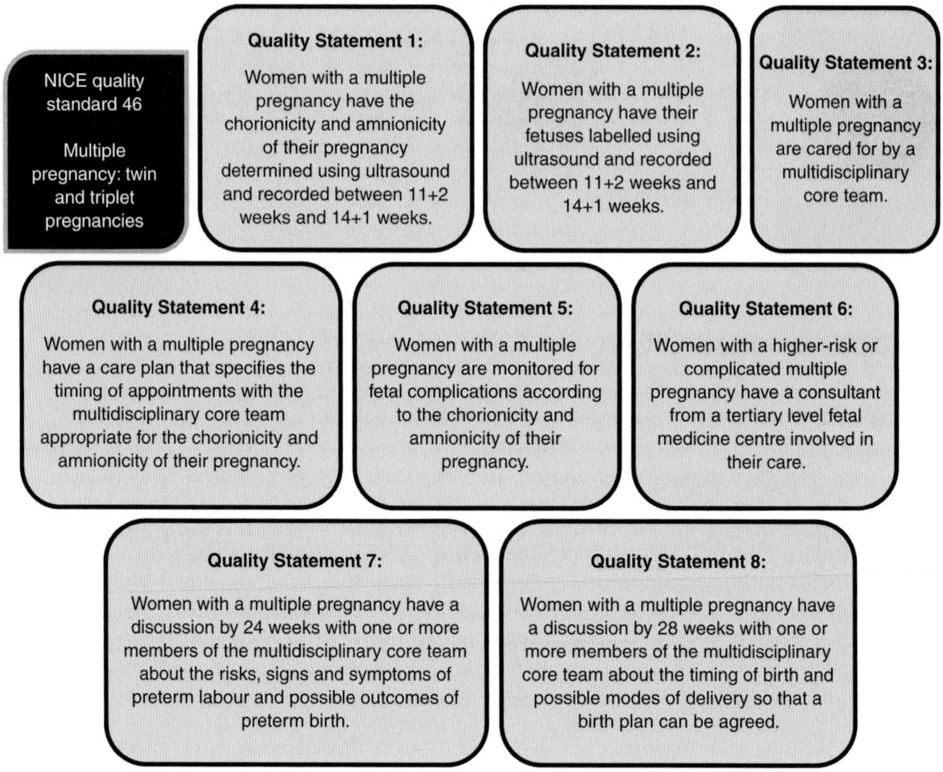

Figure 30.1 NICE Quality Standard 46 for Twin and Triplet Pregnancies[5]

appointments rather than recounting their pregnancy details each time and it allows concerns or changes to be quickly picked up. Having access to a knowledgeable specialist team reassures parents that the professionals caring for them have the knowledge to deliver their babies safely and at the right time. Parents who are kept informed feel positively about their pregnancy and towards the staff caring for them, while those who feel uninformed become anxious and may feel they need to do their own research to compensate.

In order to continue improving outcomes, it is vital that maternity units increase their adherence to NICE guidelines, as well as improving the overall patient experience, and resources are available to help achieve this.

Support for Healthcare Professionals

Multiple pregnancies require additional monitoring and specialist care, and despite its importance, some may find particular aspects difficult to implement. Through learning opportunities, free resources and practical support to improve care and address potential barriers, most charities are committed to supporting professionals to ensure the best-quality care is given to parents with a multiple pregnancy and to ensure parents are supported during the pregnancy, through birth and in the postnatal period.

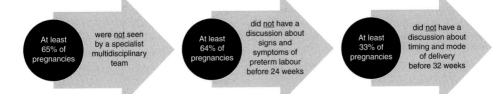

Figure 30.2 Parents' experiences of care from Twins Trust's BeCOME survey[10]

Maternity Engagement Quality Improvement Project

The Maternity Engagement team works with maternity units across the UK to ensure families expecting a multiple pregnancy receive the correct level of clinical care. The aim is to improve outcomes for twin and other multiple pregnancies by ensuring multiple pregnancy care is delivered consistently and in line with national guidance – specifically NICE Quality Standard 46. Unit adoption of this standard has proven to be an indicator of good practice and has been shown to reduce stillbirths, neonatal admissions, neonatal deaths and emergency caesarean section rates.

The team works alongside specialist midwives who visit maternity units and conduct an audit to assess local practice. An action plan is created to provide a platform for improving care and support is provided throughout the year, along with access to a wide range of resources. After 12 months a re-audit is conducted to assess changes made and their impact. In just 12 months the 30 units that participated in the first phase of the project saw a 5.8% reduction in neonatal admissions, equating to a cost saving of £51,000 per unit and a 3.1% reduction in emergency caesarean sections. After two years this increased to a 23% reduction in neonatal admissions, an 18% reduction in neonatal deaths, a 7% reduction in stillbirths and a 6% reduction in emergency caesarean sections.

NICE-Endorsed Multiple Pregnancy Care Pathway and Parents' Proforma

Twins Trust has worked very closely with several hospitals to develop a multiple pregnancy care pathway that healthcare professionals can use for all permutations of multiple pregnancy and covers the eight statements within the NICE guideline. It clearly identifies the appointment schedule for each type of pregnancy and the number of appointments that should take place with a specialist consultant. The pathway was endorsed by NICE in 2018 and was subsequently updated and re-endorsed to reflect the amendments to the guideline that took place in September 2019. The care pathway features on the NICE website, where they refer to it to give the appointment schedule for each variation of multiple pregnancy. In addition to the care pathway for healthcare professionals, the charity has produced a version for parents. This enables parents to understand the appointment schedule they should be following and what will happen at each appointment. It is a useful prompt to have the relevant discussions about being of aware of the risks and symptoms that may occur with a multiple pregnancy and the timing and mode of delivery.

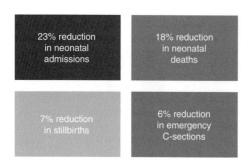

Figure 30.3 Results of the Twins Trust Maternity Engagement programme after one year[9]

Twins Trust Continuing Professional Development Area

There is a dedicated area on the Twins Trust website (www.twinstrust.org) for healthcare professionals. It offers a suite of video-recorded presentations that provide CPD learning on antenatal, intra-partum and neonatal care, as well as best practice in areas such as multiple midwives and sonography for multiples. It also focuses on certain complications that occur in multiple pregnancies such as twin–twin transfusion syndrome (TTTS), twin-reversed arterial perfusion (TRAP) sequence and twin anaemia-polycythaemia sequence (TAPS). Viewers can add a certificate to their CPD portfolio for each video watched. As well as these videos, a range of other resources are available.

Study Days

As part of the Maternity Engagement project, Twins Trust has run study days to encourage sharing of knowledge and multiple-birth expertise among the healthcare professionals who care for these pregnancies. This has covered areas such as

- NICE Guidance
- The sonographer's role in multiple pregnancy
- Reducing preterm birth
- The role of the specialist midwife
- Timing and mode of birth
- Intra-partum and postnatal care
- Neonatal care of multiple pregnancies

  The team is now working to provide more of these study days over the coming years.

Postnatal Support

The parents in the BeCOME study reported very poor postnatal care once their twins or higher-order multiples were born. They felt staff, although well-intentioned, were too stretched to support them adequately. Leaving the specialist care of the antenatal clinic whilst still having specific needs is a huge challenge, as many parents struggle to care for more than one baby during their recovery. Parents face additional challenges with feeding their babies, but often there is nowhere to turn for support as services are not made available and staff are unable to dedicate the time to establish feeding with multiple babies, sometimes recommending that parents use formula rather than breastfeeding. They often find that they are unable to feed in the way they wish to because of this lack of support. Some parents also reported complications following the birth which were not appropriately managed and led to additional hospital admissions later on.

Families with babies in neonatal care typically report care of their babies to be of a very high level, but they struggle to understand how the neonatal wards work and how they can become involved in the care of their babies in order to bond with the babies and feel like a parent. Some also report that communication between the postnatal and neonatal wards is poor and they find it difficult to balance the different routines and time spent on each ward.

Once the family are home, they can struggle to get out of the house, being unable to attend check-ups, clinics or social groups. Additionally, parents of multiples are more likely to experience mental health difficulties and postnatal depression, compounded by sleep deprivation, financial worries and social isolation. It is vital that families access specialist support during the early days, weeks and months to protect the well-being of the whole family.

Resources and Services for Parents

When considering how to support parents of multiples, professionals should remember their needs are very different to parents of singletons and they are likely to need extra support during and after pregnancy. Twins Trust has a range of resources available to support parents at every stage with common worries and difficulties, many of which are free to access online (with the exception of courses and webinars). More information about all the support available can be found on the Twins Trust website. Some of the common areas in which parents need support or information are listed in what follows, with suggestions of help available to address these particular concerns.

Pregnancy

It often comes as a shock to parents when their pregnancy is diagnosed as twins, triplets or more. As well as the worry of a high-risk pregnancy (with increased risk of stillbirth and neonatal death compared to a singleton pregnancy), parents have to navigate specialist antenatal care and cope with the increased risk of sick leave or hospitalisation. All this happens while they are getting ready to welcome their babies home and finding the finances and the space to accommodate their new arrivals. The Pregnancy Countdown tool available on the Twins Trust website allows parents to see what is happening during each week of

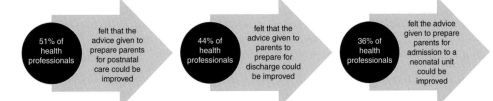

Figure 30.4 Healthcare professionals' experiences of postnatal care from Twins Trust's BeCOME survey[10]

pregnancy as well as informs them about the care they can expect to receive and the discussions they should be having with their care providers. It covers physical and emotional changes, babies' development, antenatal care pathways and signposting to other resources.

The Healthy Multiple Pregnancy Guide provides an overview of multiple pregnancies from conception, throughout pregnancy, to after birth. It is designed to complement the antenatal care parents receive and enable them to become more informed and reassured at what can be a stressful time. The guide is available to download for free online or as a paid-for physical copy. It covers topics such as

- Pregnancy and preparing for the babies' arrival
- Types of available support and how to access them
- Looking after babies in hospital
- Going home and establishing life with the babies
- Keeping babies safe
- Common illnesses and how to manage them
- Further information and sources of support

Twins Trust's antenatal courses are specifically designed to answer questions around the birth of two or more babies. Since multiple pregnancies follow their own antenatal care pathways, the timing and mode of delivery may be different from a singleton birth, and they differ based on the number of babies, chorionicity and amnionicity as well. This course will inform parents about the factors which can affect timing and mode of delivery, as well as the increased risk of premature birth and the practical aspects of caring for more than one baby in the early days.

Neonatal Care

Twins and higher-order multiples are more likely to be born early and in need of neonatal care. Having two or more babies' needs to consider can be difficult at the best of times, but when babies are split between hospitals, units or the family home, parents can feel anxious and guilty about dividing their time between their babies. Visiting the neonatal unit can be daunting and parents may need time to adjust to the particular way of working and how they can best be involved in care of their babies at this time. The guide to neonatal care offers information on preparation for premature birth, what to expect from neonatal care, how they might consider feeding multiple babies, the transition from hospital to home and the support available to parents who are struggling. The guide provides an invaluable insight into one of the most common challenges for multiple-birth families, caring for two or more babies born prematurely or with additional complications.

Bereavement

The death of any baby is devastating for a family, but in the case of twins, triplets or more it can be a very complex situation. Alongside the loss of one or more babies comes the loss of the special feeling of being a parent of multiples and the loss of the multiple relationship for the children. Grief can be difficult to manage, especially if there is a surviving multiple to care for and bond with. Specialist support is vital to help these parents through this difficult time and the mixed emotions it brings.

Twins Trust offers support to families facing a bereavement through its Bereavement Support Group, a closed online group for parents to meet others affected by the loss of one or more babies, offer peer support and share experiences in a safe space. The group also offers a newsletter which keeps the community informed of events and provides an opportunity for parents to share their stories.

The Bereavement Support booklet is a collection of personal stories, suggestions and sources of support for families who have lost babies from a multiple set. Parents may find comfort in knowing others have faced similar experiences and this guide can also help parents to plan for the birth, funeral and remembering their babies in the future. It offers anecdotes of parents' fundraising efforts and perspectives from families in many different situations. This booklet can be downloaded from the Twins Trust website or requested as a physical copy. Twins Trust also offers a befriending service to bereaved parents who wish to access individual peer support. Parents or grandparents are matched to a befriender who may have had a similar experience. This is not a counselling service but can nonetheless be beneficial to parents looking for someone to talk to about their loss.

Practical Challenges

The practical challenges of caring for two or more babies should not be underestimated. Parents have to learn to divide their time between all their babies, finding ways to engage them all in playtime or feed them together, whilst providing two or three times the care of a singleton parent. There is the challenge of funding equipment, clothes and toys for more than one baby and finding space for it all. Multiple parents benefit from all the support available to them. The Practical Preparing for Parenthood course, which is also available as a webinar, is an opportunity for expectant parents to meet each other, learn about what to expect from having more than one baby and prepare for the journey that lies ahead. These courses take place over two hours for an in-person course or as a webinar online, and cover topics such as those listed in what follows.

Similar topics are covered in the Preparing for Parenthood booklet, which guides parents through the different aspects of parenting they might need to consider and the things they need to organise, do or buy before the arrival of their babies and in the early days. For some parents, affording two or three times the equipment can be a concern. Where it is safe to do so, parents can acquire second-hand equipment from a local baby bank. Another need of some parents may be practical support. Home-Start is an organisation with branches across the country which offer around two hours per week of volunteer-led support at home to families with young children. A map on the Home-Start website (www.home-start .org.uk) shows all active branches as provision varies dependent on location. For families who experience additional circumstances, such as a bereavement, serious illness or postnatal depression, which tip them into desperate need or crisis, Twins Trust offers support through the Family Crisis Support service. Families who meet eligibility criteria are offered short-term, tailored support at home with multiple-specific challenges such as establishing a routine, getting out of the house, behaviour, feeding or sleep. Families can also be referred to other Twins Trust or external services, be given free resources or be offered remote support by

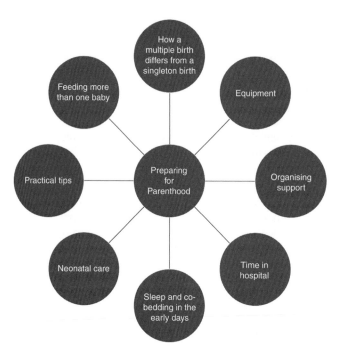

Figure 30.5 Multiple-birth parents' experiences of postnatal depression

phone or email. Families can self-refer or be referred by a healthcare professional on the Twins Trust website.

Feeding

Parents of twins, triplets and more often find that there is a lack of support when it comes to feeding, something which is more complex when there are multiple mouths to feed. Parents may have in mind their preferred method of feeding their babies, yet need some support to achieve it. Many are left feeling lost and disheartened when professionals are too stretched to give them the attention they need to succeed, and competing opinions of how parents should feed their multiples can add to the pressure. The Twins Trust website offers parents a wealth of information on breastfeeding, bottle feeding, mixed feeding and expressing, which is designed to help them achieve their feeding goals, whichever method they use. Twins Trust's breastfeeding booklet and webinar also provide invaluable information for parents and their partners who wish to breastfeed multiple babies full-time or in combination with other methods. These resources answer common questions and offer different techniques and tips for success. For those who need a bit of extra support with any aspect of breastfeeding or mixed feeding, peer supporters can offer information and support via phone and email.

Sleep

Sleep deprivation can be one of the biggest challenges new parents face, and having multiple babies with different sleep patterns can further complicate the situation.

Exhaustion can severely impact a parent's physical and mental well-being and this can have an effect on their ability to cope day to day. Twins and higher-order multiples are more likely to have been born prematurely and to have spent time in the neonatal unit, and they may now be separated between home and hospital, cared for by multiple adults or sharing a cot or bedroom. This unique set of circumstances has the potential to affect their sleep as well. The Sleep Top Tips for Multiples factsheet explains how babies sleep and how sleep cycles, associations, routines and environment can all play a part in babies' sleep. The Sleep Expectations factsheet explains how much sleep babies need at each stage and the different factors that might affect their sleep as they grow.

The Safer Sleeping factsheet explains the guidance for keeping babies safe and at a lower risk of sudden infant death syndrome (SIDS). It includes general advice for all babies and specific advice for twins and more. The Lullaby Trust also offers information and support about safer sleep to families of singletons and twins and is a good source of information for questions about reducing the risk of SIDS. For babies who are more than a year old, the sleep webinar is available to offer advice on why babies may struggle with sleep at this age and how parents can create environments and routines to encourage regular sleep. It also gives parents an opportunity to have their questions answered by sleep experts.

Mental Health

The issue of mental health is key for multiple-birth parents, who are at higher risk of postnatal depression and poor mental well-being. In addition to the specialist services and organisations which support families experiencing mental health difficulties, Twins Trust provides information for multiple birth families, their partners and the professionals caring for them.

Perinatal Mental Health: Top Tips for Multiples offers advice to those experiencing mental health difficulties on how to cope with a mental health condition and caring for multiple babies. How Partners, Family and Friends can help those with postnatal depression is a guide for those who want to support someone with postnatal depression to know how they can help the whole family and themselves.

Conclusion and Further Support

Twins Trust is committed to support families of twins, triplets and more, and the professionals who care for them, by ensuring that the care provided aligns with current guidance, and that services and resources are freely available to families in need.

All the resources and support services listed earlier in this chapter can be found on the Twins Trust website. Professionals who wish to learn more about the Maternity Engagement project findings or how they can improve their care should contact MaternityEngagement@twinstrust.org. Families in need of additional support can access Twinline on 0800 138 0509 (Monday–Friday, 10am–1pm and 7pm–10pm), Ask Twinline at AskTwinline@twinstrust.org, or the Twins Trust Support Team at support-team@twinstrust.org.

References

1. Draper ES, Gallimore ID, Kurinczuk JJ et al. MBRRACE-UK Perinatal Mortality Surveillance Report, UK Perinatal Deaths for Births from January to December 2016. [Internet]. Leicester: The Infant Mortality and Morbidity Studies, Department of

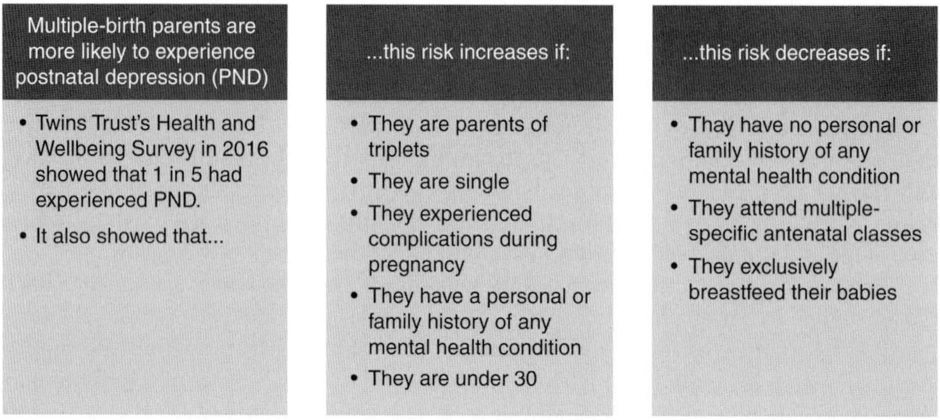

Multiple-birth parents are more likely to experience postnatal depression (PND)	...this risk increases if:	...this risk decreases if:
• Twins Trust's Health and Wellbeing Survey in 2016 showed that 1 in 5 had experienced PND. • It also showed that...	• They are parents of triplets • They are single • They experienced complications during pregnancy • They have a personal or family history of any mental health condition • They are under 30	• Thay have no personal or family history of any mental health condition • They attend multiple-specific antenatal classes • They exclusively breastfeed their babies

Figure 30.6 Twins and Multiple Births Association. Perinatal Mental Health for Multiple Birth Families. Aldershot: Tamba, 2017. Available from https://twinstrust.org/uploads/assets/ce32ec05-6501-4da6-b3621f9b8bb54b40/PND-for-Health-Professionals.pdf

Health Sciences, University of Leicester; 2018. Available from www.npeu.ox.ac.uk/downloads/files/mbrrace-uk/reports/MBRRACE-UK%20Perinatal%20Surveillance%20Full%20Report%20for%202016%20-%20June%202018.pdf

2. Draper ES, Gallimore ID, Smith LK et al. MBRRACE-UK Perinatal Mortality Surveillance Report, UK Perinatal Deaths for Births from January to December 2017 [Internet]. Leicester: The Infant Mortality and Morbidity Studies, Department of Health Sciences, University of Leicester; 2019. Available from www.npeu.ox.ac.uk/downloads/files/mbrrace-uk/reports/MBRRACE-UK%20Perinatal%20Mortality%20Surveillance%20Report%20for%20Births%20in%202017%20-%20FINAL%20Revised.pdf

3. Khalil A, Rodgers M, Baschat A et al. ISUOG Practice Guidelines: role of ultrasound in twin pregnancy. Ultrasound Obstet Gynecol 2016;47(2):247–63.

4. Kilby MD, Bricker L on behalf of the Royal College of Obstetricians and Gynaecologists. Management of monochorionic twin pregnancy. BJOG 2016;12(4):e1–e45.

5. National Institute for Health and Care Excellence. Multiple pregnancy: twin and triplet pregnancies: quality standard [Internet]. London: NICE; 2019. Available from http://nice.org.uk/guidance/qs46/resources/multiple-pregnancy-twin-and-triplet-pregnancies-pdf-2098670068933

6. National Institute for Health and Care Excellence. Twin and triplet pregnancy: NICE guideline [Internet]. London: NICE; 2019. Available from www.nice.org.uk/guidance/ng137/resources/twin-and-triplet-pregnancy-pdf-66141724389829

7. National Maternity Review. Better births: improving outcomes of maternity services in England – a five year forward view for maternity care [Internet]. London: NHS England; 2016. Available from www.england.nhs.uk/wp-content/uploads/2016/02/national-maternity-review-report.pdf

8. NHS England. Saving Babies' Lives Version Two: a care bundle for reducing perinatal mortality [Internet]. London: NHS England; 2019. Available from www.england.nhs.uk/wp-content/uploads/2019/07/saving-babies-lives-care-bundle-version-two-v5.pdf

9. Twins and Multiple Births Association. NICE Works: The Final Report. Aldershot: Tamba, 2019.

10. Twins Trust. Better Care of Multiple Pregnancies in the UK: An Exploration. Aldershot: Twins Trust, 2020.

Obstetric Anaesthesia in Multiple Pregnancy

Tarek Ansari

Introduction

Multiple pregnancy is associated with an increased risk of maternal and fetal morbidity and mortality. A successful outcome requires a multidisciplinary approach involving obstetricians, neonatologists, obstetric anaesthetists and midwives. The obstetric anaesthetist may be involved in antenatal assessment, care planning and counselling of parturients with multiple gestation. This is particularly important in pregnant women with medical comorbidities associated with special care needs and increased risk of perinatal complications or adverse outcomes. In twin vaginal delivery, effective epidural in labour is crucial for adequate analgesia, but it may also increase the chances of successful delivery of the second twin. Providing safe and effective spinal anaesthesia, or general anaesthesia when indicated, for caesarean delivery is essential. A multimodal approach to postoperative analgesia enables enhanced recovery and early discharge after caesarean section. The role of the anaesthetist is crucial in managing critically ill pregnant women including those with pre-eclampsia and its complications. This chapter covers the anaesthetist's role in the context of multiple pregnancy.

Maternal Physiological Changes in Multiple Gestation

The maternal physiological adaptation to multiple gestation is far more exaggerated than that of singleton pregnancies. Twin gestation is associated with significantly higher cardiac output than singleton pregnancy due to the increase in both stroke volume and heart rate. By 20 weeks of gestation the blood volume in twin pregnancy increases by 50–70% compared to 20% in singleton pregnancy. This is reflected in increased left atrial diameter and left ventricular end-diastolic diameter, indicating a rise in the cardiac preload in twin pregnancy. In contrast to the increase in blood volume, twin pregnancy is associated with only a 25% increase in erythrocyte volume, which leads to haemodilution anaemia, a decrease in albumin and water-soluble vitamin concentration.

Increased uterine size in multiple gestation, particularly in the third trimester, leads to reduction in total lung capacity and functional residual capacity. This predisposes to a more rapid development of hypoxemia after a brief period of apnoea. After 30 weeks of gestation, women with multiple pregnancies have an increased tendency for weight gain. The large size of the uterus displaces the stomach and reduces the competency of the lower oesophageal sphincter, increasing the risk of passive regurgitation of stomach contents. These changes combine to significantly increase the risk of difficult intubation and pulmonary aspiration during general anaesthesia for women with multiple gestation.

Risk of Maternal Morbidity and Mortality in Multiple Gestation

The risk of severe maternal morbidity in multiple pregnancies is 28 per 1,000 deliveries, while that of singleton pregnancies is 6.5 in 100,000 deliveries. Higher-order gestation further increases the risk. The relative risk of severe maternal morbidity compared to singleton pregnancy is 4.3 in twins and 6.2 in triplets. The risk of morbidity increases with a maternal age of more than 40 years, the use of assisted reproductive technology and non-spontaneous onset of labour.[1] This increased risk necessitates the involvement of the obstetric anaesthetist as part of the multidisciplinary team, including where high-dependency or intensive care is required, to optimise outcome.

Pre-eclampsia

Pre-eclampsia remains a leading cause of maternal morbidity and mortality. Twin pregnancy doubles the risk of pre-eclampsia compared to singleton pregnancy. The larger placental volume in multiple gestation may be partly responsible for this association. Multiple gestation resulting from assisted reproductive technology carries twice the risk of pre-eclampsia compared to spontaneous twin conception. Pre-eclampsia develops earlier in multiple gestation and is often more severe. The risk of developing haemolysis, elevated liver enzymes and low platelets (HELLP) syndrome is four times higher than in singleton pregnancy.[2]

The anaesthetic management of pre-eclampsia may include neuraxial block for vaginal delivery or caesarean section. Severe generalised oedema over the lower back may increase the technical difficulty of spinal or epidural anaesthesia. If general anaesthesia is required for caesarean section, airway oedema may significantly increase the risk of difficult intubation. Uncontrolled hypertension may predispose to the increased risk of cerebrovascular accidents during general anaesthesia and endotracheal intubation. The role of the anaesthetist is crucial in the critical care management of parturients with fulminating pre-eclampsia. This may include invasive monitoring, control of hypertension and the management of cardio-respiratory, cerebral and renal complications.[3]

Post-partum Haemorrhage

The risk of post-partum haemorrhage in multiple gestation is two to four times that of singleton pregnancy. Contributing factors may include greater uterine distension that predisposes to uterine atony, increased maternal blood volume and uterine blood flow. The use of tocolytic agents during vaginal twin delivery, placenta praevia and placental abruption further increase the risk.

Women with multiple gestation are more likely to suffer from iron-deficiency anaemia and are at greater risk of requiring blood transfusion. A multivariable logistic regression model identified a low platelet count (< 100,000/ microliter), haematocrit < 30% and general anaesthesia as predictors of post-partum haemorrhage requiring blood transfusion in women with twin pregnancies.[4] The anaesthetist is fundamental during the management of post-partum haemorrhage, taking the lead in cardiovascular resuscitation and replacement of blood products.

Risk of Fetal Complications

Multiple gestation is associated with a significant increase in the risk of perinatal morbidity and mortality. The perinatal mortality rate is two and a half times higher in twin pregnancy, while that of triplet pregnancy is five times higher than that of singleton pregnancy.

In all dizygotic twins (two separate fertilised ova) the placenta is dichorionic and diamniotic, while in monozygotic twins (single fertilised ovum, dividing into two distinct individuals) the placenta can be monochorionic or dichorionic, depending on the time of embryonic cleavage. Seventy-five per cent of monozygotic twins are monochorionic and diamniotic. Vascular communications occur in almost all monochorionic placentas and may result in fetal complications such as twin–twin transfusion syndrome and intrauterine fetal death (IUFD). Other fetal complications associated with multiple gestation include preterm labour, congenital anomalies, polyhydramnios, fetal growth restriction and multiple presentation.

Twin–Twin Transfusion

Monochorionic twins with deep arterio-venous vascular anastomosis may suffer from twin–twin transfusion. The donor twin will be at risk of fetal growth restriction and anaemia, while the recipient twin will be at risk of polycythaemia, polyuria, polyhydramnios, fetal hydrops and hypertrophic cardiomyopathy. Twin–twin transfusion can be managed by amnioreduction, amniotic septostomy or selective fetoscopic laser photocoagulation (SFLP). Selective fetoscopic laser photocoagulation is associated with the highest birth survival rate, with 62% mean survival rate for both twins and 88% for at least one twin.

Anaesthesia for SFLP procedures can be provided by local anaesthetic infiltration of the anterior abdominal wall. This is usually sufficient to reduce maternal discomfort; however, supplemental analgesia or sedation can be provided using a short-term opioid such as fentanyl or a hypnotic such as midazolam. A low-dose propofol infusion can also be used for sedation. Neuraxial block is occasionally used but general anaesthesia is rarely needed. When providing neuraxial block it in this clinical scenario, it is essential to avoid maternal hypotension as the compromised fetuses are cardiovascularly unstable and very sensitive to placental hypoperfusion, which may result in fetal death. General anaesthesia where the woman is intubated and ventilated is not ideal because the deep breathing movement results in exaggerated movement of the uterus and placenta and makes accurate visualisation of anastomoses and laser coagulation technically difficult. As with other anaesthesia for non-obstetric surgery, the anaesthetist should perform a full preoperative anaesthetic assessment and decide with the mother and the surgeon on the most appropriate anaesthetic technique.

Fetal hydrops secondary to twin–twin transfusion may be associated with a rare but potentially life-threatening maternal complication. Mirror syndrome is diagnosed when maternal and placental oedema develop secondary to fetal hydrops. Other causes of mirror syndrome include Rh-isoimmunisation, intrauterine infection or placental tumours. Patients with mirror syndrome will present with severe generalised oedema, ascites and pulmonary oedema. It can be associated with elevation of blood pressure and proteinuria, mimicking pre-eclampsia. The definitive treatment of mirror syndrome is the delivery of the fetus and placenta. In cases of twin–twin transfusion syndrome, resolution of the maternal signs and symptoms can be achieved by artificial feticide or fetoscopic laser photocoagulation. The anaesthetic management of mirror syndrome is similar to that of severe pre-eclampsia.[3]

Delivery of Women with Multiple Gestation

The overall rate of caesarean section for twin delivery is 75%, while the caesarean delivery rate for twins with a cephalic presenting first twin is 68%. The term breech trial published in

2000 concluded that planned caesarean section for breech presentation in singleton pregnancy reduces the risk of perinatal mortality and serious morbidity by threefold.[5] This study had a profound impact on obstetric practice. The almost unanimous and universal acceptance of its results meant most obstetricians completely abandoned planned vaginal breech delivery in favour of caesarean section. This also resulted in a general consensus that twin pregnancies where the first twin's presentation is breech should be delivered by caesarean section. However, the extrapolation of the term breech trial findings to twin pregnancies with a cephalic presenting first twin and a non-vertex presenting second twin led to a progressive increase in caesarean section rate for all twin deliveries. In 2013 the first large randomised controlled multicentre study on the mode of delivery for twin pregnancy with a cephalic presenting first twin (Twin Birth Study) was published. The study found that in twin pregnancies between 32 and 38+6 weeks of gestation there was no significant difference in fetal or neonatal outcome between planned vaginal delivery and planned caesarean section.[6]

The recent guidelines from the National Institute for Health and Care Excellence (NICE) recommend that planned vaginal delivery should be offered to women with uncomplicated dichorionic-diamniotic or monochorionic-diamniotic twin pregnancies if the presentation of the first twin is cephalic and there is no significant size discordance between the twins.[7] Planned caesarean section is indicated for the following: monoamniotic twin pregnancies, non-cephalic presentation of the first twin at the time of planned birth, triplets and higher-order pregnancies

Planned Vaginal Delivery

Women with a twin pregnancy are at increased risk of intervention in labour, particularly for the delivery of the second twin. This may include external cephalic version, internal podalic version and total breech extraction, instrumental vaginal cephalic delivery or emergency caesarean section.

In the Twin Birth Study 43.8% of women in the planned vaginal delivery group had emergency caesarean sections during labour and 4.2% had an emergency section for delivery of the second twin.[6] Only 30% of women in the planned vaginal delivery group had epidural analgesia in labour.

In a retrospective cohort study comparing outcomes of twin pregnancies with planned vaginal delivery and active second-stage management to the outcomes of planned caesarean delivery, all women in the planned vaginal delivery group had epidural analgesia: 15.4 % had emergency caesarean sections for both twins, while 84.6% delivered both twins vaginally. None of the women had emergency caesarean sections for the delivery of the second twin. All deliveries took place in the operating theatre with the anaesthesiologist in attendance.[8]

Despite the paucity of evidence on the effect of epidural analgesia on the outcome of vaginal twin delivery, the consensus is that effective labour analgesia would facilitate prompt delivery of the second twin in an emergency, reducing the risk of fetal or neonatal morbidity and mortality. The recent NICE guidelines recommended offering epidural analgesia to all women with a twin or triplet pregnancy who choose to have a vaginal birth. By providing better analgesia and relaxation of the abdominal wall and pelvic floor muscles, an effective epidural increases the chances of success for internal podalic version and total breech extraction of the second twin. If further uterine relaxation is required to facilitate the delivery of the second twin, a tocolytic agent such as nitroglycerine can be given intravenously in a dose of 150–250 micrograms.

A combination of excessive weight gain and large uterine size in multiple gestation might lead to difficulty in identifying anatomical landmarks and in positioning the mother for epidural catheter placement. The use of a pre-procedure ultrasound to guide epidural catheter insertion was shown to double the first attempt success rate compared to the traditional landmark technique in obese patients or those with difficult backs. It is postulated that identifying the depth of the dura using ultrasound may reduce the risk of accidental dural puncture and post-dural puncture headache. Applying a low-frequency curvilinear ultrasound probe using the longitudinal paramedian sagittal approach, followed by the transverse midline interspinous approach, provides information that allows the anaesthetist to determine the level of the desired intervertebral space and the optimum puncture site. It also helps to determine the depth of the dura and the best angle for the needle approach.[9] See Figures 31.1 and 31.2.

Successful management of vaginal twin delivery relies on the presence of an experienced obstetrician skilled and comfortable with the active management of the second stage of labour. This may include internal podalic version and total breech extraction. Other essential elements include continuous fetal monitoring and routine epidural analgesia. Performing twin vaginal delivery in the operating theatre with the anaesthesiologist in attendance is routine in some centres but not a universal practice. The anaesthesiologist should ensure that the epidural catheter is working effectively, and in case of any doubt, should have a low threshold for re-siting the catheter. The combination of a low-dose local anaesthetic and a lipophilic narcotic (such as ropivacaine 0.1% plus fentanyl 0.2%) is routinely used to provide effective epidural analgesia with minimal motor block. Prompt conversion of epidural analgesia into surgical anaesthesia is an essential skill to reduce the need for general anaesthesia in case of emergency caesarean section. This can be achieved using 15–20 mls of lidocaine 2% with epinephrine 1/200,000 to extend the surgical sensory block up to T4 dermatome. Every effort should be made to ensure that

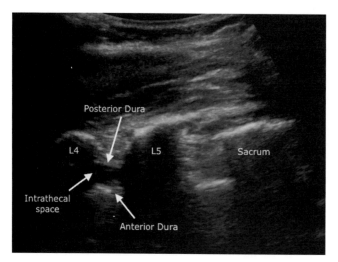

Figure 31.1 Ultrasound-guided neuraxial scan. Paramedian sagittal oblique approach

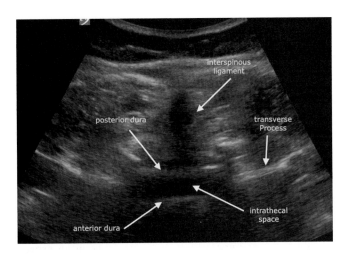

Figure 31.2 Ultrasound guided neuraxial scan. Transverse interspinous approach

the epidural top-up produces adequate surgical anaesthesia before the start of surgery. If the epidural top-up fails, a spinal or a general anaesthetic can be administered depending on the urgency of the caesarean section. Predictors for failed conversion of epidural analgesia to epidural anaesthesia include the degree of urgency of caesarean section, the need for frequent epidural top-ups during labour and the experience of the anaesthesiologist. Effective team communication between obstetricians, anaesthesiologists and midwives can help in anticipating the need for intra-partum caesarean delivery, allowing sufficient time to achieve epidural anaesthesia. A retrospective study found that 44% of general anaesthesia for caesarean section can be avoided and that a low hospital use of labour epidural analgesia is a strong predictor of potentially avoidable use of general anaesthesia for caesarean section.[10]

General anaesthesia for emergency caesarean section is associated with increased risk of maternal complications such as difficult intubation, regurgitation and pulmonary aspiration of gastric contents and intraoperative awareness. It is also associated with an increased risk for post-partum haemorrhage, surgical site infection and deep vein thrombosis. On the other hand, neuraxial anaesthesia-induced sympathetic blockade leads to attenuation of the inflammatory response to surgery. The associated peripheral vasodilatation improves tissue perfusion and oxygenation, reducing the risk of infection and thromboembolism.

The use of interdisciplinary simulation of vaginal twin delivery is essential in reducing maternal and neonatal risk and ensuring an optimum outcome. Team training in internal podalic version, breech extraction and emergency caesarean section may help optimise team dynamics and enhance timely and effective communication between obstetricians, midwives and anaesthesiologists in a challenging and time-sensitive scenario. This may lead to a reduction in avoidable intra-partum caesarean section and general anaesthesia.[11]

Anaesthesia for Caesarean Delivery

Forty years ago the risk of maternal mortality from general anaesthesia for caesarean section was 17 times greater than that from neuraxial anaesthesia. Nowadays the case fatality rates of general and neuraxial anaesthesia in obstetrics have converged to become statistically indistinguishable. However, it was shown that in the first post-operative week after caesarean section patients who had neuraxial anaesthesia had less pain, gastrointestinal stasis, coughing and fever than patients who received general anaesthesia. Women were also able to ambulate earlier and were less likely to experience breastfeeding difficulties. It was recently shown that general anaesthesia for caesarean section increases the odds of post-partum depression by 54%.

In the absence of contraindications, neuraxial anaesthesia, in particular single-shot spinal anaesthesia, is currently the default technique for caesarean section. It is estimated that on average only 5% of elective caesarean sections and 15% of emergency caesarean sections are performed under general anaesthesia. Spinal anaesthesia is achieved using a combination of hyperbaric bupivacaine 0.5% and a lipid-soluble opioid such as fentanyl 20 micrograms. It was believed that women with multiple gestation were more susceptible to spinal-induced hypotension than women with singleton gestation due to the larger uterine size. Similarly, it was thought that they were more likely to have a higher cephalad spread of sensory and motor blockade with spinal anaesthesia. However, several studies concluded that there is no difference in the effect of spinal anaesthesia in both groups of women. Spinal-induced hypotension, secondary to sympathetic blockade, can be successfully prevented using a combination of an infusion of a directly acting vasopressor (phenylephrine) and a rapid intravenous administration of Lactated Ringer's solution immediately after the spinal injection (co-loading).[12] The phenylephrine infusion can be titrated in order to maintain baseline blood pressure. Compared to the indirectly acting sympathomimetic ephedrine, phenylephrine is associated with lower incidence of maternal nausea, vomiting and tachycardia, and with better neonatal umbilical artery pH and base excess.

Managing Haemorrhage

Multiple gestation is associated with an increased risk of antepartum and post-partum haemorrhage. The rate of placental abruption is two to three times that of singleton pregnancy, while the rate of placenta praevia is 40% higher in twins than in singletons. An over-distended uterus doubles the rate of post-partum haemorrhage secondary to uterine atony. In the Twin Birth Study 6.9% had post-partum haemorrhage, 2.1% with blood loss >/= 1,500 mL, and 5% required blood transfusion (no significant difference between planned vaginal versus planned caesarean birth).[6]

Adopting an evidence-based massive haemorrhage protocol has been shown to improve maternal outcome. This should include a uterotonic drug cascade with a low threshold to move to the next drug in case of failure to achieve an adequate response. Intravenous oxytocin or carbetocin is usually the default uterotonic. In the absence of contraindications, this is followed by intramuscular methylergometrine and carboprost, then rectal or vaginal misoprostol.

In major obstetric haemorrhage the fibrinogen level was the parameter best correlating with the volume of blood loss. Fibrinogen concentration of less than 2 g/l was found to have a positive predictive value of 100% for severe post-partum haemorrhage, while a level of more than 4 g/l had a negative predictive value of 79%.[13] Compared to a fibrinogen level of more than 3 g/l, a fibrinogen level of between 2 and 3 grams, which is usually considered normal, doubles the risk of severe haemorrhage. In the setting of post-partum haemorrhage the anaesthesiologist should assess the fibrinogen level early and initiate its replacement aggressively. Fibrinogen concentrate provides a safe, effective and readily available source of fibrinogen. The use of a point-of-care coagulation monitor such as thromboelastometry can provide valuable information on clot initiation, propagation, clot firmness and stability and fibrinogen function. A thromboelastometry-guided algorithm for post-partum haemorrhage may reduce bleeding and the need for blood and blood-component transfusion.

A large, international, randomised, double-blind, placebo-controlled trial concluded that the early use of tranexamic acid can reduce maternal mortality from post-partum haemorrhage by more than 30% in cases of uterine atony or trauma.[14]

Historic concerns over the risk of amniotic fluid embolism prevented the use of cell saver in obstetrics. It is now believed that the use of cell saver in obstetrics is safe and can lead to a reduction in the use of allogeneic blood and in the overall number of patients who receive blood or blood-component transfusions. Routine cell saver use for all caesarean section patients is not recommended due to concerns over its cost-effectiveness. However, its use in high-risk obstetrics including multiple gestation is recommended by the American College of Obstetricians and Gynaecologists and the Association of Anaesthetists of Great Britain and Ireland.

Post-caesarean Analgesia

Effective analgesia after caesarean delivery improves patient satisfaction and is an essential element of enhanced recovery. It enables early ambulation, reduces the risk of venous thromboembolism and facilitates breastfeeding. It may also reduce the risk of developing chronic post-operative pain.

The gold standard for post-caesarean section analgesia is a multimodal approach. Multimodal techniques provide efficient analgesia by acting on different levels of the pain pathways to maximise analgesia while limiting side effects. At the centre of this approach lies the use of intrathecal morphine, a lipophilic long-acting opioid. Intrathecal morphine in a dose of 50–100 micrograms provides effective, long-acting analgesia. Side effects include pruritus, nausea and vomiting, urinary retention and rarely respiratory depression. Other components of the multimodel approach are regular or scheduled paracetamol and non-steroidal anti-inflammatory drugs (NSAID) such as diclofenac or ibuprofen. Both groups of drugs have an opioid-sparing effect of 20% and 50%, respectively. Intramuscular morphine may be used for breakthrough pain.

Abdominal Fascial Plane Blocks

Ultrasound-guided abdominal fascial plane blocks are a relatively recent addition to the elements of multimodal post-operative analgesia for abdominal surgeries including cesarean sections. The most commonly used techniques are transversus abdominis plane block (TAP) and quadratus lumborum block (QLB).

In TAP the local anaesthetic is injected in a fascial plane between the internal oblique and transversus abdominis muscles, blocking the somatic fibres supplying the lower abdominal wall. Although intrathecal morphine provides superior analgesia, TAP block may be used as part of a multimodal post-operative analgesic approach if caesarean delivery is done under general anaesthesia, or when intrathecal morphine is contraindicated.

Quadratus lumborum block is a posterior abdominal wall block that is a modification of TAP block. While the patient is in the supine position with a lateral tilt, a curvilinear ultrasound probe is placed transversely at the midaxillary line above the iliac crest at the

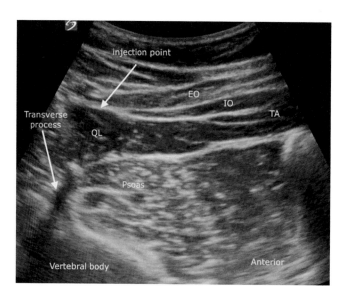

Figure 31.3 Quadratus lumborum block. TA: transversus abdominis muscle; IO: internal oblique muscle; EO: external oblique muscle; QL: quadratus lumborum muscle

level of the umbilicus. The quadratus lumborum muscle (QL) is identified as a hypoechoic muscle posterolateral to the anterior abdominal muscles (external oblique, internal oblique and transversus abdominis) and anteromedial to the psoas major muscle at the tip of the lumbar transverse process. The local anaesthetic is injected under ultrasound guidance at the posterior border of the QL. Although several injection points are proposed for QLB, the posterior approach is the default technique in our institution. We routinely use bupivacaine 0.125% in a dose of 0.4 ml/kg on both sides. After injection the local anaesthetic spreads posteriorly along the thoracolumbar fascia with its network of sympathetic fibres, blocking both somatic and visceral pain. Further spread into the paravertebral space may explain its longer-lasting analgesia effect. Quadratus lumborum block is considered a safer technique than TAP block as the tip of the needle is separated from the peritoneum by the QL, thus reducing the risk of intraperitoneal injection and bowel injury. Compared to TAP block, and as one component of a multimodal approach, QLB seems to offer superior post-operative analgesia with significant reductions in morphine consumption and pain scores. This effect lasts for up to 48 hours after the caesarean section.[15] See Figure 31.3.

Key Points

- The rate of multiple gestation is rising exponentially due to increased use of assisted reproductive technology and older maternal age.
- Multiple gestation exaggerates the physiological changes of pregnancy compared to singleton gestation.
- Women with twins and higher-order gestation are at increased risk of maternal and fetal complications such as pre-eclampsia, post-partum haemorrhage, fetal pathology particularly if monochorionic, and intrauterine fetal death.

- Good-quality evidence suggests that in twin pregnancies with a cephalic presenting first twin and a non-vertex presenting second twin there is no significant difference in maternal and neonatal outcome between planned vaginal delivery and planned caesarean delivery.
- Despite the lack of evidence, the general consensus is that epidural analgesia in twin vaginal delivery may facilitate the active management of the second stage of labour and reduce the risk of avoidable general anaesthesia for emergency caesarean section.
- Single-shot spinal anaesthesia remains the preferred technique for caesarean delivery in multiple pregnancy. It is associated with better maternal and neonatal outcomes and reduction of perioperative complications such as post-partum haemorrhage, deep vein thrombosis and surgical site infection.
- An effective multimodal post-caesarean pain management approach should include intrathecal morphine or an abdominal fascial plane block at its core. This enables smooth recovery after caesarean section and facilitates early ambulation and successful breastfeeding.

References

1. Witteveen T, Van den Akker T, Zwart JJ et al. Severe acute maternal morbidity in multiple pregnancies: a nationwide cohort study. Am J Obstet Gynecol 2016;**214**:641. e1–641.e10.

2. Day MC, Barton JR, O'Brien JM et al. The effect of fetal number on the development of hypertensive conditions of pregnancy. Obstet Gynecol 2005;**106**:927–31.

3. Xu W, Smith C, Binstock A, Lim G. Maternal mirror syndrome masquerading as congestive heart failure: a case report. A A Pract 2019;**12**(11):447–51.

4. Blitz M, Yukhayev A, Patchman S et al. Twin pregnancy and risk of postpartum hemorrhage. J Matern Fetal Neonatal Med 2020. Nov;**33**(22):3740–5. https://doi.org/10.1080/14767058.2019.1583736.Epub 2019 Mar 5.PMID:30836810

5. Hannah ME, Hannah WJ, Hewson S et al. for the Term Breech Trial Collaborative Group. Planned caesarean section versus planned vaginal birth for breech presentation at term: a randomised multicentre trial.Lancet 2000;**356**:1375–83.

6. Barrett JF, Hannah ME, Hutton EK et al. for the Twin Birth Study Collaborative Group. A randomized trial of planned cesarean or vaginal birth for twin pregnancies. N Engl J Med 2013;**369**:1295–1305.

7. National Institute for Health and Care Excellence. 2019 Twin and triplet pregnancy (NICE guideline 137). Available at www.nice.org.uk/guidance/ng137

8. Fox NS, Silverstein M, Bender S, Klauser CK, Saltzman DH, Rebarber A. Active second-stage management in twin pregnancies undergoing planned vaginal delivery in a U.S. population. Obstet Gynecol 2010;**115**(2 Pt 1):229–33.

9. Chin KJ, Perlas A. Ultrasonography of the lumbar spine for neuraxial and lumbar plexus blocks. Curr Opin Anaesthesiol 2011 Oct;**24**(5):567–72.

10. Guglielminotti J, Landau R, Li G. Adverse events and factors associated with potentially avoidable use of general anesthesia in cesarean deliveries. Anesthesiology 2019;**130**:912–22.

11. Lepage J, Ceccaldi PF, Remini SA, Plaisance P, Voulgaropoulos A, Luton D. Twin vaginal delivery: to maintain skill simulation is required. Eur J Obstet Gynecol Reprod Biol 2019 Mar;**234**:195–9.

12. Ngan Kee WD. The use of vasopressors during spinal anaesthesia for caesarean section. Curr Opin Anaesthesiol 2017 Jun;**30**(3):319–25. https://doi.org/10.1097/ACO.0000000000000453. PMID: 28277383.

13. Charbit B, Mandelbrot L, Samain E et al. The decrease of fibrinogen is an early predictor of the severity of postpartum hemorrhage. J Thromb Haemost 2007;**5**:266–73.

14. Woman Trial Collaborators. Effect of early tranexamic acid administration on mortality, hysterectomy, and other morbidities in women with post-partum haemorrhage (WOMAN): an international, randomised, double-blind, placebo-controlled trial. Lancet 2017;**389**:2105–16.

15. Blanco R, Ansari T, Riad W, Shetty N. Quadratus lumborum block versus transversus abdominis plane block for postoperative pain after cesarean delivery: a randomized controlled trial. Reg Anesth Pain Med 2016;**41**:757–62.

Index

Note: Page numbers followed by *f* indicate a figure on the corresponding page. Page numbers followed by *t* indicate a table on the corresponding page.